T0226669

Portal Hypertension

Editor

JORGE L. HERRERA

CLINICS IN
LIVER DISEASE

www.liver.theclinics.com

Consulting Editor
NORMAN GITLIN

May 2014 • Volume 18 • Number 2

ELSEVIER

1600 John F. Kennedy Boulevard • Suite 1800 • Philadelphia, Pennsylvania, 19103-2899

http://www.theclinics.com

CLINICS IN LIVER DISEASE Volume 18, Number 2
May 2014 ISSN 1089-3261, ISBN-13: 978-0-323-29711-0

Editor: Kerry Holland
Developmental Editor: Casey Jackson

© **2014 Elsevier Inc. All rights reserved.**

This periodical and the individual contributions contained in it are protected under copyright by Elsevier, and the following terms and conditions apply to their use:

Photocopying

Single photocopies of single articles may be made for personal use as allowed by national copyright laws. Permission of the Publisher and payment of a fee is required for all other photocopying, including multiple or systematic copying, copying for advertising or promotional purposes, resale, and all forms of document delivery. Special rates are available for educational institutions that wish to make photocopies for non-profit educational classroom use. For information on how to seek permission visit www.elsevier.com/permissions or call: (+44) 1865 843830 (UK)/ (+1) 215 239 3804 (USA).

Derivative Works

Subscribers may reproduce tables of contents or prepare lists of articles including abstracts for internal circulation within their institutions. Permission of the Publisher is required for resale or distribution outside the institution. Permission of the Publisher is required for all other derivative works, including compilations and translations (please consult www.elsevier.com/permissions).

Electronic Storage or Usage

Permission of the Publisher is required to store or use electronically any material contained in this periodical, including any article or part of an article (please consult www.elsevier.com/permissions). Except as outlined above, no part of this publication may be reproduced, stored in a retrieval system or transmitted in any form or by any means, electronic, mechanical, photocopying, recording or otherwise, without prior written permission of the Publisher.

Notice

No responsibility is assumed by the Publisher for any injury and/or damage to persons or property as a matter of products liability, negligence or otherwise, or from any use or operation of any methods, products, instructions or ideas contained in the material herein. Because of rapid advances in the medical sciences, in particular, independent verification of diagnoses and drug dosages should be made.

Although all advertising material is expected to conform to ethical (medical) standards, inclusion in this publication does not constitute a guarantee or endorsement of the quality or value of such product or of the claims made of it by its manufacturer.

Clinics in Liver Disease (ISSN 1089-3261) is published quarterly by Elsevier Inc., 360 Park Avenue South, New York, NY 10010-1710. Months of issue are February, May, August, and November. Business and Editorial Offices: 1600 John F. Kennedy Blvd., Ste. 1800, Philadelphia, PA 19103-2899. Customer Service Office: 3251 Riverport Lane, Maryland Heights, MO 63043. Periodicals postage paid at New York, NY and additional mailing offices. Subscription prices are $295.00 per year (U.S. individuals), $145.00 per year (U.S. student/resident), $401.00 per year (U.S. institutions), $395.00 per year (foreign individuals), $200.00 per year (foreign student/ resident), $498.00 per year (foreign instituitions), $340.00 per year (Canadian individuals), $200.00 per year (Canadian student/resident), and $498.00 per year (Canadian institutions). Foreign air speed delivery is included in all Clinics subscription prices. All prices are subject to change without notice. **POSTMASTER:** Send address changes to Clinics in Liver Disease, Elsevier Health Sciences Division, Subscription Customer Service, 3251 Riverport Lane, Maryland Heights, MO 63043. **Customer Service: Telephone: 1-800-654-2452 (U.S. and Canada); 314-447-8871 (outside U.S. and Canada). Fax: 314-447-8029. E-mail: journalscustomer service-usa@elsevier.com (for print support); journalsonlinesupport-usa@elsevier.com (for online support).**

Reprints. For copies of 100 or more of articles in this publication, please contact the Commercial Reprints Department, Elsevier Inc., 360 Park Avenue South, New York, NY 10010-1710. Tel.: 212-633-3874; Fax: 212-633-3820; E-mail: reprints@elsevier.com.

Clinics in Liver Disease is covered in MEDLINE/PubMed (Index Medicus), Science Citation Index Expanded, Journal Citation Reports/Science Edition, and Current Contents/Clinical Medicine.

Printed and bound by CPI Group (UK) Ltd, Croydon, CR0 4YY

Contributors

CONSULTING EDITOR

NORMAN GITLIN, MD, FRCP (LONDON), FRCPE (EDINBURGH), FACG, FACP
Formerly, Professor of Medicine, Chief of Hepatology, Emory University; Currently, Consultant, Atlanta Gastroenterology Associates, Atlanta, Georgia

EDITOR

JORGE L. HERRERA, MD
Professor of Medicine, Division of Gastroenterology, University of South Alabama College of Medicine, Mobile, Alabama

AUTHORS

AGUSTÍN ALBILLOS, MD, PhD
Professor of Medicine, Head, Department of Gastroenterology and Hepatology, Hospital Universitario Ramón y Cajal, CIBERehd, IRYCIS, University of Alcalá, Madrid, Spain

ANNALISA BERZIGOTTI, MD, PhD
Hepatic Hemodynamic Laboratory, Liver Unit, Hospital Clinic-IDIBAPS, Centro de Investigación Biomédica en Red de Enfermedades Hepáticas y Digestivas (CIBERehd), University of Barcelona, Barcelona, Spain

JAIME BOSCH, MD, PhD, FRCP
Hepatic Hemodynamic Laboratory, Liver Unit, Hospital Clinic-IDIBAPS, Centro de Investigación Biomédica en Red de Enfermedades Hepáticas y Digestivas (CIBERehd), University of Barcelona, Barcelona, Spain

STEPHEN CALDWELL, MD
Division of Gastroenterology and Hepatology, University of Virginia Health System, Charlottesville, Virginia

RODRIGO CARTIN-CEBA, MD
Assistant Professor of Medicine, Division of Pulmonary and Critical Care Medicine, Mayo Clinic, Rochester, Minnesota

ROBERTO DE FRANCHIS, MD, AGAF
Professor of Gastroenterology, Head, Gastroenterology Unit, Department of Clinical and Biomedical Sciences, Luigi Sacco University Hospital, University of Milan, Milan, Italy

ALESSANDRA DELL'ERA, MD, PhD
Assistant Professor of Gastroenterology, Senior Registrar, Gastroenterology Unit, Department of Clinical and Biomedical Sciences, Luigi Sacco University Hospital, University of Milan, Milan, Italy

MARCELO E. FACCIUTO, MD
Assistant Professor of Surgery, Icahn School of Medicine at Mount Sinai, The Mount Sinai Medical Center, Recanati/Miller Transplantation Institute, New York, New York

MICHAEL B. FALLON, MD
Division of Gastroenterology, Hepatology and Nutrition, Department of Internal Medicine, The University of Texas Medical School at Houston, Houston, Texas

ZACHARY HENRY, MD
Division of Gastroenterology and Hepatology, University of Virginia Health System, Charlottesville, Virginia

JORGE L. HERRERA, MD
Professor of Medicine, Division of Gastroenterology, University of South Alabama College of Medicine, Mobile, Alabama

GENE Y. IM, MD
Assistant Professor of Medicine, Icahn School of Medicine at Mount Sinai, The Mount Sinai Medical Center, Recanati/Miller Transplantation Institute, New York, New York

YASUKO IWAKIRI, PhD
Associate Professor of Medicine, Section of Digestive Diseases, Department of Internal Medicine, Yale University School of Medicine, New Haven, Connecticut

PATRICK S. KAMATH, MD
Professor of Medicine, Gastroenterology Research Unit, Division of Gastroenterology and Hepatology, Department of Physiology, Advanced Liver Disease Study Group, Fiterman Center for Digestive Diseases, Mayo Clinic, Rochester, Minnesota

RAJEEV KHANNA, MD, PDCC
Assistant Professor, Department of Pediatric Hepatology, Institute of Liver and Biliary Sciences, New Delhi, India

DAVID G. KOCH, MD, MSCR
Division of Gastroenterology and Hepatology, Department of Internal Medicine, Medical University of South Carolina, Charleston, South Carolina

MICHAEL J. KROWKA, MD
Professor of Medicine, Division of Pulmonary and Critical Care Medicine, Mayo Clinic, Rochester, Minnesota

NIR LUBEZKY, MD
Clinical Instructor of Surgery, Icahn School of Medicine at Mount Sinai, The Mount Sinai Medical Center, Recanati/Miller Transplantation Institute, New York, New York

JOHN PAUL NORVELL, MD
Assistant Professor of Medicine, Department of Digestive Diseases; Department of Medicine, Emory Transplant Center, Emory University, Atlanta, Georgia

RICHARD PARKER, MBChB, MRCP
NIHR Centre for Liver Research, University of Birmingham, Birmingham, United Kingdom

DON C. ROCKEY, MD
Chairman, Department of Internal Medicine, Medical University of South Carolina, Charleston, South Carolina

WAEL SAAD, MD
Division of Vascular and Interventional Radiology, University of Virginia Health System, Charlottesville, Virginia

SHIV K. SARIN, MD, DM, FNA, DSc
Director and Head, Department of Hepatology, Institute of Liver and Biliary Sciences, New Delhi, India

THOMAS D. SCHIANO, MD
Professor of Medicine, Icahn School of Medicine at Mount Sinai, The Mount Sinai Medical Center, Medical Director of Adult Liver Transplantation and Director of Clinical Hepatology and Intestinal Transplantation, Recanati/Miller Transplantation Institute, New York, New York

VIJAY H. SHAH, MD
Professor of Medicine, Gastroenterology Research Unit, Division of Gastroenterology and Hepatology, Department of Physiology, Advanced Liver Disease Study Group, Fiterman Center for Digestive Diseases, Mayo Clinic, Rochester, Minnesota

DOUGLAS A. SIMONETTO, MD
Instructor in Medicine, Gastroenterology Research Unit, Division of Gastroenterology and Hepatology, Department of Physiology, Advanced Liver Disease Study Group, Fiterman Center for Digestive Diseases, Mayo Clinic, Rochester, Minnesota

JAMES R. SPIVEY, MD
Associate Professor of Medicine, Division of Digestive Diseases, Department of Medicine, Medical Director of Liver Transplant, Emory Transplant Center, Emory University, Atlanta, Georgia

MARTA TEJEDOR, MD
Gastroenterology and Hepatology Specialist, Research Associate, Department of Gastroenterology and Hepatology, Hospital Universitario Ramón y Cajal, Madrid, Spain

DUSHANT UPPAL, MD
Division of Gastroenterology and Hepatology, University of Virginia Health System, Charlottesville, Virginia

NATHALIE H. URRUNAGA, MD, MS
Division of Gastroenterology and Hepatology, University of Maryland School of Medicine, Baltimore, Maryland

Contents

Portal hypertension is a major complication of liver disease that results from a variety of pathologic conditions that increase the resistance to the portal blood flow into the liver. As portal hypertension develops, the formation of collateral vessels and arterial vasodilation progresses, which results in increased blood flow to the portal circulation. Hyperdynamic circulatory syndrome develops, leading to esophageal varices or ascites. This article summarizes the factors that increase (1) intrahepatic vascular resistance and (2) the blood flow in the splanchnic and systemic circulations in liver cirrhosis. In addition, the future directions of basic/clinical research in portal hypertension are discussed.

Assessing the presence of clinically significant portal hypertension and esophageal varices is clinically important in cirrhosis. The reference standard techniques to assess the presence of portal hypertension and varices are the measurement of the hepatic vein pressure gradient and esophagogastroduodenoscopy, respectively. Some newer methods have shown a good performance, but none have been proven precise enough to replace hepatic vein pressure gradient measurement or esophagogastroduodenoscopy for the diagnosis of portal hypertension or the presence and grade of esophageal varices.

Progress in the knowledge of the pathophysiology of portal hypertension has disclosed new targets for therapy, resulting in a larger spectrum of drugs with a potential role for clinical practice. This review focuses on pharmacologic treatments already available for reducing portal pressure and summarizes drugs currently under investigation in this field.

A transjugular intrahepatic portosystemic shunt (TIPS) is an expandable metal stent inserted via the jugular vein that creates a shunt from the portal vein to the systemic circulation via an artificial communication through the liver. It is used to treat complications of portal hypertension. In addition to rescue treatment in variceal bleeding, TIPS can play an important role in prevention of rebleeding. TIPS can improve symptoms if medical treatment of ascites or hepatic hydrothrorax has failed, but may not improve survival. Selected cases of Budd-Chiari syndrome improve with TIPS. This article discusses the indications, evidence, and complications of TIPS.

Primary prevention of variceal bleeding is an important and long-debated topic in the management of patients with cirrhosis and esophageal varices. Prophylaxis is recommended for high-risk patients with small esophageal varices (advanced liver disease and/or presence of red wale marks) and those with medium/large varices. Nonselective β-blockers and endoscopic band ligation have been shown to be equally effective in primary prevention of variceal bleeding and are the only currently recommended therapies. Controversy still exists, however, regarding which one of these strategies is preferred. This article reviews the established recommendations and recent advances in the prevention of first esophageal variceal bleeding.

 Endoscopic Band Ligation (EBL) of esophageal varices accompanies the article

Acute variceal bleeding (AVB) is the most common cause of upper gastrointestinal hemorrhage in patients with cirrhosis. Advances in the management of AVB have resulted in decreased mortality. To minimize mortality, a multidisciplinary approach addressing airway safety, prompt judicious volume resuscitation, vasoactive and antimicrobial pharmacotherapy, and early endoscopy to obliterate varices is necessary. Placement of a transjugular intrahepatic portosystemic shunt (TIPS) has been used as rescue therapy for patients failing initial attempts at hemostasis. Patients who have a high likelihood of failing initial attempts at hemostasis may benefit from a more aggressive approach using TIPS earlier in their management.

Combination therapy with beta-blockers and endoscopic band ligation (EBL) is the standard prophylaxis of esophageal variceal rebleeding in cirrhosis. Beta-blockers are the backbone of combination therapy, since their benefits extend to other complications of portal hypertension. EBL carries the risk of post-banding ulcer bleeding, which explains why overall rebleeding is reduced when beta-blockers are added to EBL, and not when EBL is added to beta-blockers. TIPS is the rescue treatment, but it could be considered as first choice in patients that first bleed while on beta-blockers, those with contraindications to beta-blockers or with refractory ascites, and those with fundal varices.

Although often considered together, gastric and ectopic varices represent complications of a heterogeneous group of underlying diseases. Commonly, these are known to arise in patients with cirrhosis secondary to portal hypertension; however, they also arise in patients with noncirrhotic portal hypertension, most often secondary to venous thrombosis of the portal venous system. One of the key initial assessments is to define the underlying condition leading to the formation of these portal-collateral pathways to guide management. In the authors' experience, these patients can be grouped into distinct although sometimes overlapping conditions, which can provide a helpful conceptual basis of management.

Portal hypertensive gastropathy (PHG) and colopathy (PHC) are considered complications of portal hypertension. Both entities are clinically relevant because they may cause insidious blood loss or even acute massive gastrointestinal hemorrhage. Endoscopic evaluation is necessary for the diagnosis of PHG and PHC. The existence of different endoscopic criteria for PHG and PHC makes consensus difficult and results in a broad range of reported prevalence. Therapy targeted at reduction of portal pressure and mucosal blood flow has been used to treat acute bleeding; nonselective β-blockers are the most frequently used agents. Further studies are needed to clarify the natural history, pathogenesis, and treatment of PHG and PHC.

The hepatopulmonary syndrome (HPS) is a pulmonary complication of cirrhosis and/or portal hypertension whereby patients develop hypoxemia as a result of alterations in pulmonary microvascular tone and architecture. HPS occurs in up to 30% of patients with cirrhosis. Although the degree of hypoxemia does not reliably correlate with the severity of liver disease, patients with HPS have a higher mortality than do patients with cirrhosis without the disorder. There has been progress into defining the mechanisms that lead to hypoxemia in HPS, but to date there are no therapeutic options for HPS aside from liver transplantation.

Portopulmonary hypertension (POPH) is the presence of pulmonary arterial hypertension in patients with portal hypertension. Among liver transplant (LT) candidates, reported incidence rates of POPH range from 4.5% to 8.5%. In patients with LT, intraoperative death and immediate post-LT mortality are feared clinical events when transplantation is attempted in the setting of untreated, moderate to severe POPH; therefore, POPH precludes LT unless the mean pulmonary artery pressure can be reduced to a safe level and right ventricular function optimized. Specific

CLINICS IN LIVER DISEASE

FORTHCOMING ISSUES

August 2014
Liver Transplantation: Update of
Concepts and Practice
Kalyan Ram Bhamidimarri and
Paul Martin, *Editors*

November 2014
Interventional Procedures in
Hepatobiliary Diseases
Andres Cardenas and Paul Thuluvath,
Editors

February 2015
Consultations in Liver Disease
Steven L. Flamm, *Editor*

RECENT ISSUES

February 2014
The Impact of Obesity and Nutrition
on Chronic Liver Diseases
Zobair M. Younossi, *Editor*

November 2013
Drug Hepatotoxicity
Nikolaos T. Pyrsopoulos, *Editor*

August 2013
Hepatitis B Virus
Tarik Asselah and Patrick Marcellin,
Editors

RELATED INTEREST

Clinics in Liver Disease
August 2014 (Vol. 18, No. 3)
Liver Transplantation: Update of Concepts and Practice
Kalyan Ram Bhamidimarri and Paul Martin, *Editors*

DOWNLOAD Free App!

Review Articles
THE CLINICS

NOW AVAILABLE FOR YOUR iPhone and iPad

Preface

Portal Hypertension

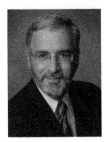

Jorge L. Herrera, MD
Editor

Portal hypertension is a universal consequence of cirrhosis and some noncirrhotic chronic liver diseases. Once portal hypertension develops, a cascade of events follow, leading to complications commonly associated with chronic liver disease. This issue reviews recent advances that have led to a better understanding of the pathophysiology of portal hypertension, its complications, and their management.

Dr Iwakiri provides an overview of the latest research on the mechanisms leading to portal hypertension and discusses current and future therapies. The diagnosis of portal hypertension is not always easy to establish and Dr De Franchis and associates review new tests and procedures that promise to simplify the process of confirming portal hypertension. While not common in Western clinical practice, noncirrhotic portal hypertension can be a vexing clinical problem; this subject is reviewed by Dr Sarin, who presents a comprehensive overview of noncirrhotic portal hypertension, its diagnosis, and its management.

The remainder of the issue focuses on the evaluation and current pharmacologic, endoscopic, and radiologic management of the complications of portal hypertension, including gastrointestinal bleeding, hepatic hydrothorax, hepatopulmonary syndrome, and portopulmonary hypertension, among others, providing a comprehensive guide for practitioners who take care of these challenging patients.

The issue ends with an extensive review of the perioperative risk assessment of patients with cirrhosis, a common scenario in clinical practice. Drs Im, Schiano, and colleagues present the current state-of-the-art on this topic and provide practical guidelines on how to best complete this challenging task.

Clin Liver Dis 18 (2014) xiii–xiv
http://dx.doi.org/10.1016/j.cld.2014.02.001
1089-3261/14/$ – see front matter © 2014 Elsevier Inc. All rights reserved.

liver.theclinics.com

We hope that you will find this issue informative and a useful reference tool as you face the ever-increasing challenge of caring for patients with advanced liver disease.

Jorge L. Herrera, MD
Professor of Medicine
Division of Gastroenterology
University of South Alabama College of Medicine
Gastroenterology Academic Offices
75 University Boulevard South, UCOM 6000
Mobile, AL 36688, USA

E-mail address:
jherrera18@gmail.com

Pathophysiology of Portal Hypertension

Yasuko Iwakiri, PhD

KEYWORDS

- Hyperdynamic circulation • Fibrosis • Cirrhosis • Nitric oxide • Lymphatic system
- Splenomegaly

KEY POINTS

- The primary cause of portal hypertension in liver cirrhosis is increased intrahepatic vascular resistance.
- A reduction of intrahepatic vascular resistance could ameliorate portal hypertension.
- Arterial vasodilatation in the splanchnic and systemic circulations worsens portal hypertension.

INTRODUCTION

Portal hypertension is a detrimental complication resulting from obstruction of portal blood flow, such as cirrhosis or portal vein thrombosis.[1,2] In liver cirrhosis, increased intrahepatic vascular resistance to the portal flow increases portal pressure and leads to portal hypertension (**Fig. 1**). Once portal hypertension develops, it influences extra-hepatic vascular beds in the splanchnic and systemic circulations, causing collateral vessel formation and arterial vasodilation. This process helps to increase the blood flow into the portal vein, which exacerbates portal hypertension and eventually brings the hyperdynamic circulatory syndrome.[1,2] As a result, esophageal varices or ascites develops. This article discusses recent advances in understanding of factors that contribute to an increase in intrahepatic vascular resistance and an increase in blood flow in the splanchnic and systemic circulations, and the future directions of basic/clinical research in portal hypertension.

INTRAHEPATIC CIRCULATION
An Overview

The primary cause of portal hypertension in cirrhosis is an increase in intrahepatic vascular resistance. In cirrhosis, increased intrahepatic vascular resistance is a result

Disclosure: The author has nothing to disclose.
Funding: This work was supported by grant R01DK082600 from the National Institutes of Health.
Section of Digestive Diseases, Department of Internal Medicine, Yale University School of Medicine, 1080 LMP, 333 Cedar Street, New Haven, CT 06520, USA
E-mail address: yasuko.iwakiri@yale.edu

Clin Liver Dis 18 (2014) 281–291
http://dx.doi.org/10.1016/j.cld.2013.12.001 **liver.theclinics.com**
1089-3261/14/$ – see front matter © 2014 Elsevier Inc. All rights reserved.

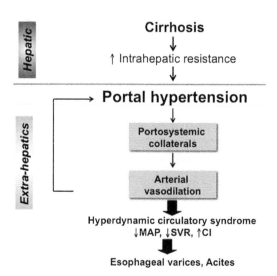

Fig. 1. Portal hypertension leads to the development of the hyperdynamic circulatory syndrome, characterized by decreased mean arterial pressure (MAP), decreased systemic vascular resistance (SVR), and increased cardiac index (CI).

of massive structural changes associated with fibrosis/cirrhosis and intrahepatic vasoconstriction.[2–4] It is reported that intrahepatic vasoconstriction accounts for at least 25% of increased intrahepatic vascular resistance.[5] Phenotypic changes in hepatic cells, such as hepatic stellate cells (HSCs) and liver sinusoidal endothelial cells (LSECs), are known to play pivotal roles in increased intrahepatic vascular resistance and have been studied intensively. This article summarizes important factors that increase intrahepatic vascular resistance in liver fibrosis/cirrhosis.

Endothelial cell dysfunction

LSECs are the first line of defense protecting the liver from injury,[2] and the cells exert diverse effects on liver functions including blood clearance, vascular tone, immunity, hepatocyte growth,[6] and angiogenesis/sinusoidal remodeling.[7,8] Therefore, LSEC dysfunction could lead to impaired vasomotor control (primarily vasoconstrictive), inflammation, fibrosis, and impaired liver regeneration,[1,9] all of which facilitate the development of liver cirrhosis and portal hypertension.

Decreased vasodilators Nitric oxide (NO) is likely the most potent vasodilator molecule known today. In cirrhotic livers, NO production/bioavailability is significantly diminished, which contributes to increased intrahepatic vascular resistance.[2,9–12] At least 2 mechanisms explain the decreased NO production. First, the NO synthesizing enzyme endothelial NO synthase (eNOS) is inhibited by negative regulators (such as caveolin-1), which are upregulated during cirrhosis; as a result, NO production decreases.[11] Details regarding eNOS regulation in liver cirrhosis can be found elsewhere.[2,12] Second, oxidative stress is increased in cirrhosis. LSECs receive oxidative stress in response to a wide variety of agents, such as bacterial endotoxins, viruses, drugs, and ethanol.[13–15] During cirrhosis, increased superoxide radicals spontaneously react with NO to form peroxynitrite (ONOO−), an endogenous toxicant,[16] thereby decreasing NO's bioavailability as a vasodilator.[13] Antioxidant molecules such as vitamin C,[14] vitamin E,[17] superoxide dismutase,[15,18] and N-acetylcysteine[19] have been shown to ameliorate intrahepatic vascular resistance and portal hypertension.

Increased vasoconstrictors In cirrhosis, not only are vasodilators decreased, but vasoconstrictors, such as thromboxane A2 (TXA_2), are also increased. TXA_2 is produced by the action of cyclooxygenase-1 (COX-1) in LSECs.[20] The activity of COX-1 increases in cirrhotic livers, which results in greater quantities of TXA_2 and thereby increased intrahepatic vascular resistance. Inhibition of TXA_2 by the prostaglandin H_2/TXA_2 receptor blocker, SQ-29548, or blocking COX-1 activity by the COX-1 inhibitor, SC-560, attenuates the increased intrahepatic vascular resistance.[20,21] Endothelin-1 (ET-1) is another important vasoconstrictor when it binds to receptors on HSCs.[22–24]

Activated HSCs

HSCs are perisinusoidal and pericytelike cells, and reside in the space between LSECs and hepatocytes. In response to liver injury, HSCs are activated and transformed into myofibroblasts, which start to express several proinflammatory and fibrotic genes. HSCs become contractile in an activated state.[22,25–27] Increased recruitment of these activated HSCs around newly formed sinusoidal vessels increases intrahepatic vascular resistance in cirrhosis (**Fig. 2**).[8,28,29] Therefore, activated HSCs play a crucial role in the development of portal hypertension because of their contractile phenotype.

Furthermore, activated HSCs display a decreased response to vasodilators, such as NO.[30] In addition, ET-1, which is increased in cirrhosis, enhances the contractions of HSCs.[25–27] Increased ET-1 production and decreased NO production in cirrhotic livers therefore augment intrahepatic resistance to the portal blood flow through activated HSCs, which facilitates the development of portal hypertension. However, the manipulation of ET receptors with ET receptor antagonists is complex because of their differential vasoactive effects based on their cellular locations.

Angiogenesis in the liver

In portal hypertension, angiogenesis plays a crucial role in intrahepatic circulation. An increased number of vessels in the fibrotic septa and the surrounding regenerative

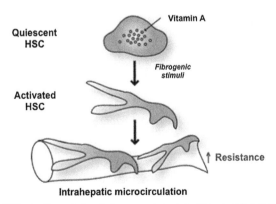

Fig. 2. Activated HSCs in liver cirrhosis increase intrahepatic vascular resistance. Quiescent HSCs are vitamin A storage cells and are found in normal livers. In response to fibrogenic stimuli, such as transforming growth factor beta, HSCs are activated to become myofibroblasts, which have a contractile and fibrogenic (collagen-producing) phenotype. These activated HSCs, located underneath LSECs, exert a contractile effect on the hepatic microcirculation, resulting in an increase in intrahepatic resistance.

nodules has been observed in cirrhotic livers.[31] Activated HSCs and/or other myofibroblasts, such as portal myofibroblasts, are thought to promote angiogenesis in liver cirrhosis. Activated HSCs activate LSECs by releasing angiogenic factors, such as angiopoietin[8,32,33] and vascular endothelial growth factor (VEGF).[34]

Irregular flow patterns, which are generated as a result of splitting (or intussusceptive) angiogenesis, may contribute to an increase in intrahepatic vascular resistance. In splitting angiogenesis, the two opposing walls of a capillary stretch and connect to each other, forming an intraluminal pillar. The junctions of the opposing endothelial cells are restructured, and the growth of the pillar is promoted. In addition, the capillary splits into 2 new vessels.[35] It has been reported that conditional Notch 1 knockout mice develop splitting angiogenesis, nodular regenerative hyperplasia, and portal hypertension. LSECs from these knockout mice show reduced endothelial fenestrae. These observations indicate that Notch 1 is necessary for LSEC fenestration, and that the absence of Notch 1 leads to pathologic angiogenesis, the development of nodular regenerative hyperplasia, and portal hypertension.[36]

EXTRAHEPATIC CIRCULATION
An Overview

Once portal hypertension develops, portosystemic collateral vessels form. Blood from the digestive organs diverts into these collateral vessels, but portal blood flowing from the splanchnic circulation increases to compensate for the blood escaping into the collateral vessels. Increased portal blood flow exacerbates portal hypertension. Furthermore, arterial vasodilatation in the splanchnic and systemic circulations observed in cirrhosis helps to increase the blood flow to the portal vein. Therefore, reducing the collateral vessel formation alone does not ameliorate portal hypertension. Inhibiting arterial vasodilation in the splanchnic circulation to reduce blood flow to portal vein is important in the treatment of portal hypertension.[2] The mechanisms of collateral vessel formation and arterial vasodilation in the splanchnic and systemic circulations in cirrhosis with portal hypertension are discussed later.

Collateral vessel formation

Portosystemic collateral vessels develop in response to an increase in portal pressure. These collateral vessels form through the opening of preexisting vessels or angiogenesis,[37,38] and are known to cause serious complications, including variceal bleeding and hepatic encephalopathy.[2,39,40] A change in portal pressure is thought to be detected first by the intestinal microcircular vascular bed, followed by arteries of the splanchnic circulation.[41] These vascular beds subsequently generate various angiogenic factors, such as VEGF[42–44] and placental growth factor (PIGF),[45] which promote the formation of portosystemic collaterals.

Studies in experimental models of portal hypertension and cirrhosis have shown that portosystemic collaterals are reduced by 18% to 78% with treatment by anti-VEGFR2,[46] a combination of anti-VEGF (rapamycin)/anti-PDGF (Gleevec),[47] anti-PIGF,[45] apelin antagonist,[48] sorafenib,[49,50] and a cannabinoid receptor 2 agonist.[51] However, the reduction of these collaterals does not necessarily decrease portal pressure because it does not substantially change the blood flow to the portal vein. Therefore, the concomitant mitigation of arterial vasodilation is also needed to reduce portal pressure.

Arterial vasodilation in the splanchnic and systemic circulations

Vasodilation NO is the most important vasodilator molecule that contributes to excessive vasodilatation observed in the arterial splanchnic and systemic circulations in portal hypertension. Experimental models of portal hypertension with or without cirrhosis have shown that other vasodilator molecules, such as carbon monoxide (CO), prostacyclin, endocannabinoids, and endothelium-derived hyperpolarizing factor (EDHF) are also induced.[2,9,12] The identity of EDHF is currently unknown, and the candidates include arachidonic acid metabolites epoxyeicosatrienoic acid, potassium ions (K$^+$), components of gap junctions, or hydrogen peroxide.[2]

An increase in portal pressure triggers eNOS activation and subsequent NO overproduction. Changes in portal pressure are detected at different vascular beds depending on the severity of portal hypertension.[41] A small increase in portal pressure is sensed first by the intestinal microcirculation and increases VEGF production with a subsequent increase in eNOS levels in the intestinal microcirculation. When portal pressure further increases and reaches a certain level, vasodilatation develops in the arterial splanchnic circulation (ie, the mesenteric arteries). It is postulated that mechanical forces including cyclic strains and shear stress, which are caused by an increased blood flow associated with an increased portal pressure, activate eNOS and lead to NO production.[41,46,52–54] Vasodilation subsequently develops in the arterial systemic circulation (ie, the aorta).

Hypocontractility Hypocontractility, decreased contractility to vasoconstrictors, is a characteristic of the arterial splanchnic and systemic circulations in portal hypertension. This phenomenon occurs largely because of the presence of excessive vasodilator molecules (ie, NO) and the resulting excessive arterial vasodilation, but is to some degree attributable to various molecules produced in smooth muscle cells and neurons. Those molecules include endocannabinoids (vasodilators),[55,56] neuropeptide Y,[57] urotensin II,[58,59] angiotensin,[60] and bradykinin[61,62] (all vasoconstrictors), with the vasodilators increased and the vasoconstrictors decreased.

Neural factors Neural factors are postulated to be involved in the development of the hyperdynamic circulatory syndrome, especially through the sympathetic system.[57,63,64] It is reported that sympathetic nerve atrophy/regression observed in the mesenteric arteries of portal hypertensive rats contributes to vasodilation and/or hypocontractility of those arteries.[65,66] The role of neural factors in decreased contractile responses is not yet fully understood and is an important area to be explored.

Structural changes of arteries The thinning of arterial walls is observed in the splanchnic and systemic circulations of rats with cirrhotic livers.[67,68] Although this arterial thinning results from hemodynamic changes caused by portal hypertension, it may also sustain arterial vasodilatation and worsen portal hypertension.[2,24] Although NO plays a role at least in part, the molecular mechanisms responsible for arterial thinning remain to be fully elucidated.

FUTURE DIRECTIONS
An Overview

Four important areas in the study of portal hypertension that have not been sufficiently explored are specified.

Microflora/bacterial translocation
In recent years, an accumulating body of evidence suggests the importance of gut microflora and bacterial translocation for the pathogenesis of a variety of diseases. Because of the anatomically close location and the connection through the vascular system, the liver is continuously exposed to microbial products from the gut.[69] Bacterial translation is closely related to the development of ascites.[70] In addition, small

changes in portal pressure are first sensed in the intestinal microcirculation. Increased portal pressure caused by portal hypertension may influence the gut-liver axis, further advance the disorders of liver fibrosis/cirrhosis, and exacerbate portal hypertension. Therefore, gut microflora may have an important role in a pathologic loop that develops and maintains portal hypertension. In addition, microflora may influence cytokine/chemokine production in the liver, which may also exacerbate portal hypertension.

Stem cell therapy

Stem cell therapy has received considerable attention as an alternative to liver transplantation. Studies have shown that stem cell transplantation improved liver functions in cirrhotic patients[71,72] as well as experimental models of liver cirrhosis.[73,74] Although stem cell therapy has shown promising effects on the amelioration of liver fibrosis and portal hypertension, more studies are needed.

The lymphatic system

The lymphatic system plays a central role in ascites and edema formation.[75] Further, an association between lymphangiogenesis and portal hypertension has been reported.[76] However, the detailed role and mechanisms of the lymphatic system in liver cirrhosis and portal hypertension are largely unknown, and these are important areas to be explored.[77,78]

Splenomegaly

Spleen stiffness has recently received considerable attention as an indicator of portal hypertension[79] because it can be examined by noninvasive imaging systems such as transient elastrography[80] and acoustic radiation force impulse imaging.[79,81] Some studies also suggest that spleen stiffness could predict the presence of varices[79–81] or ascites.[82] An experimental model of cirrhosis with portal hypertension has shown that portal pressure positively correlated with the spleen size.[42] In addition, a study using rats with partial portal vein ligation (PVL) showed that fibrosis and angiogenesis in the spleen were accompanied by splenomegaly induced by PVL, and that administration of rapamycin, an immunosuppressive agent, reduced splenomegaly as well as fibrosis and angiogenesis in the spleen.[83] At present, the detailed mechanisms through which portal pressure induces splenomegaly remain to be fully elucidated.

SUMMARY

With knowledge of vascular biology, understanding of the pathogenesis of portal hypertension has significantly advanced, revealing how vascular abnormalities both inside and outside the liver contribute to portal hypertension.[84] To ameliorate portal hypertension, first and foremost, a decrease in intrahepatic vascular resistance in cirrhotic liver is needed. Therefore, an increased production of vasodilator molecules in LSECs and a decrease in HSC contraction are important. For example, induction of apoptosis of enhanced activated HSCs,[85,86] thereby decreasing contractile HSCs, could be a useful therapeutic strategy to decrease portal pressure.

REFERENCES

1. Bosch J. Vascular deterioration in cirrhosis: the big picture. J Clin Gastroenterol 2007;41(Suppl 3):S247–53.
2. Iwakiri Y, Groszmann RJ. The hyperdynamic circulation of chronic liver diseases: from the patient to the molecule. Hepatology 2006;43:S121–31.

3. Rockey DC. Cell and molecular mechanisms of increased intrahepatic resistance and hemodynamic correlates. Totowa (NJ): Humana Press; 2005.

4. Pinzani M, Vizzutti F. Anatomy and vascular biology of the cells in the portal circulation. Totowa (NJ): Humana Press; 2005.

5. Wiest R, Groszmann RJ. The paradox of nitric oxide in cirrhosis and portal hypertension: too much, not enough. Hepatology 2002;35:478–91.

6. Ding BS, Nolan DJ, Butler JM, et al. Inductive angiocrine signals from sinusoidal endothelium are required for liver regeneration. Nature 2010;468:310–5.

7. Jagavelu K, Routray C, Shergill U, et al. Endothelial cell toll-like receptor 4 regulates fibrosis-associated angiogenesis in the liver. Hepatology 2010;52: 590–601.

8. Thabut D, Shah V. Intrahepatic angiogenesis and sinusoidal remodeling in chronic liver disease: new targets for the treatment of portal hypertension? J Hepatol 2010;53:976–80.

9. Iwakiri Y, Groszmann RJ. Vascular endothelial dysfunction in cirrhosis. J Hepatol 2007;46:927–34.

10. Shah V, Haddad FG, Garcia-Cardena G, et al. Liver sinusoidal endothelial cells are responsible for nitric oxide modulation of resistance in the hepatic sinusoids. J Clin Invest 1997;100:2923–30.

11. Shah V, Toruner M, Haddad F, et al. Impaired endothelial nitric oxide synthase activity associated with enhanced caveolin binding in experimental cirrhosis in the rat. Gastroenterology 1999;117:1222–8.

12. Iwakiri Y. The molecules: mechanisms of arterial vasodilatation observed in the splanchnic and systemic circulation in portal hypertension. J Clin Gastroenterol 2007;41:S288–94.

13. Gracia-Sancho J, Lavina B, Rodriguez-Vilarrupla A, et al. Increased oxidative stress in cirrhotic rat livers: a potential mechanism contributing to reduced nitric oxide bioavailability. Hepatology 2008;47:1248–56.

14. Hernandez-Guerra M, Garcia-Pagan JC, Turnes J, et al. Ascorbic acid improves the intrahepatic endothelial dysfunction of patients with cirrhosis and portal hypertension. Hepatology 2006;43:485–91.

15. Lavina B, Gracia-Sancho J, Rodriguez-Vilarrupla A, et al. Superoxide dismutase gene transfer reduces portal pressure in CCl4 cirrhotic rats with portal hypertension. Gut 2009;58:118–25.

16. Radi R. Peroxynitrite, a stealthy biological oxidant. J Biol Chem 2013;288: 26464–72.

17. Yang YY, Lee TY, Huang YT, et al. Asymmetric dimethylarginine (ADMA) determines the improvement of hepatic endothelial dysfunction by vitamin E in cirrhotic rats. Liver Int 2012;32:48–57.

18. Garcia-Caldero H, Rodriguez-Vilarrupla A, Gracia-Sancho J, et al. Tempol administration, a superoxide dismutase mimetic, reduces hepatic vascular resistance and portal pressure in cirrhotic rats. J Hepatol 2011;54:660–5.

19. Yang YY, Lee KC, Huang YT, et al. Effects of N-acetylcysteine administration in hepatic microcirculation of rats with biliary cirrhosis. J Hepatol 2008;49: 25–33.

20. Gracia-Sancho J, Lavina B, Rodriguez-Vilarrupla A, et al. Enhanced vasoconstrictor prostanoid production by sinusoidal endothelial cells increases portal perfusion pressure in cirrhotic rat livers. J Hepatol 2007;47:220–7.

21. Graupera M, March S, Engel P, et al. Sinusoidal endothelial COX-1-derived prostanoids modulate the hepatic vascular tone of cirrhotic rat livers. Am J Physiol Gastrointest Liver Physiol 2005;288:G763–70.

22. Kawada N, Tran-Thi TA, Klein H, et al. The contraction of hepatic stellate (Ito) cells stimulated with vasoactive substances. Possible involvement of endothelin 1 and nitric oxide in the regulation of the sinusoidal tonus. Eur J Biochem 1993; 213:815–23.

23. Bauer M, Bauer I, Sonin NV, et al. Functional significance of endothelin B receptors in mediating sinusoidal and extrasinusoidal effects of endothelins in the intact rat liver. Hepatology 2000;31:937–47.

24. Iwakiri Y. Endothelial dysfunction in the regulation of cirrhosis and portal hypertension. Liver Int 2012;32:199–213.

25. Kawada N, Seki S, Kuroki T, et al. ROCK inhibitor Y-27632 attenuates stellate cell contraction and portal pressure increase induced by endothelin-1. Biochem Biophys Res Commun 1999;266:296–300.

26. Pinzani M, Milani S, De Franco R, et al. Endothelin 1 is overexpressed in human cirrhotic liver and exerts multiple effects on activated hepatic stellate cells. Gastroenterology 1996;110:534–48.

27. Rockey DC, Weisiger RA. Endothelin induced contractility of stellate cells from normal and cirrhotic rat liver: implications for regulation of portal pressure and resistance. Hepatology 1996;24:233–40.

28. Medina J, Arroyo AG, Sanchez-Madrid F, et al. Angiogenesis in chronic inflammatory liver disease. Hepatology 2004;39:1185–95.

29. Kim MY, Baik SK, Lee SS. Hemodynamic alterations in cirrhosis and portal hypertension. Korean J Hepatol 2010;16:347–52.

30. Perri RE, Langer DA, Chatterjee S, et al. Defects in cGMP-PKG pathway contribute to impaired NO-dependent responses in hepatic stellate cells upon activation. Am J Physiol Gastrointest Liver Physiol 2006;290:G535–42.

31. Rappaport AM, MacPhee PJ, Fisher MM, et al. The scarring of the liver acini (cirrhosis). Tridimensional and microcirculatory considerations. Virchows Arch A Pathol Anat Histopathol 1983;402:107–37.

32. Taura K, De Minicis S, Seki E, et al. Hepatic stellate cells secrete angiopoietin 1 that induces angiogenesis in liver fibrosis. Gastroenterology 2008;135: 1729–38.

33. Thabut D, Routray C, Lomberk G, et al. Complementary vascular and matrix regulatory pathways underlie the beneficial mechanism of action of sorafenib in liver fibrosis. Hepatology 2011;54:573–85.

34. Novo E, Cannito S, Zamara E, et al. Proangiogenic cytokines as hypoxia-dependent factors stimulating migration of human hepatic stellate cells. Am J Pathol 2007;170:1942–53.

35. Nagy JA, Morgan ES, Herzberg KT, et al. Pathogenesis of ascites tumor growth: angiogenesis, vascular remodeling, and stroma formation in the peritoneal lining. Cancer Res 1995;55:376–85.

36. Dill MT, Rothweiler S, Djonov V, et al. Disruption of Notch1 induces vascular remodeling, intussusceptive angiogenesis, and angiosarcomas in livers of mice. Gastroenterology 2012;142:967–77.e2.

37. Sumanovski LT, Battegay E, Stumm M, et al. Increased angiogenesis in portal hypertensive rats: role of nitric oxide. Hepatology 1999;29:1044–9.

38. Sieber CC, Sumanovski LT, Stumm M, et al. In vivo angiogenesis in normal and portal hypertensive rats: role of basic fibroblast growth factor and nitric oxide. J Hepatol 2001;34:644–50.

39. Groszmann RJ, Kotelanski B, Cohn JN. Different patterns of porta-systemic shunting in cirrhosis of the liver studied by an indicator dilution technique. Acta Gastroenterol Latinoam 1971;3:111–6.

40. Bosch J, Pizcueta P, Feu F, et al. Pathophysiology of portal hypertension. Gastroenterol Clin North Am 1992;21:1–14.

41. Abraldes JG, Iwakiri Y, Loureiro-Silva M, et al. Mild increases in portal pressure upregulate vascular endothelial growth factor and endothelial nitric oxide synthase in the intestinal microcirculatory bed, leading to a hyperdynamic state. Am J Physiol Gastrointest Liver Physiol 2006;290:G980–7.

42. Huang HC, Haq O, Utsumi T, et al. Intestinal and plasma VEGF levels in cirrhosis: the role of portal pressure. J Cell Mol Med 2012;16:1125–33.

43. Fernandez M, Vizzutti F, Garcia-Pagan JC, et al. Anti-VEGF receptor-2 monoclonal antibody prevents portal-systemic collateral vessel formation in portal hypertensive mice. Gastroenterology 2004;126:886–94.

44. Geerts AM, De Vriese AS, Vanheule E, et al. Increased angiogenesis and permeability in the mesenteric microvasculature of rats with cirrhosis and portal hypertension: an in vivo study. Liver Int 2006;26:889–98.

45. Van Steenkiste C, Geerts A, Vanheule E, et al. Role of placental growth factor in mesenteric neoangiogenesis in a mouse model of portal hypertension. Gastroenterology 2009;137:2112–24.e1–6.

46. Fernandez M, Mejias M, Angermayr B, et al. Inhibition of VEGF receptor-2 decreases the development of hyperdynamic splanchnic circulation and portalsystemic collateral vessels in portal hypertensive rats. J Hepatol 2005;43:98–103.

47. Fernandez M, Mejias M, Garcia-Pras E, et al. Reversal of portal hypertension and hyperdynamic splanchnic circulation by combined vascular endothelial growth factor and platelet-derived growth factor blockade in rats. Hepatology 2007;46:1208–17.

48. Tiani C, Garcia-Pras E, Mejias M, et al. Apelin signaling modulates splanchnic angiogenesis and portosystemic collateral vessel formation in rats with portal hypertension. J Hepatol 2009;50:296–305.

49. Mejias M, Garcia-Pras E, Tiani C, et al. Beneficial effects of sorafenib on splanchnic, intrahepatic, and portocollateral circulations in portal hypertensive and cirrhotic rats. Hepatology 2009;49:1245–56.

50. Reiberger T, Angermayr B, Schwabl P, et al. Sorafenib attenuates the portal hypertensive syndrome in partial portal vein ligated rats. J Hepatol 2009;51:865–73.

51. Huang HC, Wang SS, Hsin IF, et al. Cannabinoid receptor 2 agonist ameliorates mesenteric angiogenesis and portosystemic collaterals in cirrhotic rats. Hepatology 2012;56:248–58.

52. Iwakiri Y. The systemic and splanchnic circulation. In: Gines P, Kamath PS, Arroyo V, editors. Chronic liver failure, mechanisms and management. New York: Humana Press; 2011. p. 305–20.

53. Tsai MH, Iwakiri Y, Cadelina G, et al. Mesenteric vasoconstriction triggers nitric oxide overproduction in the superior mesenteric artery of portal hypertensive rats. Gastroenterology 2003;125:1452–61.

54. Iwakiri Y, Tsai MH, McCabe TJ, et al. Phosphorylation of eNOS initiates excessive NO production in early phases of portal hypertension. Am J Physiol Heart Circ Physiol 2002;282:H2084–90.

55. Moezi L, Gaskari SA, Liu H, et al. Anandamide mediates hyperdynamic circulation in cirrhotic rats via CB(1) and VR(1) receptors. Br J Pharmacol 2006;149:898–908.

56. Batkai S, Jarai Z, Wagner JA, et al. Endocannabinoids acting at vascular CB1 receptors mediate the vasodilated state in advanced liver cirrhosis. Nat Med 2001;7:827–32.

57. Moleda L, Trebicka J, Dietrich P, et al. Amelioration of portal hypertension and the hyperdynamic circulatory syndrome in cirrhotic rats by neuropeptide Y via pronounced splanchnic vasoaction. Gut 2011;60(8):1122–32.

58. Trebicka J, Leifeld L, Hennenberg M, et al. Hemodynamic effects of urotensin II and its specific receptor antagonist palosuran in cirrhotic rats. Hepatology 2008; 47:1264–76.

59. Kemp W, Krum H, Colman J, et al. Urotensin II: a novel vasoactive mediator linked to chronic liver disease and portal hypertension. Liver Int 2007;27: 1232–9.

60. Hennenberg M, Trebicka J, Kohistani AZ, et al. Vascular hyporesponsiveness to angiotensin II in rats with CCl(4)-induced liver cirrhosis. Eur J Clin Invest 2009; 39:906–13.

61. Chu CJ, Wu SL, Lee FY, et al. Splanchnic hyposensitivity to glypressin in a haemorrhage/transfused rat model of portal hypertension: role of nitric oxide and bradykinin. Clin Sci (Lond) 2000;99:475–82.

62. Chen CT, Chu CJ, Lee FY, et al. Splanchnic hyposensitivity to glypressin in a hemorrhage-transfused common bile duct-ligated rat model of portal hypertension: role of nitric oxide and bradykinin. Hepatogastroenterology 2009;56: 1261–7.

63. Heinemann A, Wachter CH, Fickert P, et al. Vasopressin reverses mesenteric hyperemia and vasoconstrictor hyporesponsiveness in anesthetized portal hypertensive rats. Hepatology 1998;28:646–54.

64. Song D, Liu H, Sharkey KA, et al. Hyperdynamic circulation in portal-hypertensive rats is dependent on central c-fos gene expression. Hepatology 2002;35:159–66.

65. Coll M, Martell M, Raurell I, et al. Atrophy of mesenteric sympathetic innervation may contribute to splanchnic vasodilation in rat portal hypertension. Liver Int 2010;30:593–602.

66. Ezkurdia N, Coll M, Raurell I, et al. Blockage of the afferent sensitive pathway prevents sympathetic atrophy and hemodynamic alterations in rat portal hypertension. Liver Int 2012;32:1295–305.

67. Fernandez-Varo G, Ros J, Morales-Ruiz M, et al. Nitric oxide synthase 3-dependent vascular remodeling and circulatory dysfunction in cirrhosis. Am J Pathol 2003;162:1985–93.

68. Fernandez-Varo G, Morales-Ruiz M, Ros J, et al. Impaired extracellular matrix degradation in aortic vessels of cirrhotic rats. J Hepatol 2007;46:440–6.

69. Seo YS, Shah VH. The role of gut-liver axis in the pathogenesis of liver cirrhosis and portal hypertension. Clin Mol Hepatol 2012;18:337–46.

70. Frances R, Chiva M, Sanchez E, et al. Bacterial translocation is downregulated by anti-TNF-alpha monoclonal antibody administration in rats with cirrhosis and ascites. J Hepatol 2007;46:797–803.

71. Terai S, Ishikawa T, Omori K, et al. Improved liver function in patients with liver cirrhosis after autologous bone marrow cell infusion therapy. Stem Cells 2006; 24:2292–8.

72. Jang YO, Kim YJ, Baik SK, et al. Histological improvement following administration of autologous bone marrow-derived mesenchymal stem cells for alcoholic cirrhosis: a pilot study. Liver Int 2014;34(1):33–41.

73. Sakamoto M, Nakamura T, Torimura T, et al. Transplantation of endothelial progenitor cells ameliorates vascular dysfunction and portal hypertension in carbon tetrachloride-induced rat liver cirrhotic model. J Gastroenterol Hepatol 2013;28: 168–78.

74. Sakaida I, Terai S, Yamamoto N, et al. Transplantation of bone marrow cells reduces CCl4-induced liver fibrosis in mice. Hepatology 2004;40:1304–11.
75. Cardenas A, Bataller R, Arroyo V. Mechanisms of ascites formation. Clin Liver Dis 2000;4:447–65.
76. Barrowman JA, Granger DN. Effects of experimental cirrhosis on splanchnic microvascular fluid and solute exchange in the rat. Gastroenterology 1984;87: 165–72.
77. Chung C, Iwakiri Y. The lymphatic vascular system in liver diseases: its role in ascites formation. Clin Mol Hepatol 2013;19:99–104.
78. Ribera J, Pauta M, Melgar-Lesmes P, et al. Increased nitric oxide production in lymphatic endothelial cells causes impairment of lymphatic drainage in cirrhotic rats. Gut 2013;62:138–45.
79. Takuma Y, Nouso K, Morimoto Y, et al. Measurement of spleen stiffness by acoustic radiation force impulse imaging identifies cirrhotic patients with esophageal varices. Gastroenterology 2013;144:92–101.e2.
80. Colecchia A, Montrone L, Scaioli E, et al. Measurement of spleen stiffness to evaluate portal hypertension and the presence of esophageal varices in patients with HCV-related cirrhosis. Gastroenterology 2012;143:646–54.
81. Berzigotti A, Seijo S, Arena U, et al. Elastography, spleen size, and platelet count identify portal hypertension in patients with compensated cirrhosis. Gastroenterology 2013;144:102–11.e1.
82. Mori K, Arai H, Abe T, et al. Spleen stiffness correlates with the presence of ascites but not esophageal varices in chronic hepatitis C patients. Biomed Res Int 2013;2013:857862.
83. Mejias M, Garcia-Pras E, Gallego J, et al. Relevance of the mTOR signaling pathway in the pathophysiology of splenomegaly in rats with chronic portal hypertension. J Hepatol 2010;52:529–39.
84. Iwakiri Y, Grisham M, Shah V. Vascular biology and pathobiology of the liver: report of a single-topic symposium. Hepatology 2008;47:1754–63.
85. Tashiro K, Satoh A, Utsumi T, et al. Absence of Nogo-B (reticulon 4B) facilitates hepatic stellate cell apoptosis and diminishes hepatic fibrosis in mice. Am J Pathol 2013;182:786–95.
86. Zhang D, Utsumi T, Huang HC, et al. Reticulon 4B (Nogo-B) is a novel regulator of hepatic fibrosis. Hepatology 2011;53:1306–15.

Invasive and Noninvasive Methods to Diagnose Portal Hypertension and Esophageal Varices

Roberto de Franchis, MD*, Alessandra Dell'Era, MD, PhD

KEYWORDS

- Portal hypertension • Esophageal varices • Hepatic vein pressure gradient
- Esophagogastroduodenoscopy • Transient elastography

KEY POINTS

- The reference standard methods to measure portal pressure and to diagnose the presence of esophagogastric varices are the measurement of the hepatic vein pressure gradient (HVPG) and esophagogastroduodenoscopy.
- Several methods have been tested as potential surrogates of HVPG: none of them has proven accurate enough to predict the numerical value of HVPG.
- With all methods proposed as noninvasive tests to predict the presence of varices, a certain number of patients with varices will be missed, and a variable number of unnecessary endoscopies will still be done.
- If one decides to adopt a noninvasive method to replace HVPG measurement or esophagogastroduodenoscopy, the potential benefits in terms of cost saving, availability, and patient acceptance must be weighted against the potential risks of misdiagnosis and inappropriate therapeutic decisions.

INTRODUCTION

The development of portal hypertension (PH) is a crucial event in the evolution of cirrhosis and is defined by an increase in portal pressure above the normal range of 1 to 5 mm Hg, as measured by the hepatic vein pressure gradient (HVPG). When the HVPG increases further to ≥ 10 mm Hg, PH is defined as clinically significant. The occurrence of clinically significant portal hypertension (CSPH) is a crucial turning point in the natural history of cirrhosis, because it opens the way to the development of esophageal varices and hepatic decompensation. It is therefore important from

---

The authors declare that they have no conflict of interest.

Gastroenterology Unit, Department of Clinical and Biomedical Sciences, Luigi Sacco University Hospital, University of Milan, Via G. B. Grassi 74, Milan 20157, Italy

* Corresponding author.

E-mail address: roberto.defranchis@unimi.it

Clin Liver Dis 18 (2014) 293–302

http://dx.doi.org/10.1016/j.cld.2013.12.002

1089-3261/14/$ – see front matter © 2014 Elsevier Inc. All rights reserved.

a clinical standpoint to assess the presence of CSPH and of esophageal varices. Indeed, international guidelines[1] state that, "In centers where adequate resources and expertise are available, HVPG measurement should be routinely used for diagnostic and therapeutic indications" and that "All cirrhotic patients should be screened for varices at diagnosis." The reference standard technique to assess the presence and severity of PH is the measurement of HVPG, whereas esophagogastroduodenoscopy (EGD) is the gold-standard method for the diagnosis of esophageal varices. Both these methods are costly and invasive and perceived as unpleasant, and in addition, HVPG measurement is available in specialized centers only. For these reasons, in the last 10 years, methods aimed at determining noninvasively the presence of CSPH and of esophageal varices have been increasingly investigated.

In this article, the technique of HVPG measurement for the assessment of portal pressure and of EGD for the diagnosis of varices is described; also the performance of several methods that have been proposed as noninvasive alternatives to HVPG and EGD is analyzed.

INVASIVE METHODS TO DIAGNOSE PH AND ESOPHAGEAL VARICES
Measurement of HVPG

Since 1951,[2] HVPG measurement has replaced more invasive methods to assess portal pressure, such as splenic pulp manometry and percutaneous transhepatic or transvenous catheterization of the portal vein, which were used previously.

HVPG measurement is performed under local anesthesia via the internal jugular or femoral vein using a balloon catheter. The catheter is advanced into a hepatic vein, and HVPG is obtained by measuring the difference between the wedged (WHVP) and the free (FHVP) hepatic venous pressures. The WHVP is obtained by inflating the balloon, thus occluding the hepatic vein, while the FHVP is measured with the catheter floating freely in the vein lumen. The occlusion of one hepatic vein stops blood flow in the hepatic veins and in the sinusoids, equalizing the pressure in the occluded position to the pressure in the sinusoids. In the normal liver the WHVP is slightly lower than the portal pressure but in cirrhosis of viral or alcoholic cause, the WHVP gives an accurate estimate of portal pressure.[3,4] In cirrhosis, HVPG equals portal pressure, whereas in presinusoidal PH (eg, schistosomiasis, idiopathic PH) or in prehepatic PH (eg, portal vein thrombosis) HVPG is normal or slightly increased.[3-6]

Accurate measurement of the HVPG is crucial, because inaccuracy can lead to inappropriate clinical decisions. Therefore, several guidelines have been published on how to measure HVPG properly.[7,8]

The required equipment to measure HVPG is composed of a recorder with the capability of producing permanent tracings of pressure values (with an upper limit of about 30–40 mm Hg), a quartz pressure transducer that can detect even subtle changes in venous pressure, and an occlusion balloon catheter. When measuring the WHVP or the FHVP, the operators should wait for stabilization of the venous pressure and all measurements should be repeated at least 3 times to check reproducibility. Complete occlusion of the hepatic vein by the inflated balloon and the absence of venovenous shunts distally to the balloon should be routinely checked, to avoid an underestimation of the WHVP; this is usually done by injecting 5 mL of contrast medium through the tip of the catheter. All pressure tracings should be recorded and printed so that they can be reviewed by independent observers. HVPG must be measured as the difference between WHVPs and FHVPs: this prevents the measurement from being influenced by changes in intra-abdominal pressure (eg, for ascites) and by inadequate positioning of the external zero reference point. The hepatic-atrial pressure gradient, suggested by some authors to reflect the variceal hemodynamics better, should not be used because it has been shown[9] that this parameter does not correlate with HVPG and does not provide the excellent prognostic information HVPG gives when used to evaluate the response to drug therapy.

The measurement of the WHVP should be done by inflating the balloon at the tip of a balloon catheter in a large hepatic vein, as first described by Groszmann and colleagues,[10] and not by wedging the catheter in a small venule to block the blood flow[5,11]; in fact, the balloon allows measuring the pressure in a larger volume of the liver, and thus more reproducibly.[12–16]

HVPG measurement is a safe procedure with 0 to 1% minor complications in a large series of patients.[17,18] Nevertheless, the technique has limited applicability because it is available only in specialized centers and is regarded as unpleasant and potentially dangerous by the patients or their physicians.[19]

Endoscopic Evaluation of Esophageal Varices

Upper gastrointestinal (GI) endoscopy is a suitable tool for screening because it is widely available; in addition, because the risk of bleeding is related to the size of varices and the presence of red signs,[20] it can be estimated by endoscopy, and finally, besides esophageal varices, endoscopy can identify other potentially bleeding lesions related to PH, such as gastric varices, portal hypertensive gastropathy, and gastric antral vascular ectasia.

Upper GI endoscopy may be performed with or without light sedation and should include a complete examination of the esophagus, stomach, and proximal duodenum, because portal-hypertension related lesions can be found in all 3 sites. The adoption of simple rules will help improve the quality of the examination, increase the amount of information obtained, and decrease interobserver variability: (1) the evaluation must be done at the end of the examination, on the way out, after removing as much air as possible from the stomach by suction; (2) the size of varices must be assessed with the esophagus fully distended by air; (3) the worst finding present must be recorded; (4) a validated classification of esophageal varices must be used. Two widely adopted classifications are that of the Japanese Research Society for Portal Hypertension[21] and that of the Italian Liver Cirrhosis Project.[22] As stated in the introduction, international guidelines[1] state that, "All cirrhotic patients should be screened for varices at diagnosis." However, at a given point in time, a variable proportion of patients will not have varices; in fact, the reported prevalence of esophageal varices is variable,[23] ranging in different series between 24% and 80%. Thus, screening all cirrhotic patients with upper GI endoscopy to detect the presence of varices implies several unnecessary endoscopies, which increase the workload of endoscopy units. In addition, compliance with endoscopic screening recommendations may be suboptimal, because they require patients who are often totally asymptomatic to repeatedly undergo a procedure that is perceived as unpleasant.[24]

NONINVASIVE METHODS PROPOSED FOR THE DIAGNOSIS OF BOTH PH AND ESOPHAGEAL VARICES

The search for a practical "splanchnic sphygmomanometer" is challenging because the ideal noninvasive method to diagnose PH should be safe, cheap, easy to perform, accurate, and reproducible. In addition, it should be able to give objective numerical results in real-time and be predictive of significant "hard" endpoints, to allow prognostic stratification. As stated in the introduction, several methods have been examined in the hope of finding such a tool.

Laboratory Tests

Laboratory tests evaluating the degree of protein-synthetic function of the liver (albumin, international normalized ratio, bilirubin) correlate with the HVPG and the presence and grade of esophageal varices in patients with compensated as well as decompensated cirrhosis[25]; however, the correlation is not good enough to allow these tests to be used for diagnosing PH or esophageal varices.

Abdominal Imaging (Ultrasound Scan, Magnetic Resonance Imaging, Computed Tomography)

Splenomegaly is a sensitive but nonspecific imaging sign of PH.[25] Therefore, CSPH can be only suspected if splenomegaly is identified by imaging techniques, but requires confirmation by other means. On the other hand, abdominal portosystemic collaterals are specific signs of PH,[26] and when they are observed on ultrasound scan (US), magnetic resonance imaging, or computed tomography (CT), a diagnosis of CSPH can be made with confidence. The sensitivity of portosystemic collaterals, however, is limited, because only 20% to 54% of compensated cirrhotic patients with CSPH show abdominal collaterals on imaging. Therefore, imaging techniques are not accurate enough to be routinely used to diagnose or rule out PH.

Liver Stiffness Alone or in Combination

Liver stiffness (LS) is measured by means of transient elastography, an US technique that uses pulse-echo US acquisitions. The use of transient elastography in patients with liver disease is based on the assumption that fibrosis results in increased stiffness of the liver parenchyma. LS is measured in kilopascals. Transient elastography is attractive because it is noninvasive and measures stiffness in a volume of the liver that is approximately 100 times bigger than that of liver biopsy and thus might be less prone than biopsy to sampling error. Because fibrosis is one of the major determinants of PH, assessing the relationship between LS and portal pressure makes sense. LS has been shown to correlate strongly with portal pressure as measured by the HVPG and may predict clinical decompensation in compensated cirrhotic patients.[27,28] However, when HVPG values exceed 10 to 12 mm Hg, which are the threshold for CSPH and for the development of varices, portal pressure becomes largely independent from stiffness/fibrosis. Accordingly, the ability of LS to predict the presence and grade of esophageal varices in cirrhosis is insufficient.[27]

The combination of different noninvasive tests might provide complementary information, resulting in increased diagnostic value. In 2013, Berzigotti and colleagues[29] proposed 2 models, the PH risk score and the variceal risk score (VRS). The PH risk score is calculated with the formula: [PH risk score = $-5.953 + 0.188 \times$ LS + $1.583 \times$ sex (1: male; 0: female) + $26.705 \times$ spleen diameter/platelet count ratio]. The VRS is calculated with the formula: [VRS = $-4.364 + 0.538 \times$ spleen diameter $- 0.049 \times$ platelet count $- 0.44 \times$ LS + $0.001 \times$ (LS $\times$ platelet count)]. In 117 patients with compensated cirrhosis, the PH risk score and the VRS showed area under the receiver operated characteristic of 0.935 and 0.909, respectively. If used to select patients to undergo endoscopic screening, the VRS would have spared 65% of endoscopies.

Spleen Stiffness

Because spleen congestion is a specific feature of PH, spleen stiffness (SS) might also correlate with portal pressure. The performance of SS in diagnosing both CSPH and esophageal varices has been evaluated by transient elastography by Colecchia and colleagues[30]: the correlation of SS with the HVPG and with the presence or absence of varices was evaluated in comparison with LS, the LSPS index, and the platelet count/spleen diameter ratio (PSR). SS outperformed all other tests in both the assessment of CSPH and the presence of varices.

NONINVASIVE METHODS PROPOSED FOR THE DIAGNOSIS OF ESOPHAGEAL VARICES
PSR

The PSR is calculated by dividing the platelet number per cubic millimeter by the maximum spleen bipolar diameter in millimeters as estimated by abdominal US. The ratio is higher in patients without than in those with varices. In the original study, using a cutoff value of 909 of the PSR, the AUROC was 0.981, corresponding to positive and negative predictive values for the presence of varices of 96% and 100%, respectively (LR+ = 14.3; LR− = 0.1). Recently, a meta-analysis of 20 studies evaluating the performance of the PSR for the diagnosis of varices has been published.[31] The global performance of the PSR across studies was good (Hierarchical Summary ROC curve: 0.95), but there was statistically significant heterogeneity, and wide variability of the performance of PSR across studies. Therefore, the universal use of the PSR for diagnosing or ruling out varices cannot be recommended yet.

Liver Stiffness Platelet Spleen Index

In 2010, Kim and colleagues[32] proposed a new index, the Liver Stiffness Platelet Spleen index (LSPS, = LS × spleen diameter/platelet count) for the diagnosis of varices. The LSPS performed very well, with an AUROC of 0.954. The authors proposed an algorithm whereby patients with LSPS less than 3.5 should not undergo endoscopy; patients with an LSPS between 3.5 and 5.5 should be screened by EGD for varices, and patients with LSPS greater than 5.5 should undergo EGD or start empiric treatment. This method needs external validation.

Spleen Stiffness

The correlation of SS with the presence and size of varices was evaluated by transient elastography by Sharma and colleagues[33] and compared with LS, LSPS, and the PSR. Again, SS outperformed all other tests, and the authors suggested that combining SS+LS gave the best prediction of the presence of varices. SS can also be measured by acoustic radiation force impulse imaging (ARFI). ARFI is based on the measurement of the velocity of shear waves generated by mechanical excitement of liver tissue by ultrasonic impulses. ARFI is incorporated into conventional US machines and can be performed during a standard US examination. At variance with transient elastography, the region of interest whereby stiffness is measured is chosen under visual control in B-mode. These technical features and the physical principle of ARFI allow overcoming some of the limitations of transient elastography, such as the frequent technical failures in measuring SS, and in assessing LS in obese or ascitic patients. ARFI is expressed in meters per second. In a study by Takuma and colleagues,[34] ARFI measurement of SS outperformed LS and platelet count in the prediction of varices, with an AUROC of 0.933. However, a recent meta-analysis of 12 studies that compared the accuracy of SS with that of EGD in the diagnosis of esophageal varices[35] concluded that "the accuracy of SS in diagnosing esophageal varices is limited, and this precludes its widespread use in clinical practice, at this time."

Videocapsule Endoscopy

Videocapsule endoscopy (VCE), originally developed for the study of the small bowel, has become suitable for the esophagus with the development of a video capsule specifically designed to image this organ. The largest study that evaluated VCE for the screening and surveillance of esophageal varices[36] included 288 patients, of whom 62.5% had esophageal varices. The study had a noninferiority design, the assumption being that the difference (+SEM) between VCE and EGD, which was used as the gold standard, would be less than 10%. Although VCE performed well (positive predictive value 92%; negative predictive value 77%, LR+ 7; LR− 0.18), the study failed to meet the assumption, because there was a 16% difference in sensitivity in favor of EGD.

CT Esophagography

The use of single-detector and multidetector CT scanning has been evaluated as a screening modality for esophageal varices in 3 studies.[37–39] In all 3 studies the performance of CT esophagography was compared with that of EGD, which served as the gold standard. When considering all varices, across studies, CT esophagography had sensitivity ranging between of 64% and 93%, and specificity between 76% and 96.6%, respectively. For the detection of large varices, sensitivity ranged between 56% and 92%, and specificity between 84% and 92%. In the study giving the best results, air was insufflated into the esophagus (mean volume 1300 mL) via a catheter passed through the mouth.

WHAT DO THE CLINICIANS REALLY NEED TO KNOW?
Diagnosis of PH

Two crucial questions need to be answered to decide whether a noninvasive method can be used to replace HVPG measurement:

a. Is this method good enough to rule in or rule out CSPH?
b. Can this method be used to monitor the effect of drug therapy on portal pressure?

Concerning the first question, LS measurement has been shown to perform well in discriminating between patients with and without CSPH. Nevertheless, none of the proposed noninvasive alternatives to HVPG measurement is accurate enough to predict the numerical value of HVPG.

As far as the second question is concerned, it has been shown that LS is not currently capable of providing accurate information on the hemodynamic response to β-blockers (eg, LS changes do not correlate with HVPG changes during therapy).[40] Whether SS will perform better than LS remains to be ascertained.

Presence and Grade of Esophageal Varices

In deciding which method (if any) to adopt to select patients for EGD screening for varices, the following questions must be answered:

a. How many endoscopies would be spared by this method?
b. How many patients with varices would be missed?
c. How many unnecessary endoscopies would still be done?

Table 1 shows the answers to these questions for the various methods proposed.
In addition, one also must keep in mind that most studies were performed in patients with a high pretest probability of esophageal varices, not reflecting the clinical scenario of screening, that some of the methods proposed are not validated yet, and that, whatever the method, the number of endoscopies spared will have to be weighted against a proportion of missed varices and of residual unnecessary endoscopies. All the above facts should be considered in making the decision.

Table 1
Trade-offs of different methods proposed for selecting patients for the endoscopic screening of esophageal varices

Method	VCE	PSR	LS	LSPS	SS	VRS	ARFI
Author	de Franchis et al[36]	Ying et al[31]	Colecchia et al[30]	Kim et al[32]	Sharma et al[33]	Berzigotti et al[29]	Takuma et al[34]
No. of patients	288	3063	100	280	174	117	340
With varices, n (%)	181 (63)	1905 (62)	53 (53)	124 (44)	124 (71)	37 (32)	132 (39)
Endoscopies spared, n (%)	123 (43)	1088 (36)	29 (29)	157 (56)	45 (26)	76 (65)	144 (42)
Varices missed, n (%)	29 (16)	115 (6)	2 (4)	15 (12)	7 (6)	7 (23)	2 (1.5)
Unnecessary EGD, n (%)	13 (8)	185 (16)	20 (42)	14 (9)	12 (24)	11 (16)	66 (32)

SUMMARY

In summary, although HVPG measurement and EGD, the reference standard methods to diagnose the presence and grade of PH and esophageal varices, have some drawbacks, in that they are invasive, costly, and perceived as unpleasant by patients, none of the alternative noninvasive methods to replace them has been proven to be good enough so far.

As far as the evaluation of PH is concerned, LS measurement can distinguish between patients with and without CSPH; however, it is not suitable to detect treatment-related changes in HVPG, and thus, it cannot be used to guide therapy. SS is also good in diagnosing CSPH, but its performance in evaluating treatment-related HVPG changes has not been assessed.

Concerning the diagnosis and grading of esophageal varices, the PSR has given variable results, the LSPS and SS, measured either by transient elastography or ARFI, showed overall good performances, but these methods need external validation. VCE is inferior to EGD, whereas CT esophagography has given variable results, and in addition, there is the concern of radiation exposure.

At any rate, if one decides to adopt a noninvasive method to replace HVPG measurement or EGD, the potential benefits in terms of cost-saving, availability, and patient acceptance must be weighted against the potential risks of misdiagnosis and inappropriate therapeutic decisions.

REFERENCES

1. de Franchis R, Baveno V Faculty. Revising consensus in portal hypertension. Report of the Baveno V consensus workshop on methodology of diagnosis and therapy in portal hypertension. J Hepatol 2010;53:762–8.
2. Myers J, Taylor W. An estimation of portal venous pressure by occlusive catheterization of a hepatic venule. J Clin Invest 1951;30:662–3.
3. Perello A, Escorsell A, Bru C, et al. Wedged hepatic venous pressure adequately reflects portal pressure in hepatitis C virus-related cirrhosis. Hepatology 1999;30: 1393–7.
4. Thalheimer U, Leandro G, Samonakis DN, et al. Assessment of the agreement between wedge hepatic vein pressure and portal vein pressure in cirrhotic patients. Dig Liver Dis 2005;37:601–8.
5. Viallet A, Joly JG, Marleau D, et al. Comparison of free portal venous pressure and wedged hepatic venous pressure in patients with cirrhosis of the liver. Gastroenterology 1970;59:372–5.
6. Boyer TD, Triger DR, Horisawa M, et al. Direct transhepatic measurement of portal vein pressure using a thin needle. Comparison with wedged hepatic vein pressure. Gastroenterology 1977;72:584–9.
7. Groszmann RJ, Wongcharatrawee S. The hepatic venous pressure gradient: anything worth doing should be done right. Hepatology 2004;39:280–2.
8. Bosch J, Garcia-Pagan JC, Berzigotti A, et al. Measurement of portal pressure and its role in the management of chronic liver disease. Semin Liver Dis 2006;26:348–62.
9. La Mura V, Abraldes JG, Berzigotti A, et al. Right atrial pressure is not adequate to calculate portal pressure gradient in cirrhosis: a clinical–hemodynamic correlation study. Hepatology 2010;51:2108–16.
10. Groszmann RJ, Glickman M, Blei AT, et al. Wedged and free hepatic venous pressure measured with a balloon catheter. Gastroenterology 1979;76:253–8.
11. Reynolds TB, Ito S, Iwatsuki S. Measurement of portal pressure and its clinical application. Am J Med 1970;49:649–57.

12. Garcia-Tsao G, Groszmann RJ, Fisher RL, et al. Portal pressure, presence of gastroesophageal varices and variceal bleeding. Hepatology 1985;5:419–24.
13. Bützow GH, Novak D. Clinical value of hepatic vein catheterization. Improved pracability by balloon catheter technique. Gastrointest Radiol 1977;2:153–61.
14. Koyama K, Ito K, Asanuma Y, et al. Hepatic venography in portal hypertension by balloon catheter. Tohoku J Exp Med 1983;139:349–54.
15. Zipprich A, Winkler M, Seufferlein T, et al. Comparison of balloon vs. straight catheter for the measurement of portal hypertension. Aliment Pharmacol Ther 2010; 32:1351–6.
16. Montagnese S, Cavasin L, Vezzaro R, et al. Variability of the hepatic venous pressure gradient (HVPG) within the cirrhotic liver: an issue or a technical issue? Hepatology 2009;50(Suppl 1):444A.
17. Bosch J, Abraldes JG, Groszmann R. Current management of portal hypertension. J Hepatol 2003;38(Suppl 1):S54–68.
18. Thabut D, Moreau R, Lebrec D. Noninvasive assessment of portal hypertension in patients with cirrhosis. Hepatology 2011;53:683–94.
19. Dell'Era A, Cubero Sotela J, Fabris FM, et al. Primary prophylaxis of variceal bleeding in cirrhotic patients: a cohort study. Dig Liver Dis 2008;40:936–43.
20. North Italian Endoscopic Club for the Study and Treatment of Esophageal Varices. Prediction of the first variceal hemorrhage in patients with cirrhosis of the liver and esophageal varices. A prospective multicenter study. N Engl J Med 1988;319:983–9.
21. The general rules for recording endoscopic findings on esophageal varices. Jpn J Surg 1980;10:84–7.
22. Italian Liver Cirrhosis Project. Reliability of endoscopy in the assessment of variceal features. J Hepatol 1987;4:93–8.
23. Pascal JP, Calès P, Desmorat H. Natural history of oesophageal varices. review no: 22. In: Bosch J, Rodès J, editors. Recent advances in the pathophysiology and treatment of portal hypertension. Rome (Italy): Serono Symposia; 1989. p. 127–42.
24. Hapke RZ, Benner KG, Rosen HR, et al. Prevention of first variceal hemorrhage – a survey of community practice patterns [abstract]. Hepatology 1997;26(Pt 1):A30.
25. Berzigotti A, Gilabert R, Abraldes JG, et al. Noninvasive prediction of clinically significant portal hypertension and esophageal varices in patients with compensated liver cirrhosis. Am J Gastroenterol 2008;103:1159–67.
26. Vilgrain V, Lebrec D, Menu Y, et al. Comparison between ultrasonographic signs and the degree of portal hypertension in patients with cirrhosis. Gastrointest Radiol 1990;15:218–22.
27. Castera L, Pinzani M, Bosch J. Non-invasive evaluation of portal hypertension using transient elastography. J Hepatol 2012;56:696–703.
28. Robic MA, Procopet B, Metivier S, et al. Liver stiffness accurately predicts portal hypertension related complications in patients with chronic liver disease: a prospective study. J Hepatol 2011;55:1017–24.
29. Berzigotti A, Selio S, Arena U, et al. Elastography, spleen size and platelet count identify portal hypertension in patients with compensated cirrhosis. Gastroenterology 2013;1044:102–11.
30. Colecchia A, Montrone L, Scaioli E, et al. Measurement of spleen stiffness to evaluate portal hypertension and presence of esophageal varices in patients with HCV-related cirrhosis. Gastroenterology 2012;143:646–54.
31. Ying L, Lin X, Xie ZL, et al. Performance of platelet count/spleen diameter ratio for diagnosis of esophageal varices in cirrhosis: a meta-analysis. Dig Dis Sci 2012; 57:1672–81.

32. Kim BK, Han KH, Park JU, et al. A liver stiffness measurement-based, noninvasive prediction model for high risk esophageal varices in B-viral liver cirrhosis. Am J Gastroenterol 2010;105:1382–90.

33. Sharma P, Kirnake V, Tyagi P, et al. Spleen stiffness in patients with cirrhosis in predicting esophageal varices. Am J Gastroenterol 2013;108:1101–7.

34. Takuma Y, Nouso K, Morimoto Y, et al. Measurement of spleen stiffness by acoustic radiation force impulse imaging identifies cirrhotic patients with esophageal varices. Gastroenterology 2013;144:92–101.

35. Singh S, Eaton JE, Murad MH, et al. Accuracy of spleen stiffness measurement in detection of esophageal varices in patients with chronic liver disease: systematic review and meta-analysis. Clin Gastroenterol Hepatol 2013. http://dx.doi.org/10.1016/j.cgh.2013.09.013.

36. de Franchis R, Eisen GM, Laine L, et al. Oesophageal capsule endoscopy for screening and surveillance of oesophageal varices in patients with portal hypertension. Hepatology 2008;47:1595–603.

37. Kim YJ, Raman SS, Yu NC, et al. Esophageal varices in cirrhotic patients: evaluation with liver CT. AJR Am J Roentgenol 2007;188:139–44.

38. Kim SH, Kim YJ, Lee JM, et al. Oesophageal varices in patients with cirrhosis: multidetector CT esophagography – comparison with endoscopy. Radiology 2007;242:759–68.

39. Perri RE, Chiorean MV, Fidler JL, et al. A prospective evaluation of computerized tomographic (CT) scanning as a screening modality for esophageal varices. Hepatology 2008;47:1587–94.

40. Reiberger T, Ferlitsch A, Payer BA, et al. Non-selective β-blockers improve the correlation of liver stiffness and portal pressure in advanced cirrhosis. J Gastroenterol 2012;47:561–8.

Pharmacologic Management of Portal Hypertension

Annalisa Berzigotti, MD, PhD, Jaime Bosch, MD, PhD, FRCP*

KEYWORDS

- Chronic liver disease • Portal pressure • Hepatic resistance • Splanchnic blood flow
- Drug therapy

KEY POINTS

- Drugs for portal hypertension should decrease portal pressure without adverse effects on the systemic circulation and liver function.
- Targets of pharmacologic treatment of portal hypertension include increased hepatic resistance, increased splanchnic blood flow, and hyperdynamic circulation.
- Nonselective β-blockers (NSBBs) are the mainstay of chronic oral treatment of portal hypertension, whereas terlipressin and somatostatin/somatostatin analogues are used parenterally in acute variceal bleeding and hepatorenal syndrome.
- Carvedilol is a new and increasingly used NSBB with anti-α-1 adrenergic activity that has greater portal pressure decreasing effect than standard NSBBs.
- Most drugs currently under investigation are aimed at reducing hepatic resistance (hepatic vascular tone) and include statins, antioxidants, RAAS inhibitors, as well as antifibrotic stategies (structural changes).

INTRODUCTION

Portal hypertension (PH) is a frequent and severe clinical syndrome, which almost invariably complicates liver cirrhosis and is responsible for most of its clinical consequences, such as gastroesophageal varices, ascites, hepatorenal syndrome, hepatic encephalopathy, bacteremia, and hypersplenism.[1] Longitudinal studies assessing clinical-hemodynamic correlations have demonstrated that, in patients with cirrhosis, all the complications of PH do not appear until portal pressure, estimated by its clinical equivalent the hepatic venous pressure gradient (HVPG), increases to greater than 10 mm Hg.[2] This threshold value therefore defines clinically significant portal hypertension (CSPH), whereas subclinical PH is defined by HVPG between 6 and 9 mm Hg.[2]

Disclosure: The authors declare that they have no conflict of interest to disclose in relation with the contents discussed in this publication.
Hepatic Hemodynamic Laboratory, Liver Unit, Hospital Clinic-IDIBAPS, Centro de Investigación Biomédica en Red de Enfermedades Hepáticas y Digestivas (CIBERehd), University of Barcelona, c/Villarroel 170, Barcelona 08036, Spain
* Corresponding author.
E-mail address: jbosch@clinic.ub.es

Clin Liver Dis 18 (2014) 303–317
http://dx.doi.org/10.1016/j.cld.2013.12.003
1089-3261/14/$ – see front matter © 2014 Elsevier Inc. All rights reserved.

liver.theclinics.com

The aim of therapy in patients with PH is to decrease portal pressure, because elevated portal pressure is the driving force of all the clinical consequences of the syndrome.

In pragmatic terms the goal of therapy in subclinical PH should be to avoid CSPH, whereas asymptomatic patients with CSPH should be treated to decrease portal pressure below the threshold of 10 mm Hg, as CSPH markedly increases the risk of clinical complications ("decompensation"). In compensated patients without varices, there is evidence that even a small reduction in HVPG ($\geq$10% of baseline value) is beneficial, decreasing the rate of varices formation.[3] In patients with symptomatic PH, therapy should be more aggressive, aimed at decreasing portal pressure ideally to less than 12 mm Hg or, in patients not achieving this goal, a $\geq$20% decrease in HVPG versus pretreatment value, as this decreases the risk of both bleeding/rebleeding from varices, developing clinical decompensation, and reduces mortality.[4]

Drugs for PH should be able to decrease portal pressure without decreasing mean arterial pressure, which could worsen hyperdynamic circulation and increase the risk of renal failure. In addition, pharmacologic treatments should be ideally able to maintain or even improve effective liver perfusion, because this may improve liver function.

DRUGS USED IN CLINICAL PRACTICE

Most drugs used in clinical practice are splanchnic vasoconstrictors, acting by reducing splanchnic blood flow and hyperkinetic circulation (**Fig. 1**). **Box 1** summarizes the most commonly used drugs, further described herein.

Vasopressin Derivatives

Terlipressin (triglycyl lysine vasopressin) is a synthetic analogue of vasopressin with longer biologic activity and better safety profile[5–8] that is indicated for the treatment of acute variceal bleeding (AVB) and of type 1 hepatorenal syndrome (HRS).

Its effects encompass a marked vasoconstriction of the splanchnic circulation, an increase in arterial blood pressure and systemic vascular resistance, and a decrease in cardiac output. Altogether these induce a rapid and prolonged decrease in portal pressure of about 20% after a single injection.[7] The effects are maintained up to 4 hours, allowing its administration as intermittent intravenous injections, although continuous intravenous infusion is also possible.[8–10] In adults (>40 kg of body weight) the recommended dose for variceal bleeding is 2 mg every 4 hours for the first 24 to 48 hours, followed by 1 mg every 4 hours for 2 to 5 days.[11–13] In patients with HRS terlipressin is used in combination with albumin infusion at an initial dose of 0.5 to 1 mg intravenously every 4 hours, which is increased up to 3 mg every 4 hours if there is no response[14]; therapy is maintained up to 14 days. In HRS continuous intravenous infusion (beginning from 3 mg/d) might be beneficial, reducing daily dose and severity of adverse events.[15]

The most common side effects associated with the use of terlipressin are abdominal pain and increased blood pressure that reverse after drug withdrawal. In the setting of AVB, serious side effects such as peripheral, intestinal, or myocardial ischemia occur in less than 3% of the patients.[12] In patients with HRS included in 2 recent randomized controlled trials (RCT), treatment-related serious adverse events, mostly cardiovascular and leading to treatment discontinuation, were observed in 9% to 22% of patients.[16,17] Given the risk of ischemic and arrhythmic complications, terlipressin should not be used in patients with a history of ischemic heart or cerebral disease limb or gut vascular disease,[18] and caution should be used in elderly and/or hypertensive subjects. Hyponatremia, in some cases symptomatic, can arise during treatment[19] and reverses after drug discontinuation. Interestingly, terlipressin-associated

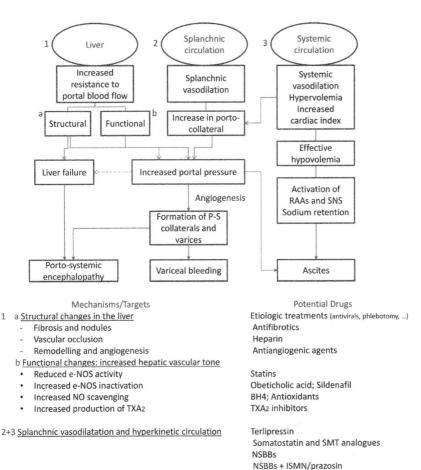

Fig. 1. Pathophysiological basis for pharmacologic therapy. PH is due to both increased hepatic resistance to portal blood flow and increased portal-collateral blood flow.[57] Hepatic resistance increases primarily by the structural changes caused by cirrhosis (fibrosis, regenerative nodules formation, vascular occlusion, and remodeling). Increased hepatic vascular tone due to sinusoidal endothelial dysfunction further increases by ~30% the hepatic resistance. As portal-systemic collaterals develop, splanchnic vasodilatation and hyperkinetic circulation contribute to maintain and worsen PH. The lower panel illustrates the multiple rational targets for the therapy for PH. These therapies include (1) increased structural resistance through the cirrhotic liver (1a in the figure); (2) increased hepatic vascular tone (1b in the figure), mainly mediated by an insufficient availability of NO due to hepatic endothelial dysfunction; (3) increased splanchnic blood flow (2 in the figure) and hyperkinetic circulation (3 in the figure). The figure further summarizes specific drugs acting on these targets. P-S, porto-systemic; SMT, somatostatin; SNS, sympathetic nervous system.

hyponatremia is more commonly observed in patients with preserved liver function and is associated with better response to treatment.[18]

Somatostatin and Long-Acting Somatostatin Analogues

Somatostatin is a 14-amino-acid peptide secreted by neural, endocrine, and enteroendocrine cells in the hypothalamus and in the digestive system (in the stomach,

Box 1
Available drugs for PH

Injection drugs used in the acute setting

Terlipressin

- Long-acting vasopressin analogue with affinity for vascular receptors higher than that of vasopressin
- Induces marked splanchnic vasoconstriction and arterial pressure increase
- Given intravenously as injections of 2 mg/4 hours for 24–48 hours, then 1 mg/4 hours for 2–5 days
- Well validated in placebo controlled RCTs and meta-analysis

Somatostatin

- Very short biologic half-life
- Induces moderate vasoconstriction due to glucagon inhibition and facilitation of adrenergic vasoconstriction
- Given as intravenous infusion of 250–500 mg/hour, after a bolus of 250 mg, for up to 5 days

Analogues of somatostatin (Octreotide, Vapreotide)

- Longer half life than somatostatin
- Short effects on portal pressure due to rapid desensitization
- Given as intravenous infusion of 50 μg/hour, after an optional bolus of 50 μg for up to 5 days
- Effective in RCTs when evaluated in addition to endoscopic sclerotherapy

Oral drugs used for chronic therapy

Propranolol

- β-1 and β-2 adrenergic receptor antagonist (NSBB)
- Induces decrease in cardiac output and splanchnic vasoconstriction
- Given orally beginning with 10–20 mg twice a day, increasing the dose every 2–3 days up to the maximum tolerated dose (provided systolic arterial pressure is >100 mm Hg and heart rate not less than 50 bpm). Dose should not exceed 320 mg/d. Should be maintained lifelong.
- Well validated in several studies
- Maximal efficacy in cirrhosis is obtained when HVPG is reduced <12 mm Hg or ≥20% versus pretreatment value

Nadolol

- β-1 and β-2 adrenergic receptor antagonist (NSBB)
- Induces decrease in cardiac output and splanchnic vasoconstriction
- Given orally once a day beginning with 20 mg a day, increasing the dose every 2–3 days up to the maximum tolerated dose (provided systolic arterial pressure is >100 mm Hg and heart rate not less than 50 bpm). Dose should not exceed 160 mg/d. Should be maintained lifelong.
- Well validated in several studies
- Maximal efficacy in cirrhosis is obtained when HVPG is reduced <12 mm Hg or ≥20% versus pretreatment value

Carvedilol

- β-1 and β-2 adrenergic receptor antagonist (NSBB), with intrinsic anti-α1 adrenergic activity
- Induces decrease in cardiac output, splanchnic vasoconstriction, and intrahepatic vasodilatation
- Given orally twice a day beginning with 6.25 mg/d, increasing the dose every 2–3 days up to a maximum of 25 mg/d (provided systolic arterial pressure is >100 mm Hg).
- Not fully validated yet

intestine, and pancreatic delta cells). It regulates the release of numerous secondary peptides, such as growth hormone, glucagon, insulin, gastrin, and secretin, and also plays a role in neural transmission. Once released, somatostatin binds to G-protein-coupled receptors (somatostatin receptor subtypes 1–5) that activate ion channels and enzymes mediating the synthesis/degradation of intracellular second messengers, including cyclic AMP, cyclic GMP, inositol trisphosphate, and diacylglycerol.[20]

The administration of somatostatin in portal hypertensive patients induces splanchnic vasoconstriction and consequently reduces portal pressure.[21] Somatostatin also blocks the brisk increase in HVPG induced by meals and blood transfusion,[22] which is considered a risk factor for rebleeding from portal hypertensive sources. The mechanisms leading to these effects are not fully known but include the inhibition of glucagon and other vasodilatory peptides, and the facilitation of adrenergic vasoconstriction.[23] Given that somatostatin has a short half-life, ranging from 1.2 to 4.8 minutes in patients with chronic liver disease,[20] it should be administered by continuous intravenous infusion to maintain an adequate plasma concentration. In AVB a dose of 250 μg/h intravenously preceded by a 250 μg intravenous bolus is empirically recommended because it slightly lowers the HVPG in stable conditions[24]; bolus injections can be repeated up to 3 times during the first hour if required. However, the use of a double infusion dose (500 μg/h) causes a greater reduction in HVPG[25] and a marked and sustained decrease in azygos blood flow. In the setting of AVB the 500 μg/h dose is required to significantly reduce the HVPG.[10] The greater hemodynamic effects of high doses translate into higher effectiveness in high-risk patients.[26] Severe side effects are rare. Usual side effects include vomiting and hyperglycemia that are usually easy to manage[20,26] and occur in about 21% of patients.

To overcome a main limitation of somatostatin, namely its short half-life, long-acting analogues have been developed.[20] Octreotide, Vapreotide, Lanreotide, and Seglitide (the latter has not been tested for PH) belong to this drug class. Their mechanism of action is probably similar to that of somatostatin, although their affinity for SMT receptors is different from that of the natural hormone. Octreotide is effective in preventing the postprandial splanchnic hyperemia in portal hypertensive patients[27,28] and this effect is long-lasting.[28,29] A single injection of octreotide and vapreotide is able to decrease portal pressure.[20] Empiric doses of octreotide and vapreotide in portal hypertensive patients are 50 μg/h as a continuous intravenous infusion with an optional initial intravenous or subcutaneous bolus of 50 μg.

Unfortunately, even though the half-life of these compounds is much longer than that of somatostatin, the duration of their hemodynamic effects on portal pressure is short. In particular, the effects on portal pressure of continuous infusion and repeated injections progressively decrease,[30] probably because of the rapid development of desensitization or tachyphylaxis.

Nonselective β-Blockers Alone and Combined with Vasodilators

Lebrec and colleagues[31] in 1980 first demonstrated that oral administration of propranolol, a nonselective β-blocker (NSBB) at doses that reduced the heart rate by ~25%, causing a sustained decrease in portal venous pressure in cirrhotic patients with PH. The same group showed that continued propranolol prevented variceal rebleeding.[32,33] Since then, NSBBs are the mainstay of chronic therapy for PH.[34] Available NSBBs include propranolol, nadolol, and timolol, the latter the less commonly used.

NSBBs decrease portal pressure by decreasing portal-collateral blood flow. They act by blocking both β-1 cardiac receptors leading to decreased cardiac output, and β-2 vascular receptors, allowing unopposed α-1 adrenergic activity that results in splanchnic vasoconstriction; this latter effect explains why selective (β-1) β-blockers are not as effective in reducing portal pressure. Other beneficial effects of NSBBs include the reduction of azygos blood flow and variceal pressure, as well as shortening the intestinal transit time which has been related to decreased bacterial overgrowth and thereby reduced risk of bacterial translocation.[34]

NSBBs are cheap, safe, and easy to use, decrease the risk of all main complications related to PH, and improve survival.[4] The recommended doses of propranolol and nadolol are listed in **Box 1**.

However, it has been shown that only 30% to 40% of the patients under long-term therapy with NSBB show a good hemodynamic response (reduction of HVPG <12 mm Hg or $\geq$20% vs pretreatment value),[24] which is a robust indicator of protection from first variceal bleeding or rebleeding.[35] In addition, up to 15% of patients have absolute or relative contraindications to therapy, and another 15% do not tolerate NSBB, requiring dose reduction or discontinuation because of side effects (ie, asthenia and shortness of breath).

The effect of NSBBs on portal pressure is potentiated by associating drugs targeting the increased hepatic vascular tone (see **Fig. 1**); this has been first tested by combining isosorbide-5-mononitrate (ISMN) with propranolol or nadolol. ISMN is an exogenous nitric oxide (NO) donor drug completely absorbed after oral administration, which causes a dose-related, significant reduction of portal pressure in patients with cirrhosis.[36–39] At relatively low doses (20 mg), ISMN has been shown to decrease portal pressure without reducing hepatic blood flow,[39] suggesting that it decreases hepatic resistance by intrahepatic NO supplementation. This finding is further supported by observing that even lower doses (10 mg) of ISMN are able to blunt the postprandial increase in HVPG that is due to intrahepatic endothelial dysfunction. In patient nonresponders to propranolol alone, the "a la carte" association of ISMN "rescues" about one-third of cases, with a corresponding decrease in their bleeding risk.[40] A second drug that has been shown to enhance even more the effects of NSBB on portal pressure is the α-adrenergic blocker prazosin.[41,42]

Carvedilol

Carvedilol is an NSBB with intrinsic anti-α adrenergic activity and capacity to enhance the release of NO that confers to this drug a mild vasodilating ability. Thus, the effects of carvedilol are quite similar to those of the combination of NSBBs and prazosin. After acute and chronic administration, carvedilol has a much greater effect decreasing HVPG (16%–43% vs pretreatment values) than propranolol or nadolol (12%–13% vs pretreatment values).[43] Carvedilol achieves a good hemodynamic response in more than 50% of patient nonresponders to standard NSBBs.[44] In a recent study in the setting of primary prophylaxis, the sequential use of propranolol followed by carvedilol in those nonresponders to propranolol achieved a good hemodynamic response in 72% of cases.[44]

In addition, carvedilol is safe in cirrhosis at low doses (<12.5 mg/d); the rate of serious adverse events reported in RCT is 0% to 13%, far lower than that of other NSBB (12%–40%).[44–47] At high doses, carvedilol may cause arterial hypotension and enhance sodium retention and ascites, bur recent evidence suggests that low doses of carvedilol (<25 mg/d) are as effective as higher doses (25–50 mg/d) in decreasing HVPG.

Evidence from RCT shows that in primary prophylaxis of variceal bleeding carvedilol appears more effective than endoscopic band ligation of esophageal varices [47]; although in prevention of rebleeding, it failed to demonstrate a benefit over nadolol plus ISMN.[46,48]

The above-mentioned data suggest that carvedilol is a very promising drug that may be the first choice in patients who are nonresponders to propranolol and are not hypotensive (ie, with a systolic blood pressure less than 100 mm Hg) or have no refractory ascites.[49,50] Further studies are needed before it definitely enters routine clinical practice.[48,50]

OTHER DRUGS THAT DECREASE PORTAL PRESSURE IN HUMANS (BUT NOT ROUTINELY USED)
Statins

As previously mentioned, insufficient NO production by endothelial cells in the liver microvessels is a major factor involved in increased hepatic resistance in cirrhosis, implying that delivering NO specifically to the liver circulation would decrease hepatic resistance. Statins (inhibitors of 3-hydroxy-3-methylglutaryl coenzyme A reductase) are lipid-lowering drugs that have pleiotropic effects. They decrease oxidative stress and inflammation at the vessel wall, have antithrombotic properties, and improve endothelial function, enhancing NO production in endothelial cells. This latter action is mediated by the phosphatidylinositol-3-kinase–dependent activation of protein kinase Akt, leading to endothelial nitric oxide synthase (eNOS) phosphorylation at Ser 1177 that induces an enhancement in eNOS function. In addition, statins improve eNOS activity by other posttranslational regulations and increase the transcription factor Kruppel-like factor 2, which is crucial for the transcription of endothelial protective genes. These observations provided evidence for testing statins for PH in cirrhosis. Studies in experimental models of PH and in patients with cirrhosis showed that statins improve intrahepatic endothelial dysfunction, reduce intrahepatic vascular resistance, and consequently, improve flow-mediated vasodilation of liver vasculature in response to meal ingestion, attenuating the postprandial peak in HVPG without reducing hepatic blood flow.[51] In cirrhosis statins induce this increase in NO availability selectively in the liver circulation,[52,53] avoiding potential detrimental effects due to systemic vasodilatation.

In a double-blind randomized placebo-controlled trial in patients with cirrhosis, oral simvastatin (20–40 mg/d for 1 month) was safe and significantly decreased portal pressure.[54] The magnitude of the effect on HVPG was moderate, greater than 10% in 40% of patients, and good ($\geq$20% or to $\leq$12 mm Hg), in one-third of treated patients. This effect was observed also in patients already on β-blockers, suggesting that adding simvastatin to NSBB may markedly increase the number of patients who are protected effectively from PH-related complications. Importantly, the decrease in HVPG was associated with improved effective liver perfusion and liver function (demonstrated by increased hepatic clearance, intrinsic clearance, and hepatic extraction of indocyanine green).[54] More recently statins have been shown to prevent intrahepatic endothelial dysfunction and reduced liver inflammation in endotoxemia.[55] A Spanish multicentric RCT (BLEPS study, EudraCT: 2009-016500-24) has included 158 patients (79 allocated to simvastatin and 79 to placebo) to verify if simvastatin on top of standard medical care could reduce the risk of rebleeding from esophageal varices in cirrhosis. Results are expected in 2014.

Renin-Angiotensin-Aldosterone System Inhibitors

Angiotensin II is associated with dynamic and static increases in hepatic resistance because of the contraction and proliferation of hepatic stellate cells leading to deposition of extracellular matrix. Several groups have studied the effects of the renin-angiotensin-aldosterone system (RAAS) antagonism in patients with cirrhotic PH with discordant results. In a recent systematic review and meta-analysis performed by the authors' group, they confirmed that antagonists of RAAS (either angiotensin receptor blockers or angiotensin-converting enzyme inhibitors) appear to be able to decrease HVPG in patients with compensated cirrhosis (Child-Pugh score, A). The magnitude of the portal hypotensive effect was smaller than that obtained by NSBB, around 10% in mean.[56] On the other hand, the activation of the systemic RAAS in patients with decompensated cirrhosis contraindicates the use of RAAS inhibitors that increase the risk of hypotension and renal failure in this population.

NEW DRUGS AND STRATEGIES IN THE HORIZON (UNDER INVESTIGATION)

Drugs currently under investigation aim primarily at preventing/correcting sinusoidal remodeling and fibrogenesis and this can be achieved by acting on several different pathogenetic mechanisms (see **Fig. 1**).[57]

Etiologic Treatments

Etiologic treatment of cirrhosis (eg, antiviral therapy in hepatitis C- and hepatitis B-related disease, alcohol withdrawal in alcoholic cirrhosis, immunosuppressants in autoimmune liver disease, iron depletion for hemochromatosis, copper chelation for Wilson disease) can modify the natural course of the disease by ameliorating fibrosis and preventing or reversing PH. In compensated viral cirrhosis achieving a sustained virological response, HVPG decreases significantly, and in some cases to less than 12 mm Hg or by more than 20% (target reduction in therapy for portal hypertensive patients).[2] If confirmed in patients with hepatitis C-related cirrhosis, the recent introduction of new interferon-free regimens with better safety/efficacy profile will probably represent a real possibility of reducing the burden of PH.

Obesity

A recent study by the authors' group showed that obesity is an independent risk factor for the development of first clinical decompensation in cirrhosis,[58] regardless of the cause. Increased body mass index after 1 year of follow-up was associated with an increase in HVPG, suggesting that a link between obesity and PH exists, whose pathophysiological mechanisms are unknown. Among possible mechanisms, leptin has been suggested[59] because this hormone is up-regulated in obesity and in cirrhosis and induces decreased NO availability, vascular dysfunction, and liver fibrosis. In a murine model of cirrhosis, the administration of a specific leptin receptor blocker (ObR antibody) significantly reduced portal pressure without modifying portal blood flow, suggesting a reduction in intrahepatic resistance,[60] which was further corroborated by finding an increased NO bioavailability and decreased oxidative stress. Drugs specifically addressing ObR might deserve further attention in patients with cirrhosis, particularly in those with concomitant obesity.

From a clinical point of view, simple weight reduction might be a novel nonpharmacologic strategy to reduce portal pressure in overweight cirrhotic patients. A study specifically designed to test this hypothesis is being conducted (SportDiet study, Clinical Trials NCT 01409356) and results are expected in late 2014.

Antifibrotic Agents

No specific antifibrotic drug is currently approved for clinical use.[61] Several compounds targeting different mechanisms of fibrogenesis are under investigation, including specific anti-TGFβ antibodies, different small molecule antagonists against toll-like receptor-4, integrins, caspases, angiotensin-1 receptor, angiotensin converting enzyme, and cannabinoid receptors 1, CB2, and FXR agonists (such as obeticholic acid). In addition, the potential of existing substances with antifibrotic activity such as curcumin, salvianolic acid, transresveratrol, silymarin, and recombinant human MnSOD is being tested. Interestingly, many natural antifibrotics also show antioxidant and anti-angiogenics properties.

Drugs Reducing Oxidative Stress

As in most chronic diseases, cirrhosis is characterized by an increase in oxidative stress,[62] causing an increase of reactive oxygen species, that are oxygen-based molecules with high chemical reactivity that include free radicals (species with one or more unpaired electrons), such as superoxide anione (O_2^-) and nonradical species such as hydrogen peroxide (H_2O_2). These free radicals promote a marked reduction in NO bioavailability by rapidly reacting with NO. Preventing NO scavenging would therefore lead to higher bioavailability of NO. Several strategies have been proposed.

Ascorbic acid (vitamin C)

Vitamin C is a potent natural antioxidant that is often reduced in patients with cirrhosis. In a study performed by the authors' group, acute intravenous administration of high doses of vitamin C improved endothelial dysfunction (as demonstrated by a reduction in postprandial peak in portal pressure) and reduced oxidative stress (as demonstrated by reduction in malondialdehyde [MDA] levels).[63]

Tetrahydrobiopterin (BH4)

Cirrhosis is associated with markedly reduced levels of BH4[64] due to a decreased activity and expression of the key enzyme in its synthesis, GTP-cyclohydrolase. Furthermore, BH4 is mostly inactivated due to oxidation. Decreased BH4 causes eNOS uncoupling, further reducing NO availability.[64] Short-term BH4 supplementation is able to correct eNOS uncoupling[65] and sets the basis for the use of BH4 for the therapy for PH.

Extracellular superoxide dismutase

Superoxide dismutases (SODs) are important antioxidant enzymes that catalyze the dismutation of superoxide (O_2^-) into oxygen and hydrogen peroxide. A decreased expression of Cytosolic and mitochondrial SOD isoforms, and a decreased SOD activity have been reported in cirrhotic livers. SOD gene transfer decreases portal pressure in murine models of PH.[66] Tempol, a SOD mimetic, increases NO in sinusoidal endothelial cells and reduces portal pressure in cirrhosis.[67]

Recently, the administration of a novel isoform of recombinant human manganese superoxide dismutase (rMnSOD) was shown to improve PH with the added effect of reducing liver fibrosis and of improving hepatic endothelial function.[68]

Intrahepatic NO availability may also be increased by 2 other strategies. The first is preventing the formation of asymmetric dimethil-arginine and endogenous eNOS antagonist that is increased in the cirrhotic liver; this can be prevented by the Farnesoid X receptor agonist, obeticholic acid, that has also been shown to decrease portal pressure in a small pilot study in patients with cirrhosis.[69] Alternatively, inhibition of phosphodiesterases that are abundant in the cirrhotic liver may also result in increased availability of NO and reduced hepatic vascular tone. However, this should be done through a liver-specific agent to prevent systemic hypotension or adverse effects, such as worsening of splanchnic vasodilatation.

Fenofibrate (peroxisome proliferator-activated receptor α activator)

Peroxisome proliferator-activated receptor α (PPARα) is a transcription factor that regulates genes related to vascular tone, oxidative stress, and fibrogenesis. The administration of fenofibrate, an activator of PPARα, induced a 30% decrease in portal pressure and increased arterial pressure in cirrhotic rats.[70] Moreover, these effects were associated with a significant reduction in hepatic fibrosis, improved vasodilatory response to acetylcholine, and increased NO bioavailability.[70] As fibrates are already used in other human diseases, this encouraging data might serve as a basis for future translational research.

Resveratrol

Resveratrol (3,5,40-trihydroxystilbene) is a polyphenol flavonoid found in several fruits and, in particular, red grapes, berries, and nuts, that shows a high hepatic uptake. Among its multiple beneficial effects (antineoplastic, anti-inflammatory, and antiplatelet aggregation activities), it is a potent antioxidant that shows protective effects on the vascular endothelium.

Among its mechanisms, it is able to reduce oxidative stress, up-regulate eNOS expression and activity, and inhibit cyclo-oxygenase-1 (COX-1) activity.

In rats with cirrhosis, resveratrol reduced portal pressure by exerting antioxidant effects that led to reduction in intrahepatic resistance.[71] Again, the effect of this drug should be tested in patients. Although safety does not seem an issue, a major limitation depends on its low stability (it oxidates on heat and light exposure) and low water solubility that limits its absorption.

Dark chocolate

Dark chocolate contains a high proportion of antioxidant cocoa flavonoids (among which are catechin and epicatechin) and increases NO availability in the systemic circulation. Data and 2 meta-analyses confirm the favorable cardiovascular profile of flavonol-rich cocoa products. In a recent phase 2 randomized study by the authors' group,[72] dark chocolate supplementation (0.55 g/kg of body weight) to a liquid meal induced a marked attenuation of the postprandial increase in portal pressure. Specifically, patients who received a meal supplemented with dark chocolate showed less than half of the increase in HVPG observed in control patients who received a meal containing white chocolate (devoid of cocoa flavonoids).

Modulation of COX-1

In cirrhosis, an increase in COX-1-derived vasoconstrictive prostanoids such as thromboxane (TXA_2) is involved in the maintenance of an increased intrahepatic vascular tone, in the setting of an insufficient availability of the vasodilator NO. COX also contributes to the increased oxidative stress of cirrhotic livers, and COX activation markedly increases the production of TXA_2 (that reduces eNOS activity) and leads to an increase in O_2^-. Altogether these effects reduce NO availability. Supporting this data, it has been proved that COX-1 inhibition improves endothelial dysfunction in animal models of cirrhosis.[73] However, detrimental effects of COX-1 inhibition on renal circulation prevent using this strategy in clinical practice. Drugs more specifically directed toward TXA_2 blockade might be the object of future studies.[74]

Antibiotics: Rifaximin

Bacterial translocation and endotoxemia further deteriorate hyperdynamic circulation in patients with decompensated cirrhosis and promote cytokine-stimulated intrahepatic release of endothelin and COX that increase portal pressure by increasing vascular resistance. Hence, bacterial translocation is a target for therapy for PH.

Rifaximin is a broad spectrum antibiotic that is unabsorbed after oral administration, acting only in the gastrointestinal tract. It is safe and US Food and Drug Administration approved for the treatment of hepatic encephalopathy in cirrhosis.[75] In a prospective study in patients with decompensated alcoholic cirrhosis, HVPG decreased significantly in most patients after intestinal decontamination with rifaximin (1200 mg/d for 28 days), in parallel with endotoxin levels.[76] In addition, in a second study, long-term rifaximin improved survival in a similar population.[77] Even if this strategy should be further evaluated in other etiologies, evidence suggests that rifaximin might be of help for decreasing portal pressure.

Antiangiogenetics

Angiogenesis actively contributes to induce and maintain PH.[78] Markers of neoangiogenesis, such as vascular endothelial growth factor and platelet-derived growth factor, are increased in animal models of PH.[78] Their inhibition by anti–vascular endothelial growth factor antibodies and antiangiogenic drugs reduces markedly splanchnic vasodilatation and collateral formation and leads to a decrease in portal pressure,[78] supporting the finding that blocking pathologic neoangionesis is a novel target of therapy of PH.[79] It has been shown that small doses of sorafenib (with low toxicity), a multikinase inhibitor used in the treatment of advanced hepatocellular carcinoma, is able to reduce liver fibrosis, portal pressure, and portal-systemic collateral formation in animal models of cirrhosis and PH.[80] Data regarding the effect of sorafenib on PH in patients are scarce, but the findings suggest that a reduction in portal pressure and portocollateral blood flow can be obtained.[81,82] Nonetheless, studies specifically focused on the use of sorafenib on PH in the absence of HCC to test its safety and efficacy at lower doses are lacking and are a field for future research.

REFERENCES

1. Bosch J. Vascular deterioration in cirrhosis. The big picture. J Clin Gastroenterol 2007;41:S247–53.
2. Bosch J, Abraldes JG, Berzigotti A, et al. The clinical use of HVPG measurements in chronic liver disease. Nat Rev Gastroenterol Hepatol 2009;6: 573–82.
3. Groszmann RJ, Garcia-Tsao G, Bosch J, et al. Beta-blockers to prevent gastroesophageal varices in patients with cirrhosis. N Engl J Med 2005;353:2254–61.
4. D'Amico G, Garcia-Pagan JC, Luca A, et al. Hepatic vein pressure gradient reduction and prevention of variceal bleeding in cirrhosis: a systematic review. Gastroenterology 2006;131:1611–24.
5. Kalambokis G, Economou M, Paraskevi K, et al. Effects of somatostatin, terlipressin and somatostatin plus terlipressin on portal and systemic hemodynamics and renal sodium excretion in patients with cirrhosis. J Gastroenterol Hepatol 2005;20:1075–81.
6. Merkel C, Gatta A, Bolognesi M, et al. Hemodynamic changes of systemic, hepatic, and splenic circulation following triglycyl-lysin-vasopressin administration in alcoholic cirrhosis. Dig Dis Sci 1988;33:1103–9.
7. Moller S, Hansen EF, Becker U, et al. Central and systemic haemodynamic effects of terlipressin in portal hypertensive patients. Liver 2000;20:51–9.
8. Narahara Y, Kanazawa H, Taki Y, et al. Effects of terlipressin on systemic, hepatic and renal hemodynamics in patients with cirrhosis. J Gastroenterol Hepatol 2009;24:1791–7.

9. Baik SK, Jeong PH, Ji SW, et al. Acute hemodynamic effects of octreotide and terlipressin in patients with cirrhosis: a randomized comparison. Am J Gastroenterol 2005;100:631–5.

10. Villanueva C, Planella M, Aracil C, et al. Hemodynamic effects of terlipressin and high somatostatin dose during acute variceal bleeding in nonresponders to the usual somatostatin dose. Am J Gastroenterol 2005;100:624–30.

11. Escorsell A, Bandi JC, Moitinho E, et al. Time profile of the haemodynamic effects of terlipressin in portal hypertension. J Hepatol 1997;27:824–9.

12. Escorsell A, Ruiz del Arbol L, Planas R, et al. Multicenter randomized controlled trial of terlipressin versus sclerotherapy in the treatment of acute variceal bleeding: the TEST study. Hepatology 2000;32:471–6.

13. Ioannou GN, Doust J, Rockey DC. Systematic review: terlipressin in acute oesophageal variceal haemorrhage. Aliment Pharmacol Ther 2003;17:53–64.

14. Gines P. Hepatorenal syndrome, pharmacological therapy, and liver transplantation. Liver Transpl 2011;17:1244–6.

15. Gerbes AL, Huber E, Gulberg V. Terlipressin for hepatorenal syndrome: continuous infusion as an alternative to i.v. bolus administration. Gastroenterology 2009;137:1179–81.

16. Martin-Llahi M, Pepin MN, Guevara M, et al. Terlipressin and albumin vs albumin in patients with cirrhosis and hepatorenal syndrome: a randomized study. Gastroenterology 2008;134:1352–9.

17. Sanyal AJ, Boyer T, Garcia-Tsao G, et al. A randomized, prospective, double-blind, placebo-controlled trial of terlipressin for type 1 hepatorenal syndrome. Gastroenterology 2008;134:1360–8.

18. Garcia-Pagan JC, Reverter E, Abraldes JG, et al. Acute variceal bleeding. Semin Respir Crit Care Med 2012;33:46–54.

19. Sola E, Lens S, Guevara M, et al. Hyponatremia in patients treated with terlipressin for severe gastrointestinal bleeding due to portal hypertension. Hepatology 2010;52:1783–90.

20. Abraldes JG, Bosch J. Somatostatin and analogues in portal hypertension. Hepatology 2002;35:1305–12.

21. Bosch J, Kravetz D, Rodes J. Effects of somatostatin on hepatic and systemic hemodynamics in patients with cirrhosis of the liver: comparison with vasopressin. Gastroenterology 1981;80:518–25.

22. Villanueva C, Ortiz J, Minana J, et al. Somatostatin treatment and risk stratification by continuous portal pressure monitoring during acute variceal bleeding. Gastroenterology 2001;121:110–7.

23. Reynaert H, Geerts A. Pharmacological rationale for the use of somatostatin and analogues in portal hypertension. Aliment Pharmacol Ther 2003;18:375–86.

24. Garcia-Tsao G, Bosch J. Management of varices and variceal hemorrhage in cirrhosis. N Engl J Med 2010;362:823–32.

25. Cirera I, Feu F, Luca A, et al. Effects of bolus injections and continuous infusions of somatostatin and placebo in patients with cirrhosis: a double-blind hemodynamic investigation. Hepatology 1995;22:106–11.

26. Moitinho E, Planas R, Bañares R, et al. Multicenter randomized controlled trial comparing different schedules of somatostatin in the treatment of acute variceal bleeding. J Hepatol 2001;35:712–8.

27. Albillos A, Rossi I, Iborra J, et al. Octreotide prevents postprandial splanchnic hyperemia in patients with portal hypertension. J Hepatol 1994;21:88–94.

28. Ludwig D, Schadel S, Bruning A, et al. 48-hour hemodynamic effects of octreotide on postprandial splanchnic hyperemia in patients with liver cirrhosis and

portal hypertension: double-blind, placebo-controlled study. Dig Dis Sci 2000; 45:1019–27.

29. Vorobioff JD, Gamen M, Kravetz D, et al. Effects of long-term propranolol and octreotide on postprandial hemodynamics in cirrhosis: a randomized, controlled trial. Gastroenterology 2002;122:916–22.

30. Escorsell A, Bandi JC, Andreu V, et al. Desensitization to the effects of intravenous octreotide in cirrhotic patients with portal hypertension. Gastroenterology 2001;120:161–9.

31. Lebrec D, Nouel O, Corbic M, et al. Propranolol–a medical treatment for portal hypertension? Lancet 1980;2:180–2.

32. Lebrec D, Nouel O, Bernuau J, et al. Propranolol in prevention of recurrent gastrointestinal bleeding in cirrhotic patients. Lancet 1981;1:920–1.

33. Lebrec D, Poynard T, Hillon P, et al. Propranolol for prevention of recurrent gastrointestinal bleeding in patients with cirrhosis: a controlled study. N Engl J Med 1981;305:1371–4.

34. Tsochatzis EA, Bosch J, Burroughs AK. New therapeutic paradigm for patients with cirrhosis. Hepatology 2012;56:1983–92.

35. Bosch J, Garcia-Pagan J. Prevention of variceal rebleeding. Lancet 2003;361: 952–4.

36. Escorsell A, Feu F, Bordas JM, et al. Effects of isosorbide-5-mononitrate on variceal pressure and systemic and splanchnic haemodynamics in patients with cirrhosis. J Hepatol 1996;24:423–9.

37. Garcia-Pagan JC, Feu F, Navasa M, et al. Long-term haemodynamic effects of isosorbide 5-mononitrate in patients with cirrhosis and portal hypertension. J Hepatol 1990;11:189–95.

38. Grose RD, Plevris JN, Redhead DN, et al. The acute and chronic effects of isosorbide-5-mononitrate on portal haemodynamics in cirrhosis. J Hepatol 1994;20:542–7.

39. Navasa M, Chesta J, Bosch J, et al. Reduction of portal pressure by isosorbide-5-mononitrate in patients with cirrhosis. Effects on splanchnic and systemic hemodynamics and liver function. Gastroenterology 1989;96: 1110–8.

40. Bureau C, Peron JM, Alric L, et al. "A la carte" treatment of portal hypertension: adapting medical therapy to hemodynamic response for the prevention of bleeding. Hepatology 2002;36:1361–6.

41. Albillos A, Lledo JL, Banares R, et al. Hemodynamic effects of alpha-adrenergic blockade with prazosin in cirrhotic patients with portal hypertension. Hepatology 1994;20:611–7.

42. Albillos A, Lledo JL, Rossi I, et al. Continuous prazosin administration in cirrhotic patients: effects on portal hemodynamics and on liver and renal function. Gastroenterology 1995;109:1257–65.

43. Banares R, Moitinho E, Piqueras B, et al. Carvedilol, a new nonselective beta-blocker with intrinsic anti-Alpha1- drenergic activity, has a greater portal hypotensive effect than propranolol in patients with cirrhosis. Hepatology 1999;30: 79–83.

44. Reiberger T, Ulbrich G, Ferlitsch A, et al. Carvedilol for primary prophylaxis of variceal bleeding in cirrhotic patients with haemodynamic non-response to propranolol. Gut 2013;62(11):1634–41.

45. Banares R, Moitinho E, Matilla A, et al. Randomized comparison of long-term carvedilol and propranolol administration in the treatment of portal hypertension in cirrhosis. Hepatology 2002;36:1367–73.

46. Lo GH, Chen WC, Wang HM, et al. Randomized, controlled trial of carvedilol versus nadolol plus isosorbide mononitrate for the prevention of variceal rebleeding. J Gastroenterol Hepatol 2012;27:1681–7.

47. Tripathi D, Ferguson JW, Kochar N, et al. Randomized controlled trial of carvedilol versus variceal band ligation for the prevention of the first variceal bleed. Hepatology 2009;50:825–33.

48. Bosch J. Carvedilol for preventing recurrent variceal bleeding: waiting for convincing evidence. Hepatology 2013;57:1665–7.

49. Bosch J. Carvedilol for portal hypertension in patients with cirrhosis. Hepatology 2010;51:2214–8.

50. Bosch J. Carvedilol: the beta-blocker of choice for portal hypertension? Gut 2013;62(11):1529–30.

51. Zafra C, Abraldes JG, Turnes J, et al. Simvastatin enhances hepatic nitric oxide production and decreases the hepatic vascular tone in patients with cirrhosis. Gastroenterology 2004;126:749–55.

52. Abraldes JG, Rodriguez-Vilarrupla A, Graupera M, et al. Simvastatin treatment improves liver sinusoidal endothelial dysfunction in CCl4 cirrhotic rats. J Hepatol 2007;46:1040–6.

53. Trebicka J, Hennenberg M, Laleman W, et al. Atorvastatin lowers portal pressure in cirrhotic rats by inhibition of RhoA/Rho-kinase and activation of endothelial nitric oxide synthase. Hepatology 2007;46:242–53.

54. Abraldes JG, Albillos A, Banares R, et al. Simvastatin lowers portal pressure in patients with cirrhosis and portal hypertension: a randomized controlled trial. Gastroenterology 2009;136:1651–8.

55. La Mura V, Pasarin M, Garcia-Pagan JC, et al. Effects of simvastatin administration on liver microvascular dysfunction induced by LPS. J Hepatol 2011;54:S48.

56. Tandon P, Abraldes JG, Berzigotti A, et al. Renin-angiotensin-aldosterone inhibitors in the reduction of portal pressure: a systematic review and meta-analysis. J Hepatol 2010;53:273–82.

57. Garcia-Pagan JC, Gracia-Sancho J, Bosch J. Functional aspects on the pathophysiology of portal hypertension in cirrhosis. J Hepatol 2012;57:458–61.

58. Berzigotti A, Garcia-Tsao G, Bosch J, et al. Obesity is an independent risk factor for clinical decompensation in patients with cirrhosis. Hepatology 2011;54:555–61.

59. Berzigotti A, Abraldes JG. Impact of obesity and insulin-resistance on cirrhosis and portal hypertension. Gastroenterol Hepatol 2013;36(8):527–33.

60. Delgado MG, Gracia-Sancho J, Marrone G, et al. Leptin receptor blockade reduces intrahepatic vascular resistance and portal pressure in an experimental model of rat liver cirrhosis. Am J Physiol Gastrointest Liver Physiol 2013;305(7):G496–502.

61. Cohen-Naftaly M, Friedman SL. Current status of novel antifibrotic therapies in patients with chronic liver disease. Therap Adv Gastroenterol 2011;4:391–417.

62. Gracia-Sancho J, Lavina B, Rodriguez-Vilarrupla A, et al. Increased oxidative stress in cirrhotic rat livers: a potential mechanism contributing to reduced nitric oxide bioavailability. Hepatology 2008;47:1248–56.

63. Hernandez-Guerra M, Garcia-Pagan JC, Turnes J, et al. Ascorbic acid improves the intrahepatic endothelial dysfunction of patients with cirrhosis and portal hypertension. Hepatology 2006;43:485–91.

64. Matei V, Rodriguez-Vilarrupla A, Deulofeu R, et al. The eNOS cofactor tetrahydrobiopterin improves endothelial dysfunction in livers of rats with CCl4 cirrhosis. Hepatology 2006;44:44–52.

65. Matei V, Rodriguez-Vilarrupla A, Deulofeu R, et al. Three-day tetrahydrobiopterin therapy increases in vivo hepatic NOS activity and reduces portal pressure in CCl4 cirrhotic rats. J Hepatol 2008;49:192–7.
66. Lavina B, Gracia-Sancho J, Rodriguez-Vilarrupla A, et al. Superoxide dismutase gene transfer reduces portal pressure in CCl4 cirrhotic rats with portal hypertension. Gut 2009;58:118–25.
67. Garcia-Caldero H, Rodriguez-Vilarrupla A, Gracia-Sancho J, et al. Tempol administration, a superoxide dismutase mimetic, reduces hepatic vascular resistance and portal pressure in cirrhotic rats. J Hepatol 2011;54:660–5.
68. Guillaume M, Rodriguez-Vilarrupla A, Gracia-Sancho J, et al. Recombinant human manganese superoxide dismutase reduces liver fibrosis and portal pressure in CCl4-cirrhotic rats. J Hepatol 2013;58:240–6.
69. Verbeke L, Farre R, Trebicka J, et al. Obeticholic acid, a farnesoid-X receptor agonist, improves portal hypertension by two distinct pathways in cirrhotic rats. Hepatology 2013 Nov 20. [Epub ahead of print]. http://dx.doi.org/10.1002/hep.26939.
70. Rodriguez-Vilarrupla A, Lavina B, Garcia-Caldero H, et al. PPARα activation improves endothelial dysfunction and reduces fibrosis and portal pressure in cirrhotic rats. J Hepatol 2012;56:1033–9.
71. Di Pascoli M, Divi M, Rodriguez-Vilarrupla A, et al. Resveratrol improves intrahepatic endothelial dysfunction and reduces hepatic fibrosis and portal pressure in cirrhotic rats. J Hepatol 2013;58:904–10.
72. de Gottardi A, Berzigotti A, Seijo S, et al. Postprandial effects of dark chocolate on portal hypertension in patients with cirrhosis: results of a phase 2, double-blind, randomized controlled trial. Am J Clin Nutr 2012;96:584–90.
73. Graupera M, Garcia-Pagan JC, Pares M, et al. Cyclooxygenase-1 inhibition corrects endothelial dysfunction in cirrhotic rat livers. J Hepatol 2003;39:515–21.
74. Rosado E, Rodriguez-Vilarrupla A, Gracia-Sancho J, et al. Terutroban, a TP-receptor antagonist, reduces portal pressure in cirrhotic rats. Hepatology 2013;58(4):1424–35.
75. Bass NM, Mullen KD, Sanyal A, et al. Rifaximin treatment in hepatic encephalopathy. N Engl J Med 2010;362:1071–81.
76. Vlachogiannakos J, Saveriadis AS, Viazis N, et al. Intestinal decontamination improves liver haemodynamics in patients with alcohol-related decompensated cirrhosis. Aliment Pharmacol Ther 2009;29:992–9.
77. Vlachogiannakos J, Viazis N, Vasianopoulou P, et al. Long-term administration of rifaximin improves the prognosis of patients with decompensated alcoholic cirrhosis. J Gastroenterol Hepatol 2013;28:450–5.
78. Fernandez M, Semela D, Bruix J, et al. Angiogenesis in liver disease. J Hepatol 2009;50:604–20.
79. Bosch J, Abraldes JG, Fernandez M, et al. Hepatic endothelial dysfunction and abnormal angiogenesis: new targets in the treatment of portal hypertension. J Hepatol 2010;53:558–67.
80. Mejias M, Garcia-Pras E, Tiani C, et al. Beneficial effects of sorafenib on splanchnic, intrahepatic, and portocollateral circulations in portal hypertensive and cirrhotic rats. Hepatology 2009;49:1245–56.
81. Coriat R, Gouya H, Mir O, et al. Reversible decrease of portal venous flow in cirrhotic patients: a positive side effect of sorafenib. PLoS One 2011;6:e16978.
82. Pinter M, Sieghart W, Reiberger T, et al. The effects of sorafenib on the portal hypertensive syndrome in patients with liver cirrhosis and hepatocellular carcinoma–a pilot study. Aliment Pharmacol Ther 2012;35:83–91.

Role of Transjugular Intrahepatic Portosystemic Shunt in the Management of Portal Hypertension

Richard Parker, MBChB, MRCP

KEYWORDS

- Transjugular intrahepatic portosystemic shunt • Portal hypertension • Varices
- Ascites

KEY POINTS

- Transjugular intrahepatic portosystemic shunt (TIPS) is an effective emergency treatment of esophageal variceal bleeding in patients who have failed conventional therapy.
- High-risk patients with advanced cirrhosis experience less rebleeding with better survival if TIPS is placed early after variceal bleeding (within 5 days of bleeding).
- TIPS prevents rebleeding more effectively than drug or endoscopic therapy after esophageal variceal bleeding.
- TIPS improves symptoms in treatment-refractory ascites or hepatic hydrothorax, but a survival benefit is yet to be conclusively shown.
- Selected cases of Budd-Chiari respond to TIPS.

INTRODUCTION: NATURE OF THE PROBLEM

A transjugular intrahepatic portosystemic shunt (TIPS) is a stent placed via the jugular vein to create a shunt from the portal vein to the systemic circulation via an artificial communication through the liver. TIPS is used to treat complications of portal hypertension by reducing portal pressure (**Table 1**). After the introduction of TIPS in 1988[1] as a treatment of uncontrolled variceal bleeding, the role of TIPS has expanded (**Table 2**). TIPS prevents rebleeding in high-risk patients, defined by measures of the severity of portal hypertension or cirrhosis. In addition to variceal bleeding, TIPS is recommended for the management of treatment-refractory or treatment-intolerant

Dr Parker is supported by a UK Medical Research Council grant (G1100448). There are no conflicts of interest to declare.
NIHR Centre for Liver Research, University of Birmingham, Birmingham B15 2TT, UK
E-mail address: richardparker@nhs.net

Clin Liver Dis 18 (2014) 319–334
http://dx.doi.org/10.1016/j.cld.2013.12.004
1089-3261/14/$ – see front matter © 2014 Elsevier Inc. All rights reserved.

liver.theclinics.com

Table 1
Hepatic venous pressure gradient (HVPG) in health and disease (see text section for explanation)

	Normal (mm Hg)	Portal Hypertension (mm Hg)	High-risk Portal Hypertension (mm Hg)	Target After Insertion of TIPS (mm Hg)
HVPG	5	5–10	>12	<12

ascites and hepatic hydrothorax, and selected cases of Budd-Chiari syndrome.[12,13] Although considered a safe procedure, TIPS has risks, the most common being provocation or exacerbation of hepatic encephalopathy. This article discusses the indications, insertion, and management of TIPS.

Table 2
Indications and outcomes for TIPS in portal hypertension

Indication	Outcome
Esophageal Varices	
Prophylaxis of first bleed	Not indicated
Treatment of acute bleeding after failure of medical and endoscopic therapy	Bleeding controlled in 90% of patients. Early rebleeding rates 6%–15%.[2,3] 50% 1-y survival[3]
Preemptive TIPS in high-risk patients (HVPG>20 mm Hg, advanced cirrhosis)	1-y mortality 14%–31% vs 39%–65% with variceal band ligation/drugs alone[4–6]
Secondary prophylaxis	More effective than drug treatment or endoscopy in prevention of rebleeding but no overall survival benefit[7,8]
Gastric Varices	
Prophylaxis of bleeding	Not indicated
Treatment of acute bleeding	TIPS as effective as cyanoacrylate glue with regard to rebleeding and survival, greater morbidity with TIPS[9]
Prevention of rebleeding	More effective in reducing rebleeding from gastric varices than cyanoacrylate glue (11% vs 38%)[10] but no improvement in overall survival
Portal hypertensive gastropathy	Control of uncontrolled acute bleeding or transfusion dependent chronic bleeding
Gastric antral vascular ectasia	Not indicated
Ascites	
Uncomplicated ascites	Not indicated
Diuretic-intolerant or diuretic-refractory ascites	TIPS significantly reduces need for paracentesis. Survival benefit unclear
Hepatic hydrothorax	60% of patients with refractory hydrothorax do not require further drainage
Budd-Chiari	Moderate Budd-Chiari syndrome unresponsive to anticoagulation; 74%–78% transplant-free survival at 5 y[11]
Pulmonary Complications of Liver Disease	
Hepatopulmonary syndrome	Not routinely indicated
Portopulmonary syndrome	Contraindicated

INDICATIONS/CONTRAINDICATIONS
Esophageal Varices

The use of TIPS for prophylaxis of variceal bleeding is not recommended.[12] Effective primary prophylaxis for varices with nonselective β-blockers or endoscopic band ligation is well documented in patients with high-risk esophageal varices.[14]

Medical and endoscopic therapy is first-line treatment of bleeding esophageal varices. Survival after esophageal variceal bleeding has improved significantly in recent years[15,16] but 1 in 5 patients still die within 6 weeks of bleeding.[17] Outcome is related to severity of cirrhosis and portal hypertension,[4,17,18] and it is patients with advanced disease who can derive most benefit from TIPS. TIPS may be used as a rescue therapy after failure of endoscopic therapy (conventionally considered after 2 endoscopic attempts at control) or to reduce the incidence of rebleeding. Rebleeding may be early (within 5 days of index bleed) or late.

Rescue Treatment of Acute Variceal Hemorrhage

TIPS used as rescue therapy brings immediate hemostasis in more than of 90% of patients, with early rebleeding seen in 6% to 15%.[2,3] In this group of severely ill patients, 1-month survival is between 60% and 74%[2] and 50% at 1 year.[3] Most studies of post-TIPS bleeding include patients who have undergone sclerotherapy and therefore have sclerotherapy-induced esophageal ulceration, which may not accurately reflect the modern practice of variceal band ligation (VBL). A more recent report of a small study described 10 patients admitted to hospital with variceal bleeding and high Child-Pugh scores[14,15] who required salvage TIPS after band ligation.[19] Bleeding was controlled in 8 cases. A retrospective study matched 19 patients undergoing TIPS after variceal bleeding with 19 controls.[6] Indication for TIPS included rescue therapy after variceal bleeding (9 patients), as well as late rebleeding (2 patients) and undergoing TIPS for secondary prophylaxis (8 patients). Participants had undergone VBL or had a Sengstaken-Blakemore tube placed before TIPS. Mortality was lower at 6 weeks and 1 year in the TIPS group (10.5% and 21.1% respectively) than in the matched controls (47.4% and 52.6%). Five patients experienced encephalopathy after TIPS, of whom 2 required revision of their stents.

Preemptive TIPS

The use of TIPS, after endoscopic therapy and within 5 days of index bleed, has been shown in randomized controlled trials to reduce treatment failure and mortality in high-risk patients. Patients at high-risk of rebleeding were defined by hemodynamic criteria (hepatic venous pressure gradient [HVPG], discussed later) or severity of cirrhosis (Child-Pugh criteria).

Fifty-two patients with acute variceal bleeding (HVPG>20 mm Hg) were treated with a single session of endoscopic sclerotherapy.[4] They were then randomized to undergo TIPS placement or conventional treatment. Treatment failure was more common in the non-TIPS group (50% vs 12%, $P<.01$), who also had greater transfusion requirements (3.7 ± 2.7 units vs 2.2 ± 2.3 units, $P<.01$), and greater need for intensive care (16% vs 3%, $P<.05$). Early TIPS placement reduced 1-year mortality (11% vs 31% respectively, $P<.05$). There was no increase in incident encephalopathy observed in this study. A more recent study examined high-risk patients (Child-Pugh score B or C but total score <13) with acute variceal bleeding and initial treatment with vasoactive drugs and endoscopic therapy. Patients were randomized to treatment with a polytetrafluoroethylene (PTFE)-covered stent within 72 hours (32 patients), or continuation of vasoactive drug therapy (32 patients).[5] The control arm patients were treated with β-blockers, VBL as required, and crossover to TIPS if these measures failed. One patient (3%) in the early-TIPS groups experienced early rebleeding, whereas this occurred in 4 patients (13%) in the control group. No patients who were treated with a TIPS experienced late rebleeding, whereas 10 control group patients did (32%). Four patients (13%) in the early-TIPS group died, compared with 12 patients (39%) in the control group ($P = .01$). No significant differences were observed between the two treatment groups with respect to serious adverse events.

Secondary Prophylaxis: Prevention of Late Rebleeding

After an episode of variceal bleeding, between 30% and 50% of patients experience another episode[20] of whom a large proportion die. TIPS prevents rebleeding more effectively than drug treatment or endoscopic procedures alone, but causes more encephalopathy without an overall survival benefit. In view of these findings, TIPS should not be considered in patients who did not receive a TIPS in the acute period of bleeding unless they have had multiple episodes of variceal bleeding or are considered at particularly high risk of rebleeding.[12]

TIPS was more effective than pharmacologic treatment in preventing rebleeding from esophageal varices in patients with advanced cirrhosis (Child-Pugh class B/C)[7]: 13% of patients with a TIPS experienced rebleeding versus 39% of the pharmacology group ($P = .07$). However, greater incidence of encephalopathy was observed in the TIPS group and survival was the same in both groups (72%). Meta-analysis of 12 randomized controlled trials comparing TIPS with endoscopic therapy showed a significant reduction in death from variceal bleeding when TIPS was used (odds ratio, 0.32, 95% confidence interval 0.24–0.43, $P<.01$) but no overall improvement in survival.[8] A higher incidence of encephalopathy was observed. This finding may not be the same in patients with advanced (Child-Pugh class C) cirrhosis, who may be more likely to benefit from TIPS.[21]

Treatment of Gastric Varices

Gastric varices have a lower risk of hemorrhage than esophageal varices, but mortality is higher if hemorrhage occurs.[22] A nonrandomized retrospective study of patients with acute gastric bleeding compared cyanoacrylate glue and TIPS as first-line treatment. They were equally effective with regard to rebleeding and survival, but morbidity requiring hospitalization was more pronounced in the TIPS group (41% vs 1.6% in cyanoacrylate arm).[9] A retrospective study of 32 patients with bleeding gastric varices unresponsive to medical and endoscopic treatment treated with TIPS reported hemostasis in 18 of 20 patients actively bleeding at the time of TIPS insertion.[23] At 1 month and 1 year, rebleeding rates were 14% and 31%, respectively, and overall survival 75% and 59% respectively.

TIPS seems to be as effective in the prevention of rebleeding from gastric varices as it is in esophageal varices.[24] In a randomized trial of TIPS (35 patients) versus cyanoacrylate glue (37 patients), glue was more effective at obliterating gastric varices, although rebleeding from gastric varices was seen in 4 patients with TIPS (11%) compared with 14 patients with cyanoacrylate (38%) ($P = .014$). Survival did not significantly differ between groups. Frequency of complications was also similar.

Clinical Outcomes: Portal Hypertensive Gastropathy

Portal hypertensive gastropathy (PHG) is a common manifestation of portal hypertension affecting the gastric mucosa, usually in the body and fundus of the stomach.[25,26] Acute bleeding may occur with PHG, particularly in severe portal hypertension, although this is rare. Chronic insidious bleeding is more common. In bleeding from

PHG, case reports and series have shown the benefit of TIPS.[27,28] In the largest series, of 54 patients, TIPS improved transfusion requirements in severe PHG, and mild PHG resolved.[29]

Clinical Outcomes: Gastric Antral Vascular Ectasia

Gastric antral vascular ectasia (GAVE) is a complication of portal hypertension that manifests as red discoloration in the gastric antrum, often in characteristic stripes.[30] It can cause chronic blood loss requiring transfusion. Two case series have shown that TIPS is ineffective in controlling blood loss from GAVE.[29,31]

Clinical Outcomes: Treatment of Ascites

Ascites is treated in the first instance with sodium restriction and diuretics.[13] If ascites fails to respond to diuretics (diuretic-refractory ascites) or the side effects of diuretics are intolerable (diuretic-intolerant ascites), TIPS may be considered as an alternative to repeated large-volume paracentesis (LVP).[12,13]

This topic has been the subject of repeated meta-analyses, as shown in **Table 3**. TIPS offers better control of refractory ascites than LVP. The benefit on survival is less clear. Meta-analyses of published data have differed with regard to survival: 3 showed no difference in survival between the TIPS and LVP groups.[32,33,35] One 2005 meta-analysis found a trend toward reduced mortality in patients treated with TIPS after having excluded an outlier trial,[34] and another meta-analysis (of patient-level data) found increased transplant-free survival in the TIPS group.[36] A trial published since the last of these meta-analyses including stable cirrhotics (Child score<11) also showed a survival benefit (58% vs 19% at 3 years, $P<.01$ by log rank).[42] The benefit in control of ascites is at the expense of increased incidence of encephalopathy. This can be so troublesome as to require narrowing or reversal of TIPS.

Clinical Outcomes: Hepatic Hydrothorax

Hepatic hydrothorax is an accumulation of fluid in the thorax (usually right sided) secondary to portal hypertension, caused by passage of ascites through the diaphragm. It occurs in approximately 5% of patients with cirrhosis[43] and is treated in the first instance with medical therapy as per abdominal ascites. TIPS may be used in cases that do not respond to treatment and require drainage.

Evidence to date is based on case reports and nonrandomized trials.[44] One-year survival is reported as up to 64%. The largest case series of 73 patients, reviewed retrospectively[45] in a single center, showed a 1-year survival of 48%. At 6 months, complete response (defined as absence of symptoms related to hydrothorax and no further requirement for thoracocentesis) was seen in 60%. No response was seen in 25% of patients. Fourteen patients died within 30 days of TIPS: 6 from liver failure, 4 from acute respiratory distress syndrome, 2 from renal failure, and 2 from sepsis. Encephalopathy occurred in 11 patients.

Clinical Outcomes: Hepatorenal Syndrome

Hepatorenal syndrome (HRS) is the development of renal impairment in a patient with cirrhosis in the absence of another cause.[13] It is known that TIPS quickly improves renal blood flow[46] and TIPS has been reported to improve HRS in case series.[47,48] However, at present there are insufficient data to support routine use of TIPS for treatment of HRS and it is not recommended.[12,13]

Table 3
Meta-analyses of TIPS for treatment of ascites

| Author, Year | Original Trials (✓ Included in Meta-analyses) | | | | | Outcomes | | |
	Lebrec et al,[37] 1996	Rossle et al,[38] 2000	Ginès et al,[39] 2002	Sanyal et al,[40] 2003	Salerno et al,[41] 2004	Recurrent Ascites	Survival	Encephalopathy
Albillos et al,[32] 2005	✓	✓	✓	✓	✓	Risk Ratio 0.56 (0.47–0.66)	0.90 (0.72–1.12)	1.36 (1.10–1.68)
Deltenre et al,[33] 2005	✓	✓	✓	✓	✓	Mean Risk Difference 35% (P<.05)	7% (P = .40)	17% (P<.05)
D'Amico et al,[34] 2005	✓	✓	✓	✓	✓	Odds Ratio 0.14 (0.08–0.26)	Mortality 0.90 (0.44–1.81)	2.34 (1.41–3.87)
Saab et al,[35] 2006	✓	✓	✓	✓	✓	Odds Ratio 0.14 (0.06–0.28)	1.29 (0.65–2.56)	2.24 (1.39–3.60)
Salerno et al,[36] 2007	Excluded because refractory ascites not defined as per International Ascites Club, and mortality not primary end point	✓	✓	✓	✓	Meta-analysis of Individual Patient Data 42.0% vs 89.4% (P<.01)	38.1% vs 28.7% at 36 mo (Kaplan-Meier log rank P = .035)	Total episodes, 1.13 vs 0.63, P<.01; severe episodes, 0.68 vs 0.24, P<.01

Clinical Outcomes: Budd-Chiari

Budd-Chiari syndrome is caused by obstruction of the venous drainage of the liver, either in the hepatic vein or the inferior vena cava, usually occurring in patients with a prothrombotic disorder.[49,50]

Budd-Chiari can be stratified into 3 classes of severity based on clinical factors (bilirubin level, encephalopathy, ascites, International Normalized Ratio),[51] and only those with intermediate (class II) disease benefited from portosystemic shunt, whereas uncomplicated disease can be managed with anticoagulation alone.[49] TIPS insertion improves liver function in Budd-Chiari[52] and is associated with an excellent outcome: 78% transplant-free survival at 5 years in a large retrospective European cohort.[11] The risk of hepatic encephalopathy after TIPS seems lower than in cirrhotic liver disease: around 21% in this cohort, compared with up to 50% of cirrhotic patients.[53,54]

Clinical Outcomes: Pulmonary Complications of Portal Hypertension

Hepatopulmonary syndrome (HPS) and portopulmonary syndrome (PPS) are complications of portal hypertension characterized by dyspnea but with differing pathogenesis.[55] Presence of these disorders confers a worse prognosis.[56]

TIPS has been used to treat HPS with varying results. Data are scarce, and are based on case reports rather than randomized trial evidence. Patients have been treated with symptomatic improvement,[57] often as a bridge to transplantation.[58–60] Data regarding pulmonary function are contradictory.[61–63] At present, TIPS is not routinely recommended for the treatment of HPS. Pulmonary hypertension is a contraindication for TIPS.

CONTRAINDICATIONS

Absolute and relative contraindications to TIPS are shown in **Table 4**.[12]

TECHNIQUE/PROCEDURE
Assessment

Candidates for TIPS should be evaluated by a gastroenterologist or hepatologist. Routine blood tests to assess liver and kidney function and clotting are necessary. In view of the effects of TIPS on cardiac function, especially in the presence of pulmonary hypertension, echocardiography should be performed before TIPS in all patients in whom there is suspicion of cardiac or respiratory disease, which may be clinically silent. Cross-sectional liver imaging is recommended to assess patency of vessels and rule out the presence of a hepatoma or cysts that may contraindicate TIPS.

Table 4
Contraindications to insertion of TIPS

Absolute Contraindication	Relative Contraindication
Congestive cardiac failure	Hepatoma (especially if central)
Multiple hepatic cysts	Hepatic vein obstruction
Uncontrolled sepsis	Portal vein thrombosis
Unrelieved biliary obstruction	Severe coagulopathy or severe thrombocytopenia ($<20 \times 10^9$/mL)
Severe pulmonary hypertension	Moderate pulmonary hypertension
Tricuspid regurgitation	Small liver

Procedure

TIPS is inserted under aseptic conditions with ultrasonography guidance, almost always via the right jugular vein,[64] although other approaches have been reported (**Fig. 1**). The procedure may be performed under local anesthetic and sedation or general anesthetic depending on the characteristics of the patient, institution, and facilities. The operator is usually an interventional radiologist but others may have the requisite training and experience to undertake TIPS insertion. A catheter is been advanced from the site of venous access to a branch of the hepatic vein, where venography delineates the venous anatomy. A needle is passed from the right or left hepatic vein to a branch of the portal vein followed by a guidewire that dilates the tract by balloon inflation (**Fig. 2**). A collapsed stent is then passed and expanded. Measurement of HVPG before and after placement of TIPS allows assessment of the success

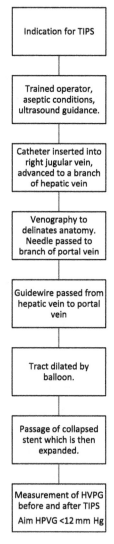

Fig. 1. Process of TIPS placement.

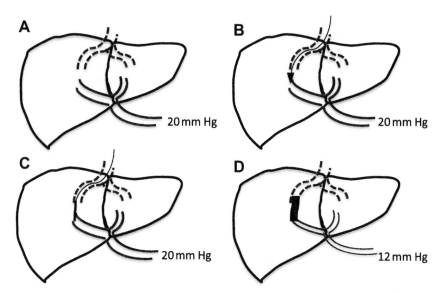

Fig. 2. Insertion of a TIPS: (*A*) portal hypertension, HVPG 20 mm Hg; (*B*) insertion of a guide wire via the jugular artery, advanced to a branch of the hepatic vein; (*C*) passage of a collapsed stent; (*D*) expansion of stent to create an artificial shunt between portal and systemic venous systems.

of the procedure (see **Table 1**). HVPG is calculated as wedged hepatic venous pressure (an indirect measurement of portal vein pressure) and the free hepatic venous pressure (without wedging the balloon catheter).[65] The aim of TIPS is to reduce the HVPG to less than 12 mm Hg. If this is achieved, there is a lower probability of developing recurrent variceal hemorrhage, ascites, spontaneous bacterial peritonitis, and death.[66,67] Embolization of collateral portosystemic vessels at the time of TIPS insertion has been shown to reduce rates of rebleeding, compared with TIPS insertion alone.[68,69] The benefit seems to be gained particularly if there is unsatisfactory reduction in post-TIPS HVPG.[70]

Bare metal stents were most widely used until recent randomized controlled studies showed the superiority of PTFE-covered stents. These PTFE-covered stents have now largely replaced bare stents because they have better performance with regard to patency, survival, and decreased risk of encephalopathy.[11,71,72] The only type of stent exclusively designed for TIPS is the Viatorr (Gore Medical), an expandable PTFE-covered device. At the portal end there is a 2-cm bare segment, which allows blood flow to side vessels of the portal vein. The bile-resistant PTFE section is placed from the portal vein through the liver to the hepatic vein ostium. A circumferential radiopaque marker at the junction between the two sections allows for radiological visualization. The diameter of the TIPS is critical for reduction of HVPG and control of symptoms: shunts with 10-mm diameter are more effective than 8-mm shunts.[73]

Postoperative Care

If no immediate complications are experienced, patients are able to leave hospital 24 hours after placement of a TIPS. Regular follow-up is mandated in the period soon after the TIPS procedure because early complications may arise and doses of drugs used to treat complications of portal hypertension may need to be adjusted.

The routine use of anticoagulants to maintain stent patency, other than in Budd-Chiari syndrome, is not recommended.

Patients should be monitored with regular Doppler ultrasonography,[12,74] although the intervals at which this should be performed are unclear and vary between centers; intervals of 6 or 12 months are commonly used. If stenosis or occlusion is suspected, confirmation with venography is warranted, which also allows an opportunity for intervention if necessary.

COMPLICATIONS AND MANAGEMENT

Mortality after a TIPS procedure is small at approximately 1.2% over a 10-year period.[53] Mortality varies depending on the indication for TIPS and the condition of the patient.[75] Immediate, early, and late complications of TIPS insertion are shown in **Table 5**.

Encephalopathy

Hepatic encephalopathy (HE) is the major complication of TIPS.[36,53] Approximately one-third to one-half of patients experience HE after insertion of TIPS, and 10% of patients experience de novo HE.[53,54] PTFE-covered stents cause significantly less HE than bare stents.[77] HE may be managed by reducing the diameter of the stent to reduce the amount of blood bypassing the liver, but this can occasionally cause bleeding.[54] However, insertion of TIPS of smaller diameter (8 mm vs 10 mm) is less effective at reducing portal hypertension and increases the likelihood of clinical events, although it does not reduce overall survival.[73]

Cardiac Complications

TIPS placement causes profound and immediate cardiodynamic changes: an increase in venous return causes an increased cardiac index and end-diastolic volume.[46,78] These changes persist for up to 6 months after TIPS placement.[79] However, observational studies have not shown significant clinical consequences of these changes; this may be a consequence of careful patient selection.

TIPS Dysfunction

TIPS dysfunction as defined by loss of decompression of the portal venous system, increase in HVPG to more than 12 mm Hg, or recurrence of complications of portal hypertension[12] may occur because of stenosis or blockage of TIPS. A TIPS may be restored to full patency with mechanical unblocking[80] or placement of another stent.[81]

Table 5
Complications of TIPS

Immediate	Early (<3 mo)	Late (>3 mo)
Hemorrhage	Hepatic encephalopathy	Hepatic encephalopathy
Perforation of gall bladder	TIPS-itis	TIPS-itis
Sepsis	Stent thrombosis	Stent stenosis
Liver laceration	Stent stenosis	—
Hemolysis (less common with coated stents)	Stent migration	—
Hepatic segmental ischemia[42,76]	—	—

TIPS-itis

Infection of a TIPS is rare, occurring in approximately 1% of TIPS.[82] It should be suspected if patients have a bacteremia without any other obvious cause. Prolonged (3 months) courses of antibiotics, tailored to isolated organisms should be used. This complication is dangerous and can precipitate decompensation or death in cirrhotic patients.

Liver Transplantation

Patients who require TIPS usually have advanced liver disease and may be considered for liver transplantation soon after placement of TIPS. TIPS may cause technical difficulties with liver transplantation, particularly if the stent has migrated, although final outcomes seem similar to patients without TIPS.[83] If liver transplantation is likely, TIPS is best avoided if possible.

SUMMARY

TIPS has become an essential therapeutic tool in the management of patients with portal hypertension. TIPS is an effective emergency treatment of esophageal bleeding in patients who have failed conventional therapy. High-risk patients (those with advanced cirrhosis) experience less rebleeding and have better survival if TIPS is placed early (within 5 days) after variceal bleeding. The other major indication for TIPS is refractory ascites, in which TIPS improves symptoms but a survival benefit is less clear. Future trials will clarify the role of TIPS, which will expand as understanding of the optimal timing and choice of patients improves.

REFERENCES

1. Rossle M, Richter GM, Noldge G, et al. Performance of an intrahepatic portocaval shunt (PCS) using a catheter technique: a case report. Hepatology 1988;8(5):1348.
2. Vangeli M, Patch D, Burroughs AK. Salvage TIPS for uncontrolled variceal bleeding. J Hepatol 2002;37(5):703–4.
3. Azoulay D, Castaing D, Majno P, et al. Salvage transjugular intrahepatic portosystemic shunt for uncontrolled variceal bleeding in patients with decompensated cirrhosis. J Hepatol 2001;35(5):590–7.
4. Monescillo A, Martinez-Lagares F, Ruiz-del-Arbol L, et al. Influence of portal hypertension and its early decompression by TIPS placement on the outcome of variceal bleeding. Hepatology 2004;40(4):793–801.
5. García-Pagán JC, Caca K, Bureau C, et al. Early use of TIPS in patients with cirrhosis and variceal bleeding. N Engl J Med 2010;362(25):2370–9.
6. Corbett C, Murphy N, Olliff S, et al. A case-control study of transjugular intrahepatic portosystemic stent shunts for patients admitted to intensive care following variceal bleeding. Eur J Gastroenterol Hepatol 2013;25(3):344–51.
7. Escorsell À, Bañares R, García-Pagán JC, et al. TIPS versus drug therapy in preventing variceal rebleeding in advanced cirrhosis: a randomized controlled trial. Hepatology 2002;35(2):385–92.
8. Zheng M, Chen Y, Bai J, et al. Transjugular intrahepatic portosystemic shunt versus endoscopic therapy in the secondary prophylaxis of variceal rebleeding in cirrhotic patients: meta-analysis update. J Clin Gastroenterol 2008;42(5): 507–16.

9. Procaccini NJ, Al-Osaimi A, Northup P, et al. Endoscopic cyanoacrylate versus transjugular intrahepatic portosystemic shunt for gastric variceal bleeding: a single-center US analysis. Gastrointest Endosc 2009;70(5):881–7.

10. Lo G-H, Liang H-L, Chen W-C, et al. A prospective, randomized controlled trial of transjugular intrahepatic portosystemic shunt versus cyanoacrylate injection in the prevention of gastric variceal rebleeding. Endoscopy 2007;39(08):679–85.

11. Garcia-Pagan JC, Heydtmann M, Raffa S, et al. TIPS for Budd-Chiari syndrome: long-term results and prognostics factors in 124 patients. Gastroenterology 2008;135(3):808–15.

12. Boyer TD, Haskal ZJ. The role of transjugular intrahepatic portosystemic shunt (TIPS) in the management of portal hypertension: update 2009. Hepatology 2010;51(1):1–16.

13. Ginès P, Angeli P, Lenz K, et al. EASL clinical practice guidelines on the management of ascites, spontaneous bacterial peritonitis, and hepatorenal syndrome in cirrhosis. J Hepatol 2010;53(3):397–417.

14. Gluud LL, Krag A. Banding ligation versus beta-blockers for primary prevention in oesophageal varices in adults. Cochrane Database Syst Rev 2012;(8):CD004544.

15. Carbonell N, Pauwels A, Serfaty L, et al. Improved survival after variceal bleeding in patients with cirrhosis over the past two decades. Hepatology 2004;40(3):652–9.

16. Taefi A, Cho WK, Nouraie M. Decreasing trend of upper gastrointestinal bleeding mortality risk over three decades. Dig Dis Sci 2013;58(10):2940–8.

17. Amitrano L, Guardascione MA, Manguso F, et al. The effectiveness of current acute variceal bleed treatments in unselected cirrhotic patients: refining short-term prognosis and risk factors. Am J Gastroenterol 2012;107(12):1872–8.

18. Moitinho E, Escorsell A, Bandi JC, et al. Prognostic value of early measurements of portal pressure in acute variceal bleeding. Gastroenterology 1999;117(3):626–31.

19. Rudler M, Rousseau G, Thabut D. Salvage transjugular intrahepatic portosystemic shunt followed by early transplantation in patients with Child C14-15 cirrhosis and refractory variceal bleeding: a strategy improving survival. Transpl Int 2013;26(6):E50–1.

20. Chalasani N, Kahi C, Francois F, et al. Improved patient survival after acute variceal bleeding: a multicenter, cohort study. Am J Gastroenterol 2003;98(3):653–9.

21. Jalan R, Bzeizi KI, Tripathi D, et al. Impact of transjugular intrahepatic portosystemic stent-shunt for secondary prophylaxis of oesophageal variceal haemorrhage: a single-centre study over an 11-year period. Eur J Gastroenterol Hepatol 2002;14(6):615–26.

22. Sarin SK, Lahoti D, Saxena SP, et al. Prevalence, classification and natural history of gastric varices: a long-term follow-up study in 568 portal hypertension patients. Hepatology 1992;16(6):1343–9.

23. Barange K, Péron J, Imani K, et al. Transjugular intrahepatic portosystemic shunt in the treatment of refractory bleeding from ruptured gastric varices. Hepatology 1999;30(5):1139–43.

24. Tripathi D, Therapondos G, Jackson E, et al. The role of the transjugular intrahepatic portosystemic stent shunt (TIPSS) in the management of bleeding gastric varices: clinical and haemodynamic correlations. Gut 2002;51(2):270–4.

25. Primignani M, Carpinelli L, Preatoni P, et al. Natural history of portal hypertensive gastropathy in patients with liver cirrhosis. Gastroenterology 2000;119(1):181–7.

26. Thuluvath PJ, Yoo HY. Portal hypertensive gastropathy. Am J Gastroenterol 2002;97(12):2973–8.

27. Mezawa S, Homma H, Ohta H, et al. Effect of transjugular intrahepatic portosystemic shunt formation on portal hypertensive gastropathy and gastric circulation. Am J Gastroenterol 2001;96(4):1155–9.
28. Urata J, Yamashita Y, Tsuchigame T, et al. The effects of transjugular intrahepatic portosystemic shunt on portal hypertensive gastropathy. J Gastroenterol Hepatol 1998;13(10):1061–7.
29. Kamath PS, Lacerda M, Ahlquist DA, et al. Gastric mucosal responses to intrahepatic portosystemic shunting in patients with cirrhosis. Gastroenterology 2000;118(5):905–11.
30. Burak KW, Lee SS, Beck PL. Portal hypertensive gastropathy and gastric antral vascular ectasia (GAVE) syndrome. Gut 2001;49(6):866–72.
31. Spahr L, Villeneuve JP, Dufresne MP, et al. Gastric antral vascular ectasia in cirrhotic patients: absence of relation with portal hypertension. Gut 1999; 44(5):739–42.
32. Albillos A, Bañares R, González M, et al. A meta-analysis of transjugular intrahepatic portosystemic shunt versus paracentesis for refractory ascites. J Hepatol 2005;43(6):990–6.
33. Deltenre P, Mathurin P, Dharancy S, et al. Transjugular intrahepatic portosystemic shunt in refractory ascites: a meta-analysis. Liver Int 2005;25(2): 349–56.
34. D'Amico G, Luca A, Morabito A, et al. Uncovered transjugular intrahepatic portosystemic shunt for refractory ascites: a meta-analysis. Gastroenterology 2005; 129(4):1282–93.
35. Saab S, Nieto JM, Lewis SK, et al. TIPS versus paracentesis for cirrhotic patients with refractory ascites. Cochrane Database Syst Rev 2006;(4):CD004889.
36. Salerno F, Camma C, Enea M, et al. Transjugular intrahepatic portosystemic shunt for refractory ascites: a meta-analysis of individual patient data. Gastroenterology 2007;133(3):825–34.
37. Lebrec D, Giuily N, Hadengue A, et al. Transjugular intrahepatic portosystemic shunts: Comparison with paracentesis in patients with cirrhosis and refractory ascites: a randomized Trial. French Group of Clinicians and a Group of Biologists. J Hepatol 1996;25(2):135–44.
38. Rossle M, Ochs A, Gulberg V, et al. A comparison of paracentesis and transjugular intrahepatic portosystemic shunting in patients with ascites. N Engl J Med 2000;342(23):1701–7.
39. Ginès P, Uriz J, Calahorra B, et al. Transjugular intrahepatic portosystemic shunting versus paracentesis plus albumin for refractory ascites in cirrhosis. Gastroenterology 2002;123(6):1839–47.
40. Sanyal AJ, Genning C, Reddy KR, et al. The North American study for the treatment of refractory ascites. Gastroenterology 2003;124(3):634–41.
41. Salerno F, Merli M, Riggio O, et al. Randomized controlled study of tips versus paracentesis plus albumin in cirrhosis with severe ascites. Hepatology 2004; 40(3):629–35.
42. Narahara Y, Kanazawa H, Fukuda T, et al. Transjugular intrahepatic portosystemic shunt versus paracentesis plus albumin in patients with refractory ascites who have good hepatic and renal function: a prospective randomized trial. J Gastroenterol 2011;46(1):78–85.
43. Cárdenas A, Kelleher T, Chopra S. Hepatic hydrothorax. Aliment Pharmacol Ther 2004;20(3):271–9.
44. Rossle M, Gerbes AL. TIPS for the treatment of refractory ascites, hepatorenal syndrome and hepatic hydrothorax: a critical update. Gut 2010;59(7):988–1000.

45. Dhanasekaran R, West JK, Gonzales PC, et al. Transjugular intrahepatic porto-systemic shunt for symptomatic refractory hepatic hydrothorax in patients with cirrhosis. Am J Gastroenterol 2009;105(3):635–41.

46. Umgelter A, Reindl W, Geisler F, et al. Effects of TIPS on global end-diastolic volume and cardiac output and renal resistive index in ICU patients with advanced alcoholic cirrhosis. Ann Hepatol 2010;9(1):40–5.

47. Brensing KA, Textor J, Perz J, et al. Long term outcome after transjugular intra-hepatic portosystemic stent-shunt in non-transplant cirrhotics with hepatorenal syndrome: a phase II study. Gut 2000;47(2):288–95.

48. Testino G, Ferro C, Sumberaz A, et al. Type-2 hepatorenal syndrome and refractory ascites: role of transjugular intrahepatic portosystemic stent-shunt in eighteen patients with advanced cirrhosis awaiting orthotopic liver transplantation. Hepatogastroenterology 2003;50(54):1753–5.

49. Murad SD, Plessier A, Hernandez-Guerra M, et al. Etiology, management, and outcome of the Budd-Chiari syndrome. Ann Intern Med 2009;151(3): 167–75.

50. Rajani R, Melin T, Björnsson E, et al. Budd-Chiari syndrome in Sweden: epidemiology, clinical characteristics and survival–an 18-year experience. Liver Int 2009; 29(2):253–9.

51. Murad SD, Valla D, De Groen PC, et al. Determinants of survival and the effect of portosystemic shunting in patients with Budd-Chiari syndrome. Hepatology 2004;39(2):500–8.

52. Qi X, Yang M, Fan D, et al. Transjugular intrahepatic portosystemic shunt in the treatment of Budd-Chiari syndrome: a critical review of literatures. Scand J Gastroenterol 2013;48(7):771–84.

53. Tripathi D, Helmy A, Macbeth K, et al. Ten years' follow-up of 472 patients following transjugular intrahepatic portosystemic stent-shunt insertion at a single centre. Eur J Gastroenterol Hepatol 2004;16(1):9–18.

54. Riggio O, Angeloni S, Salvatori FM, et al. Incidence, natural history, and risk factors of hepatic encephalopathy after transjugular intrahepatic portosystemic shunt with polytetrafluoroethylene-covered stent grafts. Am J Gastroenterol 2008;103(11):2738–46.

55. Hoeper MM, Krowka MJ, Strassburg CP. Portopulmonary hypertension and hepatopulmonary syndrome. Lancet 2004;363(9419):1461–8.

56. Schenk P, Schöniger-Hekele M, Fuhrmann V, et al. Prognostic significance of the hepatopulmonary syndrome in patients with cirrhosis. Gastroenterology 2003; 125(4):1042–52.

57. Selim KM, Akriviadis EA, Zuckerman E, et al. Transjugular intrahepatic portosystemic shunt: a successful treatment for hepatopulmonary syndrome. Am J Gastroenterol 1998;93(3):455–8.

58. Benitez C, Arrese M, Jorquera J, et al. Successful treatment of severe hepatopulmonary syndrome with a sequential use of TIPS placement and liver transplantation. Ann Hepatol 2009;8(1):71–4.

59. Riegler JL, Lang KA, Johnson SP, et al. Transjugular intrahepatic portosystemic shunt improves oxygenation in hepatopulmonary syndrome. Gastroenterology 1995;109(3):978–83.

60. Lasch HM, Fried MW, Zacks SL, et al. Use of transjugular intrahepatic portosystemic shunt as a bridge to liver transplantation in a patient with severe hepatopulmonary syndrome. Liver Transpl 2001;7(2):147–9.

61. Martínez-Pallí G, Drake BB, Garcia-Pagan JC, et al. Effect of transjugular intra-hepatic portosystemic shunt on pulmonary gas exchange in patients with portal

hypertension and hepatopulmonary syndrome. World J Gastroenterol 2005; 11(43):6858.

62. Paramesh AS, Husain SZ, Shneider B, et al. Improvement of hepatopulmonary syndrome after transjugular intrahepatic portasystemic shunting: case report and review of literature. Pediatr Transplant 2003;7(2):157–62.

63. Chevallier P, Novelli L, Motamedi JP, et al. Hepatopulmonary syndrome successfully treated with transjugular intrahepatic portosystemic shunt: a three-year follow-up. J Vasc Interv Radiol 2004;15(6):647–8.

64. Gaba RC, Khiatani VL, Knuttinen MG, et al. Comprehensive review of TIPS technical complications and how to avoid them. AJR Am J Roentgenol 2011;196(3): 675–85.

65. De Franchis R, Dell'Era A, Primignani M. Diagnosis and monitoring of portal hypertension. Dig Liver Dis 2008;40(5):312–7.

66. Bosch J, Garcia-Pagan JC. Prevention of variceal rebleeding. Lancet 2003; 361(9361):952–4.

67. Abraldes JG, Tarantino I, Turnes J, et al. Hemodynamic response to pharmacological treatment of portal hypertension and long-term prognosis of cirrhosis. Hepatology 2003;37(4):902–8.

68. Tesdal IK, Filser T, Weiss C, et al. Transjugular intrahepatic portosystemic shunts: adjunctive embolotherapy of gastroesophageal collateral vessels in the prevention of variceal rebleeding. Radiology 2005;236(1):360–7.

69. Gaba RC, Bui JT, Cotler SJ, et al. Rebleeding rates following TIPS for variceal hemorrhage in the Viatorr era: TIPS alone versus TIPS with variceal embolization. Hepatol Int 2010;4(4):749–56.

70. Xiao T, Chen L, Chen W, et al. Comparison of transjugular intrahepatic portosystemic shunt (TIPS) alone versus TIPS combined with embolotherapy in advanced cirrhosis: a retrospective study. J Clin Gastroenterol 2011;45(7):643–50.

71. Bureau C, Otal P, Pomier-Layrargues G, et al. Improved clinical outcome using polytetrafluoroethylene-coated stents for TIPS: results of a randomized study. Gastroenterology 2004;126(2):469–75.

72. Angermayr B, Cejna M, Koenig F, et al. Survival in patients undergoing transjugular intrahepatic portosystemic shunt: ePTFE-covered stentgrafts versus bare stents. Hepatology 2003;38(4):1043–50.

73. Riggio O, Ridola L, Angeloni S, et al. Clinical efficacy of transjugular intrahepatic portosystemic shunt created with covered stents with different diameters: results of a randomized controlled trial. J Hepatol 2010;53(2):267–72.

74. Engstrom BI, Horvath JJ, Suhocki PV, et al. Covered transjugular intrahepatic portosystemic shunts: accuracy of ultrasound in detecting shunt malfunction. Am J Roentgenol 2013;200(4):904–8.

75. Jalan R, Redhead DN, Allan PL, et al. Prospective evaluation of haematological alterations following the transjugular intrahepatic portosystemic stent-shunt (TIPSS). Eur J Gastroenterol Hepatol 1996;8(4):381–6.

76. Ferguson JW, Tripathi D, Redhead DN, et al. Transient segmental liver ischaemia after polytetrafluoroethylene transjugular intrahepatic portosystemic stent-shunt procedure. J Hepatol 2005;42(1):145.

77. Yang Z, Han G, Wu Q, et al. Patency and clinical outcomes of transjugular intrahepatic portosystemic shunt with polytetrafluoroethylene-covered stents versus bare stents: a meta-analysis. J Gastroenterol Hepatol 2010;25(11):1718–25.

78. Salerno F, Cazzaniga M, Pagnozzi G, et al. Humoral and cardiac effects of TIPS in cirrhotic patients with different "effective" blood volume. Hepatology 2003; 38(6):1370–7.

79. Merli M, Valeriano V, Funaro S, et al. Modifications of cardiac function in cirrhotic patients treated with transjugular intrahepatic portosystemic shunt (TIPS). Am J Gastroenterol 2002;97(1):142–8.
80. Tanaka T, Günther RW, Isfort P, et al. Pull-through technique for recanalization of occluded portosystemic shunts (TIPS): technical note and review of the literature. Cardiovasc Intervent Radiol 2011;34(2):406–12.
81. Echenagusia M, Rodriguez-Rosales G, Simo G, et al. Expanded PTFE-covered stent-grafts in the treatment of transjugular intrahepatic portosystemic shunt (TIPS) stenoses and occlusions. Abdom Imaging 2005;30(6):750–4.
82. Kochar N, Tripathi D, Arestis NJ, et al. Tipsitis: incidence and outcome-a single centre experience. Eur J Gastroenterol Hepatol 2010;22(6):729–35.
83. Tripathi D, Therapondos G, Redhead DN, et al. Transjugular intrahepatic portosystemic stent-shunt and its effects on orthotopic liver transplantation. Eur J Gastroenterol Hepatol 2002;14(8):827–32.

Prophylaxis of Variceal

to, MD, Vijay H. Shah, MD,

ᴍᴅ*

• Cirrhosis • Gastrointestinal hemorrhage • Endoscopy

of esophageal varices is recommended for patients at high risk for
phageal varices, and small varices in patients with Child-Turcotte-
/or red wale markings).

axis of varices with nonselective β-blockers is ineffective, and there-
ended.

ective β-blocker with anti–α_1-adrenergic activity, significantly reduces
the risk of first variceal hemorrhage.

kers and variceal band ligation are equally effective in preventing first

ular therapy depends on local resources, expertise, and patient pref-
ugh discussion.

a common consequence of cirrhosis, is defined as a pathologic
n to inferior vena cava pressure gradient greater than 5 mm Hg.
rhosis directly related to portal hypertension include variceal
d hepatic encephalopathy. Variceal bleeding is the most feared
al hypertension and, despite significant advances in management
des, is still associated with substantial morbidity and mortality.[1]
n of variceal hemorrhage remains an important goal in treating
geal varices.

ESOPHAGEAL VARICEAL BLEEDING

rance of varices in patients with compensated cirrhosis is associated with
ed risk of death (1.0%–3.4% per year), and the occurrence of variceal bleed
y increases this risk, with 1-year mortality rate as high as 57%. Approxi-
% of deaths occur in the first 6 weeks of a bleeding episode.[2]

hendations for primary prophylaxis for esophageal varices differ according
ociated risk of bleeding. One of the most important risk factors for variceal
ie is variceal size. Varices can be classified simply as small or large (**Fig. 1**),
ff diameter of 5 mm.[3] Patients with no varices have a risk of bleeding of 2%
hereas this risk increases to 5% per year in those with small varices, and up
those with large varices.[4]

ence of red wale markings and the severity of liver disease (Child-Turcotte-
B/C) have also been associated with increased risk of bleeding. These pa-
ave been combined in the North Italian Endoscopic Club index.[5]

element implicated on the risk of variceal rupture and bleeding is variceal
n. Wall tension is directly proportional to transmural pressure (ie, difference
travariceal pressure and esophageal lumen pressure), variceal diameter,
al wall thickness. Increase in wall tension is associated with a reduction
s of the variceal wall. Variceal size and red wale markings reflect 2 of these
s: variceal diameter and wall thickness, respectively. The third component,
essure, is the most important because it is the driver for the dilatation of
d is a direct function of portal venous pressure.[6]

venous pressure gradient (HVPG), an indirect measure of portal pressure,
hown to be an independent predictor of variceal bleeding and death.[7] Var-
ling does not occur with an HVPG of less than 12 mm Hg.[8] Moreover, an
uction to less than 12 mm Hg or by greater than 20% significantly reduces
bleeding, and a reduction greater than 20% in HVPG significantly reduces
[-11] The goal of primary prophylaxis using pharmacologic therapy, therefore,
ase HVPG.

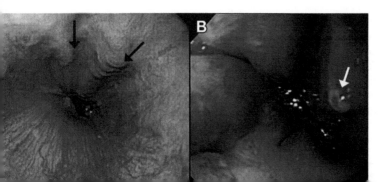

PREPRIMARY PROPHYLAXIS

Nonselective β-adrenergic blockers have been shown to significantly reduce portal pressure, as measured by HVPG, and this reduction seems to be greater in patients without varices than in those with varices.[12] Also, studies in animal models of portal hypertension have suggested a potential role for nonselective β-blockers in preventing the development of portosystemic collaterals or shunts.[13,14] These observations prompted evaluation of nonselective β-blockers for preventing the formation of esophageal varices in patients with cirrhosis.

In 1999, Cales and colleagues[15] evaluated the effect of propranolol in preventing large esophageal varices. A total of 206 patients, 38% without varices and 62% with small varices, were randomized to receive propranolol or placebo. At 2 years, 31% of patients in the propranolol group had developed large varices compared with 14% in the placebo group. The rate of variceal bleeding and death was similar in both groups. A second randomized, double-blind, placebo-controlled trial evaluated the effectiveness of timolol for the primary prevention of esophageal varices in patients with cirrhosis. This study, conducted in 4 centers, randomly assigned 213 subjects to receive timolol or placebo. At 55 months of follow-up, 39% and 40% of patients in the timolol and placebo groups, respectively, reached the primary end point (development of gastroesophageal varices or variceal hemorrhage). No difference was seen in the primary end point of the study ($P = .89$). Serious adverse events were significantly more frequent in the timolol group (19% vs 6%; $P<.01$).[16] Therefore, nonselective β-blockers cannot be recommended for the prevention of variceal formation in patients with cirrhosis.

PREVENTION OF VARICEAL GROWTH

Prevention of growth of small esophageal varices has been explored in 2 randomized trials with conflicting results. The first trial, mentioned earlier, showed a significantly higher rate of development of large varices in the propranolol group compared with the placebo group.[15] In contrast, a second multicenter, randomized, placebo-controlled trial showed that nadolol significantly reduced the progression from small to large esophageal varices at 3 years (11% vs 37%).[17] No difference in survival was observed, and again, a higher proportion of patients developed significant adverse events in the β-blocker group (11% vs 1%). Therefore, the current guidelines recommend prophylaxis with nonselective β-blockers only for patients with small gastroesophageal varices who are at high risk for bleeding, such as those with advanced liver disease (Child-Turcotte-Pugh class B/C) and/or the presence of red wale marks on varices.[3,18]

PHARMACOLOGIC PROPHYLAXIS OF VARICEAL BLEEDING

The goal of primary prophylaxis is to prevent the first bleeding episode and consequently improve survival through decreasing bleeding-related death. Nonselective β-blockers reduce portal pressure through blockade of β_1- and β_2-adrenergic receptors. Blockade of these receptors results in a decrease in the cardiac output and unopposed splanchnic vasoconstriction, respectively, which in turn leads to a reduction of the portal inflow. In contrast, β_1-selective agents lack the splanchnic vasoconstrictive effect, and are therefore not used for prophylaxis of variceal bleeding.

Nonselective β-adrenergic blockers have been extensively studied for the prevention of variceal bleeding and are considered the cornerstone therapy for primary prophylaxis. Numerous randomized studies have confirmed the effectiveness of nonselective β-blockers in reducing the risk of a first bleeding episode. A systematic review of the 11 randomized controlled trials comparing β-blockers with placebo or nonactive treatment showed a 9% absolute risk reduction of first variceal bleeding at 2 years (from 24% with nonactive treatment to 15% with β-blockers). The number needed to treat to prevent one variceal bleed was 10.[19] A significant reduction in mortality was also seen with β-blocker use. The beneficial effect of β-blockers is independent of the cause or severity of cirrhosis.[20]

Propranolol and nadolol are the most widely used nonselective β-blockers.[2] Propranolol is typically initiated at a dose of 20 mg twice a day and it is titrated up as indicated, to a maximum tolerated dose of up to 160 mg twice daily. A long-acting preparation of propranolol that can be administered once a day in the evening is preferred in practice. Nadolol has a longer half-life, allowing once-a-day administration. Nadolol is less lipid-soluble than propranolol and is less likely to cross the blood-brain barrier. It is excreted largely by the kidneys, unlike propranolol, which has hepatic excretion. Nadolol is commonly initiated at a dose of 20 mg daily and can be titrated up to a maximum tolerated dose of 240 mg once a day. Starting β-blockers at small doses and taking the medication at night may reduce side effects and improve compliance. Approximately 15% of patients require discontinuation of nonselective β-blockers because of side effects, the most common of which include lightheadedness, fatigue, dyspnea, impotence, or sleep disorders. Also, approximately 15% of patients have contraindications to the use of β-blockers, such as asthma, severe chronic obstructive pulmonary disease, severe aortic stenosis, brittle diabetes mellitus, and atrioventricular block.

Recently, nonselective β-blockers have also been associated with lower survival in patients with refractory or intractable ascites. Median survival time was 20 months in untreated patients and 5 months in those treated with propranolol (P<.0001).[21] However, a major methodological limitation of this study is that only 4% of patients not on β-blockers had esophageal varices compared with 100% in the propranolol-treated group. A subsequent study also suggested that patients with cirrhosis and refractory ascites on nonselective β-blockers may be at increased risk for paracentesis-induced circulatory dysfunction.[22] Therefore, β-blockers should be used with caution in this subset of patients with refractory ascites; however, additional studies are required to confirm these findings.

HVPG has been used to evaluate the hemodynamic response to β-blockers, with approximately 49% responders overall.[23] An HVPG reduction to less than 12 mm Hg essentially eliminates the risk of bleeding and improves survival,[10] and reductions greater than 10% or 20% significantly reduce the risk of first variceal bleed.[24] Unfortunately, HVPG is not widely available; most studies evaluating the effect of β-blockers have aimed for a 25% reduction in heart rate from baseline. However, reduction in heart rate does not correlate well with reduction in HVPG[25]; hence, β-blockers should be titrated to maximal tolerated doses. Once initiated, nonselective β-blockers should be maintained indefinitely; the bleeding risk returns to baseline when treatment is withdrawn.[26] No follow-up endoscopies are required unless the patient has a variceal bleed or variceal ligation is being considered a patient intolerant to β-blockers.

Carvedilol, a nonselective β-blocker with intrinsic anti–α_1-adrenergic activity, through its α_1-adrenergic blocking effect, also decreases the intrahepatic and portocollateral vascular resistance, resulting in further reduction in the portal pressure. Carvedilol has been shown to reduce HVPG greater than 20% from baseline or to lower than 12 mm Hg in a larger proportion of patients when compared with propranolol (64% vs 14%; P<.05).[27]

A recent study compared the hemodynamic effects of carvedilol in nonresponders to propranolol. The authors showed that carvedilol leads to a significantly greater decrease in portal pressure compared with propranolol, and was associated with reduction in the bleeding rates at 2 years of follow-up.[28] One concern, however, is that carvedilol also significantly decreases the mean arterial pressure, unlike propranolol, which causes a greater decrease in heart rate and cardiac output.[27] For that reason, carvedilol may be considered in patients with concomitant systemic hypertension.[29] The initial recommended dose of carvedilol is 6.25 mg per day, titrated up to 12.50 mg per day if well tolerated. Higher doses have demonstrated a greater decrease in HVPG but at the cost of increased adverse events, mainly symptomatic hypotension.[27]

Nitrates in experimental models decrease intrahepatic and portocollateral resistance, and consequently portal pressure.[30] In humans, the effect is more likely because of hypotension-induced reflex splanchnic vasoconstriction. Long-acting nitrates, mainly isosorbide mononitrate, have been explored in 5 randomized trials for the primary prevention of variceal bleed: in 2 as monotherapy[31,32] and 3 in combination with β-blockers.[33] The results of these studies are somewhat conflicting, and more side effects have been observed in the combination group. Therefore, isosorbide mononitrate is not currently recommended for primary prophylaxis of variceal bleed, either alone or in combination with β-blockers.[3,34,35]

Spironolactone and a low-sodium diet have been shown to reduce portal pressure through decreasing the plasma volume and, consequently, the splanchnic blood flow.[36] However, a preliminary study examining spironolactone in combination with nadolol showed no benefit over nadolol alone in primary prophylaxis.[37]

ENDOSCOPIC PROPHYLAXIS

Variceal band ligation (VBL) has become the preferred method for endoscopic prevention of variceal bleeding because it has been associated with fewer complications than endoscopic sclerotherapy.[38] A meta-analysis of 5 randomized clinical trials comparing VBL with no treatment showed a significant decrease in the risk of first variceal bleeding and lower mortality rates in the VBL group.[39] VBL is repeated every 2 to 4 weeks until the varices have been eradicated, which typically requires 2 to 4 sessions. After eradication, follow-up endoscopies should be obtained every 6 months and repeat ligation is performed on recurrence of esophageal varices. The procedure is usually fairly well tolerated, with low risk of significant adverse events. Minor complications are common, such as transient dysphagia, chest discomfort, and shallow ulcerations at the site of ligation. Mucosal tears or complete esophageal perforation have become less frequent with the advent of multiple-band ligation devices.[40] Death has been reported as a complication of VBL.

VBL has also been compared with nonselective β-blockers in 19 trials, 12 published in full, involving a total of 1483 patients (**Table 1**). Two prior meta-analyses, including 8 and 12 of these studies, respectively, had suggested VBL to be superior to β-blockers in preventing first variceal bleed.[41,42] However, most of these trials were underpowered or prematurely stopped, and the 2 largest trials comparing VBL with nadolol or propranolol for primary prophylaxis had not been included in the earlier-cited meta-analyses.[43,44] A more recent meta-analysis, including all 19 of these trials, still suggested VBL to be slightly superior to β-blockers in reducing the risk of first variceal bleeding. However, when taking into account only high-quality trials, which included 100 patients or more, the results were no longer significantly different (**Fig. 2**). No difference was seen either in bleeding-related and overall mortality compared with

Table 1
Results of 12 fully published trials comparing VBL with nonselective β-blockers for overall bleeding

Study Name	Sample Size	Odds Ratio	Confidence Interval		P Value
Schepke et al,[44] 2004	152	1.177	0.577	2.406	.654
Lay et al,[52] 2006	100	1.831	0.627	5.941	.2
Lui et al,[53] 2002	110	2.004	0.593	5.775	.404
Lo et al,[43] 2004	100	2.101	0.792	5.571	.179
Sarin et al,[49] 2005	89	3.431	1.17	10.062	.059
Perez-Ayuso et al,[54] 2010	75	2.207	0.696	7.003	.179
Drastich et al,[55] 2011	73	1.224	0.164	9.146	.544
Norberto et al,[56] 2007	62	1.0	0.188	5.313	.036
Jutabha et al,[57] 2005	62	8.194	1.096	61.158	.041
Psilopoulos et al,[58] 2005	60	4.83	1.266	16.935	.012
Thuluvath et al,[59] 2005	31	0.524	0.05	5.463	.016
De et al,[60] 1999	30	0.489	0.047	5.101	.022

Studies are ordered according to sample size. VBL was not superior to β-blockers in preventing first variceal bleeding if only the 4 trials with 100 patients or more were included, but VBL becomes significantly superior with inclusion of trials with 62 patients or fewer.

β-blockers.[45] Side effects from VBL are less frequent but more severe than those associated with β-blockers, and may lead to fatalities. Regarding its cost-effectiveness, 2 studies used a Markov model to compare VBL with β-blockers and showed β-blockers to be more cost-effective.[46,47] However, one of the studies suggested VBL to be more cost-effective when quality of life was considered.[47]

Recently, a randomized multicenter controlled trial compared carvedilol with VBL for preventing first variceal bleed. A total of 152 patients with cirrhosis and large esophageal varices were randomized to either carvedilol or VBL and followed for 20 months. Carvedilol showed significantly lower rates of first variceal bleed in an intent-to-treat analysis (10% vs 23%; $P = .04$), with no significant differences in overall or bleeding-related mortality.[48]

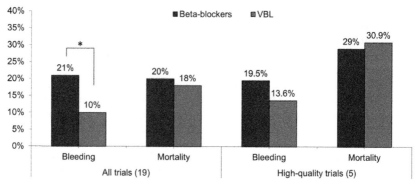

Fig. 2. Comparison of nonselective β-blockers versus variceal band ligation in the prevention of first variceal bleeding and mortality, according to a meta-analysis of 19 randomized controlled trials. *$P<.05$. (*From* Simonetto DA, Shah VH. Primary prophylaxis of esophageal variceal bleeding. Clinical Liver Disease 2012;1(5):149; with permission.)

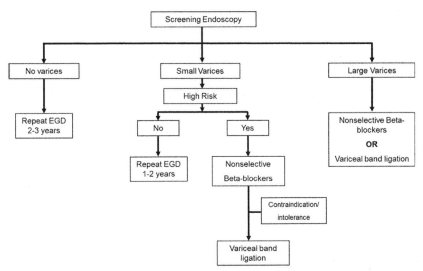

Fig. 3. Schematic diagram of current recommendations for primary prophylaxis of esophageal variceal bleeding. High risk for variceal bleeding: Child-Turcotte-Pugh class B and C or presence of red wales on varices. EGD, esophagogastroduodenoscopy.

Therefore, either nonselective β-blockers or VBLs may be an appropriate first-line choice for primary prophylaxis of variceal bleeding. The combination of the therapies has not been shown to be more effective and is associated with increased side effects.[49] Because VBL and β-blockers are essentially equivalent therapies, the choice of therapy depends on patient preference after a thorough discussion. A pilot study evaluating the predicted preference of patients and physicians showed that most patients (64%) and physicians (57%) preferred VBL over β-blockers for primary prophylaxis of variceal hemorrhage. Patients' predicted preferences were mostly influenced by the risk of dyspnea, hypotension, fatigue, or procedure-related bleeding.[50]

SUMMARY

In summary, primary prophylaxis of variceal bleeding is recommended for all patients with large esophageal varices, independently of the severity of liver disease or the presence of risk factors. Either nonselective β-blockers or VBL could be used, and the choice of treatment depends on local resources, expertise, and patient preference. Primary prophylaxis is also recommended for patients with small varices at high risk of bleeding (Child-Turcotte-Pugh class B/C or presence of red wales on varices), and nonselective β-blockers are generally preferred in this setting, unless contraindicated or not well tolerated, in which case VBL should be considered (**Fig. 3**).[51]

REFERENCES

1. D'Amico G, De Franchis R. Upper digestive bleeding in cirrhosis. Post-therapeutic outcome and prognostic indicators. Hepatology 2003;38(3): 599–612.
2. D'Amico G, Garcia-Tsao G, Pagliaro L. Natural history and prognostic indicators of survival in cirrhosis: a systematic review of 118 studies. J Hepatol 2006;44(1): 217–31.

3. de Franchis R. Evolving consensus in portal hypertension. Report of the Baveno IV consensus workshop on methodology of diagnosis and therapy in portal hypertension. J Hepatol 2005;43(1):167–76.

4. D'Amico G, Luca A. Natural history. Clinical-haemodynamic correlations. Prediction of the risk of bleeding. Baillieres Clin Gastroenterol 1997;11(2):243–56.

5. North Italian Endoscopic Club for the Study and Treatment of Esophageal Varices. Prediction of the first variceal hemorrhage in patients with cirrhosis of the liver and esophageal varices. A prospective multicenter study. N Engl J Med 1988;319(15):983–9.

6. Tiani C, Abraldes JG, Bosch J. Portal hypertension: pre-primary and primary prophylaxis of variceal bleeding. Dig Liver Dis 2008;40(5):318–27.

7. Merkel C, Bolognesi M, Bellon S, et al. Prognostic usefulness of hepatic vein catheterization in patients with cirrhosis and esophageal varices. Gastroenterology 1992;102(3):973–9.

8. Bosch J. A la carte or menu fixe: improving pharmacologic therapy of portal hypertension. Hepatology 2002;36(6):1330–2.

9. D'Amico G, Garcia-Pagan JC, Luca A, et al. Hepatic vein pressure gradient reduction and prevention of variceal bleeding in cirrhosis: a systematic review. Gastroenterology 2006;131(5):1611–24.

10. Groszmann RJ, Bosch J, Grace ND, et al. Hemodynamic events in a prospective randomized trial of propranolol versus placebo in the prevention of a first variceal hemorrhage. Gastroenterology 1990;99(5):1401–7.

11. Feu F, Garcia-Pagan JC, Bosch J, et al. Relation between portal pressure response to pharmacotherapy and risk of recurrent variceal haemorrhage in patients with cirrhosis. Lancet 1995;346(8982):1056–9.

12. Escorsell A, Ferayorni L, Bosch J, et al. The portal pressure response to beta-blockade is greater in cirrhotic patients without varices than in those with varices. Gastroenterology 1997;112(6):2012–6.

13. Lin HC, Soubrane O, Cailmail S, et al. Early chronic administration of propranolol reduces the severity of portal hypertension and portal-systemic shunts in conscious portal vein stenosed rats. J Hepatol 1991;13(2):213–9.

14. Sarin SK, Groszmann RJ, Mosca PG, et al. Propranolol ameliorates the development of portal-systemic shunting in a chronic murine schistosomiasis model of portal hypertension. J Clin Invest 1991;87(3):1032–6.

15. Cales P, Oberti F, Payen JL, et al. Lack of effect of propranolol in the prevention of large oesophageal varices in patients with cirrhosis: a randomized trial. French-Speaking Club for the Study of Portal Hypertension. Eur J Gastroenterol Hepatol 1999;11(7):741–5.

16. Groszmann RJ, Garcia-Tsao G, Bosch J, et al. Beta-blockers to prevent gastroesophageal varices in patients with cirrhosis. N Engl J Med 2005;353(21):2254–61.

17. Merkel C, Marin R, Angeli P, et al. A placebo-controlled clinical trial of nadolol in the prophylaxis of growth of small esophageal varices in cirrhosis. Gastroenterology 2004;127(2):476–84.

18. Garcia-Tsao G, Sanyal AJ, Grace ND, et al. Prevention and management of gastroesophageal varices and variceal hemorrhage in cirrhosis. Hepatology 2007;46(3):922–38.

19. D'Amico G, Pagliaro L, Bosch J. Pharmacological treatment of portal hypertension: an evidence-based approach. Semin Liver Dis 1999;19(4):475–505.

20. Poynard T, Cales P, Pasta L, et al. Beta-adrenergic-antagonist drugs in the prevention of gastrointestinal bleeding in patients with cirrhosis and esophageal varices. An analysis of data and prognostic factors in 589 patients from four

randomized clinical trials. Franco-Italian Multicenter Study Group. N Engl J Med 1991;324(22):1532–8.

21. Serste T, Melot C, Francoz C, et al. Deleterious effects of beta-blockers on survival in patients with cirrhosis and refractory ascites. Hepatology 2010;52(3):1017–22.

22. Serste T, Francoz C, Durand F, et al. Beta-blockers cause paracentesis-induced circulatory dysfunction in patients with cirrhosis and refractory ascites: a crossover study. J Hepatol 2011;55(4):794–9.

23. Albillos A, Banares R, Gonzalez M, et al. Value of the hepatic venous pressure gradient to monitor drug therapy for portal hypertension: a meta-analysis. Am J Gastroenterol 2007;102(5):1116–26.

24. Turnes J, Garcia-Pagan JC, Abraldes JG, et al. Pharmacological reduction of portal pressure and long-term risk of first variceal bleeding in patients with cirrhosis. Am J Gastroenterol 2006;101(3):506–12.

25. Garcia-Tsao G, Grace ND, Groszmann RJ, et al. Short-term effects of propranolol on portal venous pressure. Hepatology 1986;6(1):101–6.

26. Abraczinskas DR, Ookubo R, Grace ND, et al. Propranolol for the prevention of first esophageal variceal hemorrhage: a lifetime commitment? Hepatology 2001;34(6):1096–102.

27. Banares R, Moitinho E, Piqueras B, et al. Carvedilol, a new nonselective beta-blocker with intrinsic anti- Alpha1-adrenergic activity, has a greater portal hypotensive effect than propranolol in patients with cirrhosis. Hepatology 1999;30(1):79–83.

28. Reiberger T, Ulbrich G, Ferlitsch A, et al. Carvedilol for primary prophylaxis of variceal bleeding in cirrhotic patients with haemodynamic non-response to propranolol. Gut 2013;62(11):1634–41.

29. Bosch J. Carvedilol for portal hypertension in patients with cirrhosis. Hepatology 2010;51(6):2214–8.

30. Bhathal PS, Grossman HJ. Reduction of the increased portal vascular resistance of the isolated perfused cirrhotic rat liver by vasodilators. J Hepatol 1985;1(4):325–37.

31. Bosch J, Garcia-Pagan JC. Complications of cirrhosis. I. Portal hypertension. J Hepatol 2000;32(Suppl 1):141–56.

32. Angelico M, Carli L, Piat C, et al. Effects of isosorbide-5-mononitrate compared with propranolol on first bleeding and long-term survival in cirrhosis. Gastroenterology 1997;113(5):1632–9.

33. Merkel C, Marin R, Enzo E, et al. Randomised trial of nadolol alone or with isosorbide mononitrate for primary prophylaxis of variceal bleeding in cirrhosis. Gruppo-Triveneto per L'ipertensione portale (GTIP). Lancet 1996;348(9043):1677–81.

34. Angelico M, Lionetti R. Long-acting nitrates in portal hypertension: to be or not to be? Dig Liver Dis 2001;33(3):205–11.

35. Gluud LL, Langholz E, Krag A. Meta-analysis: isosorbide-mononitrate alone or with either beta-blockers or endoscopic therapy for the management of oesophageal varices. Aliment Pharmacol Ther 2010;32(7):859–71.

36. Garcia-Pagan JC, Salmeron JM, Feu F, et al. Effects of low-sodium diet and spironolactone on portal pressure in patients with compensated cirrhosis. Hepatology 1994;19(5):1095–9.

37. Abecasis R, Kravetz D, Fassio E, et al. Nadolol plus spironolactone in the prophylaxis of first variceal bleed in nonascitic cirrhotic patients: a preliminary study. Hepatology 2003;37(2):359–65.

38. Laine L, Cook D. Endoscopic ligation compared with sclerotherapy for treatment of esophageal variceal bleeding. A meta-analysis. Ann Intern Med 1995;123(4): 280–7.
39. Imperiale TF, Chalasani N. A meta-analysis of endoscopic variceal ligation for primary prophylaxis of esophageal variceal bleeding. Hepatology 2001;33(4): 802–7.
40. Bosch J, Abraldes JG, Groszmann R. Current management of portal hypertension. J Hepatol 2003;38(Suppl 1):S54–68.
41. Garcia-Pagan JC, Bosch J. Endoscopic band ligation in the treatment of portal hypertension. Nat Clin Pract Gastroenterol Hepatol 2005;2(11):526–35.
42. Khuroo MS, Khuroo NS, Farahat KL, et al. Meta-analysis: endoscopic variceal ligation for primary prophylaxis of oesophageal variceal bleeding. Aliment Pharmacol Ther 2005;21(4):347–61.
43. Lo GH, Chen WC, Chen MH, et al. Endoscopic ligation vs. nadolol in the prevention of first variceal bleeding in patients with cirrhosis. Gastrointest Endosc 2004;59(3):333–8.
44. Schepke M, Kleber G, Nurnberg D, et al. Ligation versus propranolol for the primary prophylaxis of variceal bleeding in cirrhosis. Hepatology 2004;40(1):65–72.
45. Funakoshi N, Duny Y, Valats JC, et al. Meta-analysis: beta-blockers versus banding ligation for primary prophylaxis of esophageal variceal bleeding. Ann Hepatol 2012;11(3):369–83.
46. Saab S, DeRosa V, Nieto J, et al. Costs and clinical outcomes of primary prophylaxis of variceal bleeding in patients with hepatic cirrhosis: a decision analytic model. Am J Gastroenterol 2003;98(4):763–70.
47. Imperiale TF, Klein RW, Chalasani N. Cost-effectiveness analysis of variceal ligation vs. beta-blockers for primary prevention of variceal bleeding. Hepatology 2007;45(4):870–8.
48. Tripathi D, Ferguson JW, Kochar N, et al. Randomized controlled trial of carvedilol versus variceal band ligation for the prevention of the first variceal bleed. Hepatology 2009;50(3):825–33.
49. Sarin SK, Wadhawan M, Agarwal SR, et al. Endoscopic variceal ligation plus propranolol versus endoscopic variceal ligation alone in primary prophylaxis of variceal bleeding. Am J Gastroenterol 2005;100(4):797–804.
50. Longacre AV, Imaeda A, Garcia-Tsao G, et al. A pilot project examining the predicted preferences of patients and physicians in the primary prophylaxis of variceal hemorrhage. Hepatology 2008;47(1):169–76.
51. de Franchis R. Revising consensus in portal hypertension: report of the Baveno V consensus workshop on methodology of diagnosis and therapy in portal hypertension. J Hepatol 2010;53(4):762–8.
52. Lay CS, Tsai YT, Lee FY, et al. Endoscopic variceal ligation versus propranolol in prophylaxis of first variceal bleeding in patients with cirrhosis. J Gastroenterol Hepatol 2006;21(2):413–9.
53. Lui HF, Stanley AJ, Forrest EH, et al. Primary prophylaxis of variceal hemorrhage: a randomized controlled trial comparing band ligation, propranolol, and isosorbide mononitrate. Gastroenterology 2002;123(3):735–44.
54. Perez-Ayuso RM, Valderrama S, Espinoza M, et al. Endoscopic band ligation versus propranolol for the primary prophylaxis of variceal bleeding in cirrhotic patients with high risk esophageal varices. Ann Hepatol 2010;9(1):15–22.
55. Drastich P, Lata J, Petrtyl J, et al. Endoscopic variceal band ligation compared with propranolol for prophylaxis of first variceal bleeding. Ann Hepatol 2011; 10(2):142–9.

56. Norberto L, Polese L, Cillo U, et al. A randomized study comparing ligation with propranolol for primary prophylaxis of variceal bleeding in candidates for liver transplantation. Liver Transpl 2007;13(9):1272-8.
57. Jutabha R, Jensen DM, Martin P, et al. Randomized study comparing banding and propranolol to prevent initial variceal hemorrhage in cirrhotics with high-risk esophageal varices. Gastroenterology 2005;128(4):870-81.
58. Psilopoulos D, Galanis P, Goulas S, et al. Endoscopic variceal ligation vs. propranolol for prevention of first variceal bleeding: a randomized controlled trial. Eur J Gastroenterol Hepatol 2005;17(10):1111-7.
59. Thuluvath PJ, Maheshwari A, Jagannath S, et al. A randomized controlled trial of beta-blockers versus endoscopic band ligation for primary prophylaxis: a large sample size is required to show a difference in bleeding rates. Dig Dis Sci 2005; 50(2):407-10.
60. De BK, Ghoshal UC, Das T, et al. Endoscopic variceal ligation for primary prophylaxis of oesophageal variceal bleed: preliminary report of a randomized controlled trial. J Gastroenterol Hepatol 1999;14(3):220-4.

Management of Acute Variceal Bleeding

Jorge L. Herrera, MD

KEYWORDS

- Portal hypertension • Acute variceal bleeding • Cirrhosis • Endoscopic band ligation
- Endoscopy • Vasoactive therapy

KEY POINTS

- Recent changes in the management of acute variceal bleeding (AVB) have resulted in decreased mortality.
- A structured approach incorporating airway safety, volume resuscitation, vasoactive and antimicrobial pharmacotherapy, and early endoscopy minimizes morbidity and mortality in patients presenting with AVB.
- Presenting features that indicate a high risk of failing standard vasoactive and endoscopic therapy include Child C cirrhosis, active bleeding on index endoscopy, presence of infection, or a hepatic vein pressure gradient greater than 20 mm Hg.
- Patients at high risk of failing standard therapy for AVB may benefit from more aggressive approaches such as early TIPS placement following the index endoscopy.

 Endoscopic Band Ligation (EBL) of esophageal varices accompanies the article at http://www.liver.theclinics.com/

INTRODUCTION

Acute variceal bleeding (AVB) remains one of the most dangerous complications of portal hypertension. Advances in the management of AVB have resulted in a decline in the rate of hospitalization in recent years,[1] and mortality has decreased from 50%[2] to between 15% and 20%[3,4] over the last 3 decades. Despite these advances, in-hospital mortality remains high and is related to the severity of the underlying cirrhosis, ranging from 0% in Child A to 32% in Child C disease.[5]

A prompt and standardized approach to patients with variceal bleeding is required to minimize the risk of bleeding-related mortality. This integrated and multidisciplinary approach consists of airway protection, judicious volume resuscitation, vasoactive therapy, antibiotic prophylaxis, and endoscopic intervention (**Box 1**).

Financial Disclosure: The author has no financial relationships in the subject matter or materials discussed in this article.

Division of Gastroenterology, University of South Alabama College of Medicine, Gastroenterology Academic Offices, 6000 University Commons, 75 University Boulevard S., Mobile, AL 36688-0002, USA

E-mail address: jherrera18@gmail.com

> **Box 1**
> **Approach to variceal bleeding**
>
> *Airway management*
> - Consider endotracheal intubation if:
>   - Altered mental status
>   - Massive hemorrhage requiring emergent endoscopy
>
> *Volume resuscitation*
> - Place 2 large-bore intravenous access catheters
> - Avoid excessive volume replacement
> - Maximum hemoglobin target of 7 to 8 g/dL
> - Use of FFP or platelets to correct coagulopathy may not be beneficial
>
> *Vasoactive therapy*
> - Reduce portal pressure by using one of the following:
>   - Octreotide: 50 μg IV bolus followed by 50 μg/h infusion
>   - Terlipressin[a]: 2 mg every 4 h IV for 24 to 48 h, then 1 mg every 4 h
>   - Somatostatin[a]: 250 μg IV bolus followed by 250 to 500 μg/h infusion
>   - Vasopressin: 0.4 units/min IV plus IV or transdermal nitroglycerin
>   - Vapreotide[a]: IV bolus of 50 μg followed by 50 μg/h infusion
>
> *Antibiotic prophylaxis*
> - Initiate antibiotics to reduce rebleeding risk; choose either:
>   - Ceftriaxone 1 g IV every day for up to 7 days
>   - Norfloxacin 400 mg orally once a day for up to 7 days
>
> *Endoscopic therapy*
> - Obliterate varices using band ligation
>
> *Abbreviations:* FFP, fresh frozen plasma; IV, intravenous.
> [a] Not currently available in the United States.

AIRWAY MANAGEMENT

Most patients presenting with AVB are alert, not massively bleeding, and have an intact gag reflex. In this situation, no special precautions are needed to protect the airway.[6] Patients presenting with altered mental status, often caused by hepatic encephalopathy or intoxication, are at risk of aspiration and a decision to protect the airway via endotracheal intubation should be made early in the course. Patients with massive gastrointestinal bleeding not responding to initial interventions and in need of emergent endoscopic therapy are at high risk for aspiration and should undergo endotracheal intubation before sedation and endoscopy regardless of their mental status.[7]

VOLUME RESUSCITATION

At least 2 large-bore (14–18 gauge) venous accesses should be placed on admission for rapid administration of fluids and blood products. Excessive volume replacement may lead to increased portal pressure and increases the risk for early rebleeding from varices; judicious use of volume expanders is recommended. In general, fluids should be administered to keep systolic blood pressure at 100 mm Hg and maintain renal perfusion. Saline use should be minimized because it may aggravate or precipitate the formation of ascites and edema. Red blood cell transfusions should be administered to achieve a hemoglobin no greater than 8 g/dL; higher levels have been associated with increased portal pressure, more frequent complications, and worse outcomes, particularly among patients with Child A or B cirrhosis.[8]

The routine use of platelet transfusions or fresh frozen plasma (FFP) to correct a low platelet count or prolonged international normalized ratio (INR) is not supported by data and may further contribute to volume overload and increased portal pressure. In particular, the use of FFP to normalize a prolonged INR may not result in improved coagulation, because INR results have poor correlation with bleeding risk in cirrhosis.[9] Recent studies indicate that, despite a prolonged INR, some patients with cirrhosis show a hypercoagulable state caused by a deficiency of anticoagulant factors and a relative excess of procoagulant factors,[10] a balance that is not reflected by the INR results. Likewise, increased levels of von Willebrand factor, often present in cirrhosis, enhance platelet function and may compensate for the thrombocytopenia that is commonly present in portal hypertension.[11] For these reasons, the use of blood products to correct coagulation abnormalities should be individualized on a case-by-case basis. Recombinant activated factor VII failed to achieve superiority compared with placebo in patients with variceal bleeding,[12] and should not be routinely administered, although selected patients with more severe bleeding may benefit from its use.

VASOACTIVE THERAPY

Interventions designed to decrease portal pressure should be instituted early in the management of variceal bleeding. The use of vasoactive agents has been associated with a significantly lower risk of acute all-cause mortality and transfusion requirements, improved control of bleeding, and shorter hospital stay.[13] In most cases a variceal source of bleeding can be suspected based on the patient's history, physical examination findings, or laboratory results. In this situation, empiric use of vasoactive therapy to decrease portal pressure is recommended even before the source of bleeding is confirmed.

Vasoactive drugs reduce portal pressure mainly by causing splanchnic vasoconstriction and reducing portal blood flow. Two main classes of drugs are used: (1) vasopressin or its analogue terlipressin, and (2) somatostatin or its analogues octreotide or vapreotide (see **Box 1**). In the United States, only vasopressin and octreotide are available. Vasopressin is generally not recommended because of its side effect profile and its minimal effects on decreasing rebleeding and improving survival.[14] Vasopressin infusion is associated with significant ischemic side effects including coronary artery vasoconstriction and mesenteric ischemia. To minimize side effects, it should be used in combination with intravenous or transdermal nitroglycerine[15] and only if other, safer vasoactive drugs are not available.

Terlipressin is a vasopressin analogue with an improved side effect profile. It is a selective vasoconstrictor of the splanchnic bed and does not need to be used as a continuous infusion. Terlipressin provides a 34% relative risk reduction in mortality in acute variceal hemorrhage,[16] with an improved side effect profile compared with vasopressin. At present, terlipressin is not approved by the US Food and Drug Administration for use in the United States.

The somatostatin analogue octreotide is the most commonly used vasoactive therapy to control AVB in the United States. A Cochrane Review found that administration of octreotide in AVB reduces the number of patients failing initial hemostasis, reduces the need for blood transfusion, but does not improve mortality.[17] Octreotide causes rapid splanchnic vasoconstriction, presumably by inhibiting the release of glucagon, a vasodilator hormone. Octreotide bolus injection results in a sharp decrease in portal pressure and azygous vein blood flow[18]; however, this effect is short-lived,[19] suggesting that octreotide's main benefit takes place in the first few minutes after initiating the bolus injection. Because octreotide has effects on other neurohumoral systems, prolonged intravenous infusion as is currently recommended may provide other beneficial effects such as blunting the postprandial increase in portal pressure once oral intake is resumed after an episode of variceal bleeding.[20]

Octreotide is administered intravenously; following a 50-μg bolus, an infusion of 50 μg/h is administered for a minimum of 48 hours and up to 5 days. Octreotide infusion is typically stopped after therapy with nonselective β-blockers is initiated once the patient is hemodynamically stable. Although octreotide has minimal side effects, its efficacy is inconclusive and controversial, but some have found it to be superior to vasopressin and an important adjunct in decreasing rebleeding.[21]

ANTIBIOTIC PROPHYLAXIS

Bacterial infection is independently associated with failure to control bleeding in cirrhotic patients.[22] The most common infections are spontaneous bacterial peritonitis, urinary tract infection, and pneumonia; up to 66% of cirrhotics admitted with variceal bleeding develop an infection soon after admission.[23] Infection and endotoxemia in cirrhosis further worsen the peripheral and splanchnic vasodilatation present in portal hypertension leading to increased portal blood flow and portal pressure. Infection favors variceal bleeding by increasing sinusoidal pressure, interfering with platelet aggregation, and increasing the release of heparinlike substances by endothelial cells, resulting in impaired coagulation.[24]

After an episode of variceal bleeding, the use of prophylactic antibiotics increases the probability of remaining free of rebleeding and is superior to using on-demand antibiotics in response to signs and symptoms of infection.[25] Oral norfloxacin 400 mg every 12 hours has been effective in decreasing infections in cirrhotics with gastrointestinal hemorrhage.[26] More recently, 1 g of intravenous ceftriaxone administered once a day for up to 7 days was more effective than norfloxacin in the prophylaxis of bacterial infections in patients with cirrhosis and hemorrhage.[27] On multivariate analysis, antibiotic prophylaxis has been an independent predictor of survival in patients with AVB.[5] A meta-analysis concluded that antibiotic prophylaxis for inpatients with cirrhosis is efficacious in reducing the number of deaths and bacterial infections regardless of the underlying risk factors.[28] Therefore, all patients with cirrhosis and AVB should be started on prophylactic antibiotics soon after arrival at the hospital and continued while hospitalized for up to 7 days.

ENDOSCOPIC THERAPY

Endoscopy allows confirmation of the source of bleeding and of the best therapeutic intervention. Endoscopic therapy is effective in controlling bleeding and preventing early rebleeding. Although endoscopy is considered one of the cornerstones of management of AVB, the timing of the endoscopic procedure is controversial. In general, urgent endoscopy should be performed within 12 to 24 hours of arrival, after the patient is hemodynamically stabilized and antibiotic and vasoactive therapies have been initiated.[29] Immediate endoscopy on arrival is generally discouraged because the patient is usually unstable and sufficient time has not been allowed for vasoactive therapy to take effect. In addition, a large amount of blood in the stomach increases the risk of aspiration and limits the ability to complete a diagnostic examination. If emergent endoscopy is necessary, the use of intravenous erythromycin significantly improves endoscopic visibility and shortens the duration of the index endoscopy.[30]

Endoscopic therapy for varices is designed to obliterate the varices and stop bleeding. Two commonly used endoscopic methods are sclerotherapy and endoscopic band ligation (EBL). Endoscopic sclerotherapy controls acute bleeding in 80% to 95% of cases, but sclerotherapy is associated with a significant risk of complications; its effect on early rebleeding rates is uncertain and it has no effect on survival. A meta-analysis of 10 randomized controlled trials showed an almost significant benefit of EBL compared with sclerotherapy.[31] Others studies have found that, compared with sclerotherapy, EBL has fewer complications, lower rates of rebleeding, and lower mortality.[32] As a result, EBL has largely replaced sclerotherapy as the main endoscopic therapy tool for the management of variceal hemorrhage. EBL consists of placing elastic bands at the base of the varices using commercially available banding devices that are attached to the end of the endoscope (Video 1). After the bands are placed, the varix is occluded and becomes thrombosed (**Fig. 1**). The bands subsequently fall off leaving a superficial ulcer that eventually heals, disrupting the flow of blood in the varix. Sessions are repeated every 2 to 4 weeks until all varices are eradicated. Most patients undergo a single banding session during the index hospitalization and return as outpatients for subsequent sessions.

EBL is highly effective in stopping variceal bleeding and decreasing the risk of early rebleeding. Complications are not common and include transient difficulty swallowing; chest pain, which occasionally may be severe and last hours or days; and development of strictures after healing. Five to 10 days after banding, shallow ulcers form in the esophagus that may cause bleeding. Post-EBL ulcer bleeding is more common in Child C patients, but cannot be predicted based on results of INR or platelet count.[33] The use of pantoprazole limits the size of the ulcers but has not been shown to be effective in decreasing the risk of bleeding.[34]

RESCUE THERAPIES

Most patients respond to the therapeutic maneuvers outlined earlier with cessation of bleeding soon after admission to the hospital. Approximately 20% of patients either

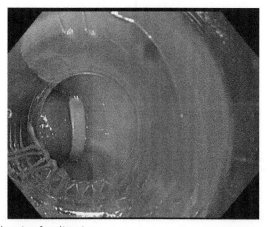

Fig. 1. Esophageal varix after ligation.

fail to respond to initial therapy or experience early rebleeding within the first 3 to 5 days.[35,36] By consensus, treatment failure is defined as failure to control AVB within 24 hours or failure to prevent clinically significant rebleeding within 5 days after treatment initiation.[29] Following the traditional approach to variceal bleeding (**Fig. 2**), rescue therapy is offered to patients who fail to stop bleeding or who rebleed soon after banding. Balloon tamponade, surgery, or placement of a transjugular intrahepatic portosystemic shunt (TIPS) are potential rescue therapies. The choice of therapy depends on the available local expertise and the magnitude of the bleeding.

Balloon tamponade is considered a temporizing option to stabilize the patient before a more definitive intervention. Two types of tubes for balloon tamponade are commercially available: the Sengstaken-Blakemore tube (SBT) and the Minnesota tube. Both tubes consist of an esophageal balloon and a gastric balloon as well as a gastric aspiration port. Compared with SBT, the Minnesota tube has a larger gastric balloon and an additional aspiration port above the esophageal balloon. In most cases, only the gastric balloon is initially inflated to provide pressure at the gastroesophageal (GE) junction, preventing blood flow to the esophageal varices. Inflation of the esophageal balloon is associated with increased risk of complications; for this reason the esophageal balloon is usually inflated only when bleeding persists despite inflation of the gastric balloon. To reduce the risk of necrosis of the GE junction, the gastric balloon should not remain continuously inflated for more than 48 hours. If the esophageal balloon is inflated, periodic deflation every 12 hours is recommended to reduce the risk of esophageal necrosis. In experienced hands, balloon tamponade is highly effective in controlling bleeding but recurrence is common after balloon deflation.[37] Complications associated with balloon tamponade occur in 20% to 30% of patients and include aspiration pneumonia and esophageal tears or rupture.[38] Despite the associated risks, balloon tamponade can be lifesaving for a patient with uncontrolled bleeding while preparations are made for more definitive therapies such as placement of a TIPS or surgery.

Surgical approaches to AVB include the creation of portosystemic shunts to decrease portal pressure or esophageal transection to disrupt blood flow into the esophageal varices. Surgery should be the last resort in the management of AVB,

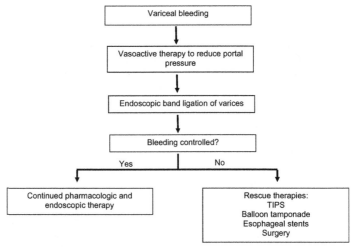

Fig. 2. Traditional approach to variceal bleeding. TIPS, transjugular intrahepatic portosystemic shunt.

because mortality is as high as 75%.[39] Surgery should be reserved for the stable patient who has recovered from an episode of massive AVB in a setting in which EBL and TIPS are not available. With the development of TIPS, the need to use emergent surgery as a rescue modality in the management of AVB has virtually disappeared. TIPS functions as a side-to-side portocaval shunt, effectively decreasing portal pressure and leading to cessation of bleeding. TIPS is a radiologic procedure that can be performed under moderate or deep sedation, avoiding the complications of general anesthesia. More details on the TIPS procedure, its indications, and complications are given elsewhere in this issue by Richard Parker.

In the acute setting, TIPS is typically considered for patients who fail to stop bleeding after initial endoscopic attempts, or who rebleed within the first 3 to 5 days after successful EBL has been performed. In this situation TIPS is highly effective; it controls bleeding in 94% of cases, with a low early rebleeding rate. However, when used as rescue therapy, hospital mortality at 6 weeks was 36%.[40] This high mortality likely reflects the severity of the bleeding and underlying liver disease in patients who are refractory to standard therapy for AVB; the urgency of TIPS is an independent predictor of early mortality.[41]

The use of a removable, covered, self-expanding esophageal stent to control variceal bleeding has been explored.[42] This specialized stent is supplied with an insertion system that includes a gastric balloon that is inflated to anchor the stent at the GE junction. Esophageal stent placement may be useful as rescue therapy in those patients for whom balloon tamponade is being considered. Covered esophageal stents were successfully placed in all subjects in a small study of 20 patients who failed pharmacologic and endoscopic therapy to arrest bleeding. After stent placement, bleeding stopped in all patients and the stents were removed in 5 to 7 days after other therapeutic interventions were completed. No significant stent-related complications or rebleeding were observed during a 30-day observation period.[37] Despite this encouraging report, the use of esophageal stents to treat refractory AVB remains experimental.

RISK STRATIFICATION TO TAILOR THERAPY

Patients presenting with variceal bleeding and Child A cirrhosis usually respond to standard pharmacologic and endoscopic therapy without rebleeding or the need for rescue therapy, and mortality in this group is typically low. In contrast, there is a high failure rate of standard therapy for AVB in Child C patients, those presenting with bacterial infection, those with evidence of renal insufficiency,[43] or in patients with high portal pressures.[4] These patients often require rescue therapy. Rescue therapy with TIPS is associated with a 30-day mortality of 29% and 60-day mortality of 35%.[44] The delay between the index bleed and TIPS placement, the number of endoscopic attempts to stop bleeding, and the need to use balloon tamponade predict increased mortality when using TIPS as a rescue modality.[38] These data suggest that a more aggressive approach may be needed for high-risk patients presenting with AVB.

The strongest predictor of a negative outcome in patients presenting with AVB is a hepatic vein portal gradient pressure (HVPG) greater than 20 mm Hg. These patients are 4 to 5.1 times more likely to fail standard therapy using vasoactive drugs and endoscopic therapy,[3,45] require more blood transfusions, are more likely to experience early rebleeding, and have longer hospitalizations. The value of a high HVPG predicting poor outcome has been prospectively validated.[46] HVPG is not commonly measured in clinical practice; however, patients presenting with HVPG greater than 20 mm Hg are more likely to be Child C, present with a systolic blood pressure less than 100 mm Hg, have a nonalcoholic cause of liver cirrhosis,[3] or show active bleeding on the initial endoscopy despite ongoing vasoactive therapy.[40] These clinical characteristics can be used to identify a group of patients at presentation who are likely to have high HVPG and a high risk of not responding to standard therapy and who may benefit from more aggressive management such as early placement of TIPS.

The efficacy of an aggressive approach to high-risk patients was shown by Garcia-Pagan and colleagues.[47] Sixty-two patients presenting with variceal bleeding, who were Child C (≤13 points) or Child B with bleeding at the initial endoscopy, were randomized to standard medical therapy with EBL and vasoactive drugs or to early TIPS after the initial endoscopic banding session. During a median follow-up of 16 months, rebleeding or failure to control bleeding occurred in 14 (45%) patients managed with EBL and vasoactive drugs compared with only 1 (3%) randomized to TIPS; 6-week mortality was reduced from 33% in the standard care group to 4% in the early TIPS group.[46] Seven of the patients in the conventional arm required rescue TIPS, but 4 died, confirming the poor prognosis of patients who fail initial attempts at hemostasis and require rescue TIPS. A retrospective review of cases admitted for AVB also found that, among Child C or Child B patients with active bleeding on the index endoscopy, early TIPS placement had superior outcomes compared with standard therapy and rescue TIPS for nonresponders.[48] The use of the recently developed covered stents for TIPS likely contributed to the positive outcomes of these trials because the risk of early thrombosis and TIPS dysfunction is lower.[49]

These preliminary data suggest that the approach to AVB should be stratified based on clinical characteristics at presentation, as shown in **Fig. 3**. All Child A and Child B patients who show no active bleeding on the index endoscopy can be managed with EBL and vasoactive drugs. In contrast, Child B patients who have active bleeding on the index endoscopy despite vasoactive therapy and Child C patients with less than or equal to 13 points may benefit from early intervention with TIPS placement using a covered stent rather than allowing them to fail initial therapy and then considering rescue TIPS.

An aggressive approach or rescue therapy may not be appropriate for all patients. Child C patients with 14 or 15 points are too ill to undergo TIPS and are unlikely to benefit from this therapy. Likewise, patients presenting with AVB in association with

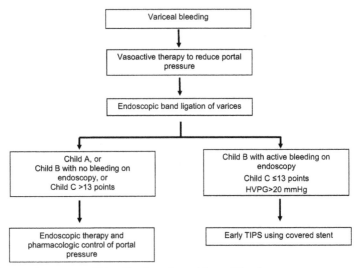

Fig. 3. Approach to variceal bleeding based on risk stratification.

hepatocellular carcinoma, serum creatinine greater than 3 mg/dL, portal thrombosis, or evidence of sepsis are not likely to benefit from rescue therapy[33] unless they are being considered for urgent liver transplantation.

SUMMARY

The approach to AVB has changed in the last few years. Newer, safer vasoactive drugs have been developed, some resulting in measurable reduction in mortality. The value of prophylactic antibiotics to decrease early rebleeding has become apparent and these are now standard of care. Endoscopic band ligation has replaced variceal sclerotherapy as the endoscopic therapy of choice to obliterate varices. Using readily available clinical parameters, a subset of high-risk patients can be identified at presentation who are less likely to respond to the traditional approach to variceal bleeding and may benefit from early TIPS placement to improve outcomes.

SUPPLEMENTARY DATA

Supplementary data related to this article can be found online at http://dx.doi.org/10.1016/j.cld.2014.01.001.

REFERENCES

1. Jamal MM, Samarasena JB, Hashemzadeh M, et al. Declining hospitalization rate of esophageal variceal bleeding in the United States. Clin Gastroenterol Hepatol 2008;6:689–95.
2. Graham DY, Smith JL. The course of patients after variceal hemorrhage. Gastroenterology 1981;80:800–9.
3. Villanueva C, Piqueras M, Aracil C, et al. A randomized controlled trial comparing ligation and sclerotherapy as emergency endoscopic treatment added to somatostatin in acute variceal bleeding. J Hepatol 2006;45:560–7.
4. Abraldes JG, Villanueva C, Bañares R, et al. Hepatic venous pressure gradient and prognosis in patients with acute variceal bleeding treated with pharmacologic and endoscopic therapy. J Hepatol 2008;48:229–36.
5. Carbonell N, Pauwels A, Serfaty L, et al. Improved survival after variceal bleeding in patients with cirrhosis over the past two decades. Hepatology 2004;40:652–9.
6. Koch DG, Arguedas MR, Fallon MB. Risk of aspiration pneumonia in suspected variceal hemorrhage: the value of prophylactic endotracheal intubation prior to endoscopy. Dig Dis Sci 2007;52:2225–8.
7. Rudolph SJ, Landsverk BK, Freeman ML. Endotracheal intubation for airway protection during endoscopy for severe GI hemorrhage. Gastrointest Endosc 2003;57:58–61.
8. Villanueva C, Colomo A, Bosch A, et al. Transfusion strategies for acute gastrointestinal bleeding. N Engl J Med 2013;368:11–21.
9. Tripodi A, Mannucci M. The coagulopathy of chronic liver disease. N Engl J Med 2011;365:147–56.
10. Tripodi A, Primignani M, Chantarangkul V, et al. An imbalance of pro- vs. anticoagulation factors in plasma from patients with cirrhosis. Gastroenterology 2008;38:1378–83.
11. Hugenholtz GG, Porte RJ, Lisman T. The platelet and platelet function testing in liver disease. Clin Liver Dis 2009;13:11–20.

12. Bosch J, Thabut D, Albillos A, et al. Recombinant factor VIIa for variceal bleeding in patients with advanced cirrhosis: a randomized controlled trial. Hepatology 2008;47:1604–14.

13. Wells M, Adams CP, Beaton M, et al. Meta-analysis: vasoactive medications for the management of acute variceal bleeds. Aliment Pharmacol Ther 2012;35:1267–78.

14. Imperiale TF, Teran JC, McCullough AJ. A meta-analysis of somatostatin versus vasopressin in the management of acute esophageal variceal hemorrhage. Gastroenterology 1995;109:1289–94.

15. Groszman RJ, Kravetz D, Bosch J, et al. Nitroglycerin improves the hemodynamic response to vasopressin in portal hypertension. Hepatology 1982;2:757–62.

16. Ioannou G, Doust J, Rockey D. Terlipressin for acute esophageal variceal hemorrhage. Cochrane Database Syst Rev 2003;(1):CD002147.

17. Gotzsche PC, Hrobjartsson A. Somatostatin analogues for acute bleeding oesophageal varices. Cochrane Database Syst Rev 2005;(1):CD000193. http://dx.doi.org/10.1002/14651858.CD000193.pub2.

18. Zironi G, Rossi C, Siringo S, et al. Short- and long-term hemodynamic response to octreotide in portal hypertensive patients: a double-blind, controlled study. Liver 1996;16:225–34.

19. Escorsell A, Bandi JC, Andreu V, et al. Desensitization to the effects of intravenous octreotide in cirrhotic patients with portal hypertension. Gastroenterology 2000;120:161–9.

20. Vorobioff JD, Gamen M, Kravetz D, et al. Effects of long-term propranolol and octreotide on postprandial hemodynamics in cirrhosis: a randomized controlled trial. Gastroenterology 2002;122:916–22.

21. Corley DA, Cello JP, Adkisson W. Octreotide for acute esophageal variceal bleeding: a meta-analysis. Gastroenterology 2001;120:946–54.

22. Goulis J, Armonis A, Patch D. Bacterial infection is independently associated with failure to control bleeding in cirrhotic patients with gastrointestinal hemorrhage. Hepatology 1998;27:1207–12.

23. Blaise M, Pateron D, Trinchet JC, et al. Systemic antibiotic therapy prevents bacterial infection in cirrhotic patients with gastrointestinal hemorrhage. Hepatology 1994;20:34–8.

24. Wong F, Bernardi M, Balk R, et al. Sepsis in cirrhosis: report on the 7th meeting of the International Ascites Club. Gut 2005;54:718–25.

25. Hou MC, Lin HC, Liu TT, et al. Antibiotic prophylaxis after endoscopic therapy prevents rebleeding in acute variceal hemorrhage: a randomized trial. Hepatology 2004;39:746–53.

26. Rimola A, Bory F, Teres J, et al. Oral, nonabsorbable antibiotics prevent infection in cirrhotics with gastrointestinal hemorrhage. Hepatology 1985;5:463–7.

27. Fernandez J, Ruiz del Arbol L, Gomez C, et al. Norfloxacin vs. ceftriaxone in the prophylaxis of infections in patients with advanced cirrhosis and hemorrhage. Gastroenterology 2006;131:1049–56.

28. Soares-Weiser K, Brezis M, Tur-Kaspa R, et al. Antibiotic prophylaxis of bacterial infections in cirrhotic inpatients: a meta-analysis of randomized controlled trials. Scand J Gastroenterol 2003;38:193–200.

29. de Franchis R. Evolving consensus in portal hypertension. Report of the Baveno IV consensus workshop on methodology of diagnosis and therapy in portal hypertension. J Hepatol 2005;43:167–76.

30. Altraif I, Handoo FA, Aljumah A, et al. Effect of erythromycin before endoscopy in patients presenting with variceal bleeding: a prospective, randomized, double blind placebo-controlled trial. Gastrointest Endosc 2011;73:245–50.

31. Garcia-Pagan JC, Bosch J. Endoscopic band ligation in the treatment of portal hypertension. Nat Clin Pract Gastroenterol Hepatol 2005;2:526–35.

32. Lo GH, Lai KH, Cheng JS, et al. Emergency banding ligation versus sclerotherapy for the control of active bleeding from esophageal varices. Hepatology 1997;25:1101–4.

33. Vieira EC, D'Amico EA, Caldwell SH, et al. A prospective study of conventional and expanded coagulation indices in predicting ulcer bleeding after variceal band ligation. Clin Gastroenterol Hepatol 2009;7:988–93.

34. Shaheen NJ, Stuart E, Schmitz SM, et al. Pantoprazole reduces the size of post-banding ulcers after variceal band ligation: a randomized controlled trial. Hepatology 2005;41:588–94.

35. Banares R, Albillos A, Rincon D, et al. Endoscopic treatment versus endoscopic plus pharmacologic treatment for acute variceal bleeding: a meta-analysis. Hepatology 2002;35:609–15.

36. Amitrano L, Guardascione MA, Manguso F, et al. The effectiveness of current acute variceal bleed treatments in unselected cirrhotic patients: refining short-term prognosis and risk factors. Am J Gastroenterol 2012;107:1872–8.

37. Pitcher JL. Safety and effectiveness of the modified Sengstaken-Blakemore tube: a prospective study. Gastroenterology 1971;61:291–8.

38. Gossat D, Bolin TD. An unusual complication of balloon tamponade in the treatment of esophageal varices: a case report and brief review of the literature. Am J Gastroenterol 1985;80:600–1.

39. Jalan R, John TG, Redhead DN, et al. A comparative study of emergency transjugular intrahepatic portosystemic stent shunt and esophageal transection in the management of uncontrolled variceal hemorrhage. Am J Gastroenterol 1995;90:1932–7.

40. Vangeli M, Patch D, Burroughs AK. Salvage TIPS for uncontrolled variceal bleeding. J Hepatol 2003;37:703–4.

41. Chalasani N, Clark WS, Martin LG, et al. Determinants of mortality in patients with advanced cirrhosis after transjugular intrahepatic portosystemic shunting. Gastroenterology 2000;118:138–44.

42. Hubmann R, Bodlaj G, Czompo M, et al. The use of self-expanding metal stents to treat acute esophageal variceal bleeding. Endoscopy 2006;38:896–901.

43. Augustin S, Muntaner L, Altamirano JT. Predicting early mortality after acute variceal hemorrhage based on classification and regression tree analysis. Clin Gastroenterol Hepatol 2009;7:1347–54.

44. Azoulay D, Castaing D, Majno P, et al. Salvage transjugular intrahepatic portosystemic shunt for uncontrolled variceal bleeding in patients with decompensated cirrhosis. J Hepatol 2001;35:590–7.

45. Moitinho E, Escrosell A, Bandi JC, et al. Prognostic value of early measurements of portal pressure in acute variceal bleeding. Gastroenterology 1999;117:626–31.

46. Monescillo A, Martinez-Lagares F, Ruiz del Arbol L, et al. Influence of portal hypertension and its early decompression by TIPS placement on the outcome of variceal bleeding. Hepatology 2004;40:793–801.

47. Garcia-Pagan JC, Caca K, Bureau C, et al. Early use of TIPS in patients with cirrhosis and variceal bleeding. N Engl J Med 2010;362:2370–9.

48. Garcia-Pagan JC, Di Pascoli M, Caca K, et al. Use of early TIPS for high risk variceal bleeding: results of a post-RCT surveillance study. J Hepatol 2013;58:45–50.

49. Bureau C, Garcia Pagan JC, Layrargues GP, et al. Patency of stents covered with polytetrafluoroethylene in patients treated by transjugular intrahepatic portosystemic shunts: long-term results of a randomized multicenter study. Liver Int 2007;27:742–7.

Secondary Prophylaxis for Esophageal Variceal Bleeding

Agustín Albillos, MD, PhD[a],*, Marta Tejedor, MD[b]

KEYWORDS

- Secondary prophylaxis • Variceal rebleeding • β-blockers
- Endoscopic band ligation • Hemodynamic responders
- Transjugular intrahepatic portosystemic shunt (TIPS)

KEY POINTS

- A combination of drug treatment with β-blockers and endoscopic therapy with band ligation is the standard first-line option for secondary prophylaxis of variceal bleeding in cirrhosis. Transjugular intrahepatic portosystemic shunt is the recommended treatment when combination therapy fails.
- β-Blockers are the backbone of combination therapy, because their benefit goes beyond their portal-pressure-lowering effect and their efficacy extends to complications of portal hypertension other than bleeding. The added value of endoscopic band ligation is rather marginal.
- In the setting of rebleeding prevention, there is a lack of robust criteria to stratify patients according to their rebleeding risk, because some patients are likely to respond to β-blockers or endoscopic band ligation, whereas others present a high risk of rebleeding despite being on combination therapy.
- Hepatic venous pressure gradient monitoring can identify responders to β-blockers ("hemodynamic responders"), who have a very low rebleeding rate while treated only with β-blockers.
- Bleeders who could benefit more from a transjugular intrahepatic portosystemic shunt than from combination therapy include patients who first bleed while on β-blockers, those with contraindications to β-blockers or with refractory ascites, and patients with fundal varices.

Portal hypertension is responsible for one of the most severe consequences of cirrhosis, variceal bleeding. Patients with cirrhosis who survive an episode of variceal hemorrhage have a risk of rebleeding greater than 60% at 2 years[1]; this risk is higher

Supported in part by grants from the Spanish Ministry of Health, Instituto de Salud Carlos III (no. PS09/00485 and PI051871, Ciberehd) and Fundación Mutua Madrileña (AP100652012).
[a] Department of Gastroenterology and Hepatology, Hospital Universitario Ramón y Cajal, CIBERehd, IRYCIS, University of Alcalá, Ctra. Colmenar km. 9.100, Madrid 28034, Spain;
[b] Department of Gastroenterology and Hepatology, Hospital Universitario Ramón y Cajal, Ctra. Colmenar km 9.100, Madrid 28034, Spain
* Correspondence author.
E-mail address: aalbillosm@meditex.es

Clin Liver Dis 18 (2014) 359–370
http://dx.doi.org/10.1016/j.cld.2014.01.007
1089-3261/14/$ – see front matter © 2014 Elsevier Inc. All rights reserved.

liver.theclinics.com

during the first 6 weeks after the index bleeding. Because mortality related to each rebleeding episode is about 15% to 20%, interventions to prevent rebleeding are mandatory.

In this article, the currently recommended first-line treatment for the prevention of variceal rebleeding (secondary prophylaxis of variceal bleeding), combination of drugs (β-blockers) and endoscopic therapy (endoscopic band ligation, EBL) is critically revised. It is hypothesized that the efficacy of combination therapy mainly relies on β-blockers, whereas the additional benefit that EBL provides is rather marginal. Besides, a major limitation of current therapy is that it is uniformly recommended for the whole population of rebleeders, as robust clinical criteria are lacking to stratify patients according to their rebleeding risk while on combination therapy. A transjugular intrahepatic portosystemic shunt (TIPS), at present considered second-line treatment, could be a better choice to prevent rebleeding than standard therapy in those subgroups of patients at high risk of rebleeding if placed on combination therapy, or in those suffering from other complications of portal hypertension, such as recurrent or refractory ascites.

CURRENT RECOMMENDATIONS FOR THE PREVENTION OF ESOPHAGEAL VARICEAL REBLEEDING

> • *β-Blockers and EBL reduce to a similar extent the rate of variceal rebleeding, but β-blockers reduce overall mortality, whereas EBL does not.*

β-Blockers and EBL are the 2 first-line therapies currently used to prevent variceal rebleeding. Both have comparable efficacy in the prevention of variceal rebleeding and bleeding-related mortality, but β-blockers reduce overall mortality, whereas EBL does not. This contention is supported by the results of the meta-analysis of the 8 trials (970 patients) that compared β-blockers plus nitrates and EBL in the prevention of variceal rebleeding. This meta-analysis showed that both treatments were similarly able to reduce upper gastrointestinal bleeding (relative risk [RR] 1.15; 95% confidence interval [CI] 0.81–1.63) and variceal rebleeding (RR 1.23; 95% CI 0.74–2.06) as well as bleeding-related mortality (RR 0.75; 95% CI 0.37–1.50), but overall mortality was only lowered with β-blockers (RR 0.78; 95% CI 0.64–0.96).[2,3] Another meta-analysis by Li and colleagues[4] found similar results.

The beneficial effect of β-blockers goes beyond the reduction in the variceal bleeding risk and is probably related to an improvement of other complications of portal hypertension. Indeed, patients in whom β-blockers achieve target reductions in hepatic venous pressure gradient (HVPG) show reduced rates of rebleeding, but also of spontaneous bacterial peritonitis and liver-related mortality.[5,6] Therefore, the observed reduction in mortality but not in rebleeding supports a nonhemodynamic effect of β-blockers in cirrhosis, which is independent of the portal pressure response and likely linked to reductions in porto-collateral blood flow and bacterial translocation.[7] This hypothesis is also supported by a meta-analysis of randomized trials and observational studies,[8] which showed that β-blockers reduce the risk of spontaneous bacterial peritonitis by 12%, independently of the hemodynamic response.

> • *A combination of drug therapy, with β-blockers, and EBL is the recommended first-line therapy for the prevention of variceal rebleeding.*

A combination of drug and endoscopic therapy is the currently recommended first-line treatment for the prevention of variceal rebleeding.[9,10] Drug treatment implies the use of nonselective adrenergic β-blockers, such as propranolol or nadolol. In some studies, organic nitrates, such as isosorbide mononitrate, are also added. Band ligation is the endoscopic therapy of choice and has replaced injection sclerotherapy because it is safer and more effective. The rationale is that β-blockers reduce portal pressure by lowering portal blood flow, considering that increased portal pressure is the driving force that promotes variceal growth and rupture, whereas EBL acts locally, causing variceal obliteration.

The greater efficacy of a combination of drug (β-blockers ± nitrates) and endoscopic therapy over each treatment alone was demonstrated by a meta-analysis that included trials using either sclerotherapy or EBL. In such a study, Gonzalez and colleagues[11] analyzed 23 trials (1860 patients) and found that combination therapy led to lower overall rebleeding rates than either drug (RR 0.71; 95% CI, 0.59–0.86) or endoscopic (RR 0.68; 95% CI, 0.52–0.89) therapy alone. Variceal rebleeding rates were also lower in the combination therapy group. The beneficial impact of combination therapy on overall and variceal rebleeding did not translate into a reduction in mortality. Subgroup analysis concluded that the benefit of combination therapy was independent of the type of endoscopic therapy, sclerotherapy in 17 trials and EBL in 6 trials. More recently, a specific meta-analysis of 9 trials (955 patients) using EBL has also confirmed that the combination of EBL and drug treatment reduces the risk of overall and variceal rebleeding, but not overall mortality, when compared with β-blockers or EBL alone.[12]

> • *Prophylaxis of variceal rebleeding should start immediately after the acute bleeding episode.*

β-blockers for prophylaxis of esophageal variceal rebleeding should start immediately after the acute bleeding episode (ie, 5 days after the index bleed) once vasoconstrictor drugs have been stopped, when the risk of rebleeding is higher, and before discharge of the patient from hospital (**Fig. 1**). β-Blockers are expected to provide protection against rebleeding during the initial phase after the index hemorrhage, while varices are being obliterated by EBL.

Propanolol is started at a dose of 20 mg orally twice a day, and this dose is titrated every 3 days to the maximum tolerated by the patient or a heart rate of 50 to 55 bpm

Prophylaxis of variceal rebleeding

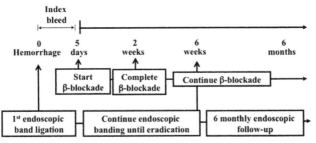

Fig. 1. For use in clinical practice of first-line therapy for the prevention of variceal rebleeding: combination of β-blockers and EBL.

(maximum dose 320 mg per day). Careful β-blocker dose titration by trained nurses results in higher maintenance doses of the drug and lower discontinuation rates than those observed in clinical trials (5% vs 15%).[13] Shortness of breath and fatigue are the most common side effects requiring drug discontinuation. In addition, up to 15% of the patients may have relative (eg, sinus bradycardia <55 bpm) or absolute (eg, heart failure, grade II heart block) contraindications to β-blockers.

The combination of β-blockers and nitrates (such as 5-isosorbide-mononitrate) has a synergistic portal pressure-reducing effect. However, in clinical trials such a combination is not different from β-blockers alone in terms of overall rebleeding or mortality and has a greater rate of side effects (38% vs 23%) and a higher discontinuation rate (15% vs 6%) than β-blockers alone.[14] It is for the latter 2 reasons that it is not routinely recommended.[9,10] If used, 5-isosorbide-mononitrate should always be combined with β-blockers at a maximal dose of 20 mg twice daily.

Banding sessions using multiband devices are repeated at 7- to 14-day intervals after the index bleeding until variceal obliteration, which usually requires 2 to 4 sessions. The first session of banding is usually performed at the diagnostic endoscopy during the bleeding episode, followed by a second one 7 to 14 days later. Once the varices have been eradicated, the first surveillance endoscopy should be done at 3 months and, if negative, repeated every 6 months to assess variceal recurrence and need for repeat banding. Complications of band ligation occur in about 14% of cases, the most common being transient dysphagia and chest discomfort. Postbanding ulcer bleeding rates are similar in the 3 trials comparing combination therapy with β-blockers alone and range from 5.0% to 6.6%.[15-17] Treatment with proton pump inhibitors after EBL reduces the sizes of postbanding ulcers, with a trend toward a lower bleeding risk.[18]

CRITICAL APPRAISAL OF CURRENT RECOMMENDATIONS TO PREVENT ESOPHAGEAL VARICEAL REBLEEDING

> • *β-Blockers are the backbone of the current standard first-line treatment for the prevention of variceal rebleeding, a combination of EBL and β-blockers.*

A closer analysis of the trials that compare a combination of β-blockers and EBL with either therapy alone shows that β-blockers are the mainstay component of treatment (**Fig. 2**). Up to now, the combination of β-blockers and EBL has been compared with β-blockers alone in 3 trials (389 patients)[15-17] and with EBL alone in 7 trials (603 patients).[17,19-24] Trials comparing combination therapy with β-blockers alone address the effect of adding EBL to β-blockers (ie, β-blockers act as a control group), whereas trials comparing combination therapy with EBL alone address the effect of adding β-blockers to EBL (ie, EBL act as a control group). Pooled analysis shows a statistically significant effect favoring combination therapy for reducing variceal rebleeding, both when EBL is added to β-blockers (35% with combination therapy vs 21% with β-blockers; risk difference [RD] −0.14, 95% CI −0.23 to −0.05) and when β-blockers are added to EBL (22% with combination therapy vs 14% with EBL; RD −0.09, 95% CI −0.15 to −0.03). Interestingly, overall rebleeding is significantly reduced when β-blockers are added to EBL (33% with combination therapy vs 19% with EBL; RD −0.14, 95% CI −0.27 to −0.02), but not when EBL is added to β-blockers (42% with combination therapy vs 32% with β-blockers; RD −0.10, 95% CI −0.21 to 0.01). The number needed to treat to prevent an episode of overall

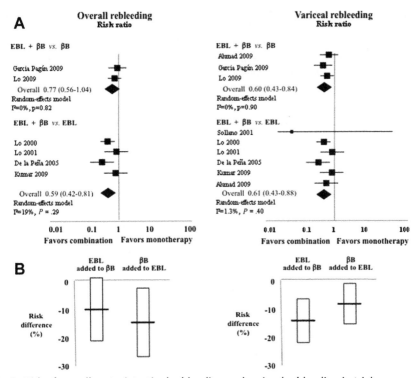

Fig. 2. Risk of overall gastrointestinal rebleeding and variceal rebleeding in trials comparing a combination of β-blockers (βB) and EBL with β-blockers or EBL alone. Meta-analysis of trials comparing combination therapy with β-blockers alone (ie, band ligation added to β-blockers) or with band ligation alone (ie, β-blockers added to band ligation). (A) Forrest plots of rebleeding events. The squares and the lines represent the relative risk for rebleeding events and mortality, and the 95% confidence interval, respectively. (B) Absolute risk differences. The horizontal lines represent the absolute risk difference and the squares represent the 95% confidence interval.

or variceal rebleeding when EBL is added to β-blockers is 10 (95% CI −21 to +2) and 7 (95% CI −23 to −5), respectively, whereas the number needed to treat when β-blockers are added to EBL is 7 (95% CI −27 to −2) and 12 (95% CI −16 to −2), for overall and variceal rebleeding, respectively. Mortality is unchanged and similar between both comparisons (RD 2.01, 95% CI −0.07 to 0.10, when EBL was added to β-blockers; RD −4.0, 95% CI −0.10 to 0.01, when β-blockers were added to EBL).

The above analysis may be limited by the small number of trials, because only 3 compared combination therapy with β-blockers alone. However, all 3 trials assessing the effect of adding EBL to β-blockers have been published in full, and 2 in high-quality journals.[15–17] Two of the 6 trials comparing combination therapy with EBL have been published in abstract form.[19,24]

Taken together, these data indicate that EBL seems more effective than β-blockers to prevent esophageal variceal rebleeding, but this benefit is offset by favoring upper gastrointestinal bleeding from other sources, such as postbanding ulcers, and its lack of impact on the natural history of portal hypertension. The combination of β-blockers and EBL should continue to be the standard of care for variceal rebleeding prevention, but clinicians should take into account that β-blockers are the mainstay component of such therapy.

STRATIFICATION OF PATIENTS ACCORDING TO THEIR RISK OF VARICEAL REBLEEDING

> • *There is a lack of robust criteria to stratify cirrhotic patients with a previous bleed by their risk of rebleeding and response to combination therapy.*

In the setting of rebleeding prevention, there is a lack of robust criteria to stratify patients according to their rebleeding risk, because some patients are likely to respond to β-blockers or EBL, whereas others present a high risk of rebleeding despite being on combination therapy. As a result, the standard of care is uniformly applied to all cirrhotic patients with a previous variceal bleed. Recognition of those criteria would allow therapy to be tailored to, for instance, identification of patients with a good response to β-blockers in whom EBL would be futile or patients unlikely to respond to combination therapy in whom TIPS could be a better choice. According to the knowledge so far, prior variceal bleeders can be stratified by hemodynamic or clinical criteria.

Stratification by Hemodynamic Criteria

> • *Hemodynamic responders to β-blockers are protected from future episodes of variceal rebleeding.*

The aim of therapy with β-blockers in cirrhosis is to achieve a target reduction in portal pressure, as estimated by hepatic vein catheterization and calculation of HVPG. Protection from bleeding in patients undergoing β-blocker treatment is related to the extent of portal pressure reduction. Patients achieving an HVPG reduction greater than 20% from baseline or a final value less than 12 mm Hg ("hemodynamic responders") have a much lower risk of rebleeding than patients not achieving these targets ("hemodynamic nonresponders").[5,6] β-Blockers achieve target reductions in HVPG in about half of the previous bleeders, and the variceal rebleeding rate at 2 years in these patients is 16%, whereas the rebleeding risk in nonresponders to β-blockers is 46%, much lower than the rate in untreated historical controls (55%–67%).[6] Interestingly, the percentage of patients on β-blockers not rebleeding is consistently higher than the hemodynamic response rate (median, 64% vs 51%, respectively).[7] Therefore, β-blockers seem to confer protection in patients with cirrhosis beyond HVPG reduction.

The effect on the rebleeding rate of adding EBL to these patient groups, classified according to the HVPG response to β-blockers, is a matter of debate. In the only multicenter randomized controlled trial in which rebleeding risk has been assessed among nonresponders to β-blockers, the probability of variceal rebleeding at 2 years was non-significantly lower in patients treated with combination therapy than in those treated only with β-blockers (20% vs 35%), whereas overall rebleeding was unchanged (32% vs 37%, respectively).[15] On the other hand, the addition of EBL to β-blockers reduced overall rebleeding in 2 series of nonresponders to β-blockers, in which the number of overall and variceal rebleeders was identical (**Fig. 3**).[25,26] The latter results should be considered with caution, because in these 2 studies the number of patients is small, they are single-center studies, and the coincidence of overall and variceal rebleeding could be explained by a low rate of postbanding ulcer bleeding. Therefore, it is controversial whether the addition of EBL reduces rebleeding

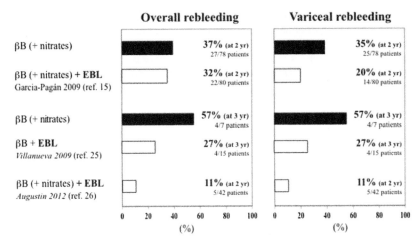

Fig. 3. Effect on overall gastrointestinal rebleeding and variceal rebleeding of adding EBL to β-blockers in hemodynamic nonresponders. The bars represent the rates of rebleeding in hemodynamic nonresponders treated only with β-blockers (βB) (*black bars*) or with a combination of β-blockers and EBL (*white bars*).

in hemodynamic nonresponders. At most, it could provide some benefit in variceal, but not in overall, rebleeding. Randomized controlled trials should address the best option to prevent rebleeding in nonresponders to β-blockers (ie, EBL addition or TIPS).

It should be highlighted that the rebleeding rate is very high in hemodynamic nonresponders switched from β-blockers to EBL or not receiving β-blockers at all (78% and 64% at 2 years, respectively),[27,28] a fact that further supports the nonhemodynamically mediated beneficial effect of β-blockade in cirrhosis. By contrast, the rebleeding rate in hemodynamic responders is 16% at 2 years,[6] and it is not further reduced by EBL addition.[15]

HVPG-guided therapy is probably the most rational approach to prevent variceal rebleeding. However, its applicability is limited because of the uncertainty about the most appropriate treatment in hemodynamic nonresponders, by the lack of evidence to suggest that tailoring therapy by HVPG response is superior to the current empiric treatment, and by the unavailability of routine hepatic vein catheterization in most centers.

Stratification by Clinical Criteria

> • Patients who bleed on primary prophylaxis with β-blockers have a high variceal rebleeding risk when placed on combination therapy.

Alternatively to the HVPG response, therapy to prevent rebleeding could be targeted to specific high-risk groups identified on clinical grounds. It is known that the worse the liver function, estimated by serum concentrations of albumin or bilirubin, and the lower the dose of β-blockers, the less likely it is that a patient will respond to these drugs.[26,29] However, this information lacks the ability to identify the individual response to β-blockers.

A subset of "nonresponders" that can be clinically identified comprises cirrhotic patients who first bleed from varices while on β-blockers ("clinical nonresponders").

In this situation, current guidelines recommend adding EBL to β-blockers.[9] However, information is meager, because these patients are excluded from most clinical trials. In fact, only 4% of the patients randomized in the trials that compare combination therapy with EBL or β-blockers alone had received primary prophylaxis with β-blockers before inclusion.[15–17,20–23] Moreover, a recent observational study has shown that the addition of EBL is particularly ineffective in this patient subset, with rates of overall and variceal rebleeding at 2 years as high as 48% and 39%, respectively, and a probability of transplant-free survival of 66%. The comparable results in the patients who presented their index episode of bleeding while not on primary prophylaxis with β-blockers were 24%, 17%, and 88%, respectively.[30] Therefore, patients who first bleed while on primary prophylaxis with β-blockers constitute a distinct high-risk subpopulation, with an especially poor response to combination therapy in terms of rebleeding risk and death.

Variceal rebleeding prophylaxis is commonly considered worthless in patients with hepatocellular carcinoma. Indeed, standard secondary prophylaxis with β-blockers and EBL is less frequently offered to these patients than to those without hepatocellular carcinoma, which leads to a greater probability of variceal rebleeding and death for the former group.[31] Interestingly, the use of secondary prophylaxis in patients with liver cancer had an independent protective effect on the risk of rebleeding and death, which highlights the relevance of using this treatment as long as the clinical condition of the patient allows it.

THE TIPS CHOICE

> • TIPS is highly effective in rebleeding prevention and is the second-line therapy for patients who fail combination treatment (β-blockers and EBL).

TIPS is very effective in preventing rebleeding, although it markedly increases the risk of hepatic encephalopathy and does not have any effect on survival, as shown in a meta-analysis of trials that compared TIPS with endoscopic treatment.[32,33] These results mirror those of the surgical trials for the prevention of variceal rebleeding. The only trial that compared TIPS with propranolol plus 5-isosorbide mononitrate to prevent rebleeding in patients with advanced cirrhosis (child B or C) showed that patients allocated to TIPS had lower rates of overall and variceal rebleeding and a lower rate of ascites, but greater rates of encephalopathy and identical survival.[34] Covered stents with lower occlusion and encephalopathy rates have largely replaced uncovered ones.[35]

Based on the above findings, TIPS is recommended as the second-line therapy for patients who have failed variceal rebleeding prevention with the combination of drug and endoscopic therapy.[9,10]

> • TIPS could be considered as the first-line therapy for rebleeding prevention in patients unlikely to respond to combination therapy or with other complications of portal hypertension.

Improvements in TIPS design make it a good first-line option for the prevention of rebleeding in those patients likely to fail standard combination therapy or who present complications of portal hypertension other than bleeding (**Table 1**):

• Patients presenting a variceal bleed while on primary prophylaxis with β-blockers ("clinical nonresponders").[30]

Table 1
Patients in whom TIPS should be considered as the first-line therapy to prevent esophageal variceal rebleeding instead of the combination of β-blockers and EBL

Patient Subgroup	Special Considerations
Variceal bleeding while on β-blockers for primary prophylaxis	Poor response to combination therapy[30]
Contraindication to β-blockers	Prophylaxis only relies on EBL Especial concern if bleeding occurs while on EBL for primary prophylaxis
Recurrent or refractory ascites	Concerns about the safety of β-blockers in refractory ascites[38] Worse response to β-blockers in advanced cirrhosis[26,29] TIPS also treats ascites[36,37]
Portal vein thrombosis	High risk of variceal rebleeding Concerns about the efficacy of β-blockers TIPS feasible in 75%–100%[39,40]
Fundal varices	Concerns about endoscopic therapy in esophageal varices with simultaneously large fundal varices

- Patients in whom β-blockers are contraindicated, especially if they bleed while on EBL for primary prophylaxis.
- Patients with recurrent or refractory ascites. TIPS eliminates the ascites in two-thirds of the patients with refractory ascites, with a trend toward improved survival.[36,37] Besides, in this population concern has recently been raised about the safety of β-blockers.[38]
- Patients with nontumoral portal vein thrombosis. Portal vein thrombosis, either occlusive or not, is found in about 15% of patients with cirrhosis and likely worsens the outcome of complications of portal hypertension. TIPS placement is feasible, safe, and effective in most of these patients, being especially valuable in those eligible for liver transplantation, because extension of the thrombosis might complicate surgery.[39,40]
- Patients with fundal varices. Patients bleeding from esophageal varices who simultaneously have large fundal varices constitute a difficult-to-treat population that can benefit from TIPS.

REFERENCES

1. D'Amico G. Esophageal varices: from appearance to rupture; natural history and prognostic indicators. In: Groszmann RJ, Bosch J, editors. Portal hypertension in the 21st century. Dordretch (The Netherlands): Kluwer Academic; 2004. p. 147–54.
2. Krag A, Wiest R, Gluud LL. Reduced mortality with non-selective β-blockers compared to banding is not related to prevention of bleeding or bleeding related mortality: systematic review of randomized trials. J Hepatol 2011;54:S72.
3. Krag A, Wiest R, Albillos A, et al. The window hypothesis: haemodynamic and non-haemodynamic effects of beta-blockers improve survival of patients with cirrhosis during a window in the disease. Gut 2012;61(7):967–9.
4. Li L, Yu C, Li Y. Endoscopic band ligation versus pharmacological therapy for variceal bleeding in cirrhosis: a meta-analysis. Can J Gastroenterol 2011;25(3):147–55.
5. D'Amico G, Garcia-Pagan JC, Luca A, et al. Hepatic vein pressure gradient reduction and prevention of variceal bleeding in cirrhosis: a systematic review. Gastroenterology 2006;131(5):1611–24.

6. Albillos A, Bañares R, González M, et al. Value of the hepatic venous pressure gradient to monitor drug therapy for portal hypertension: a meta-analysis. Am J Gastroenterol 2007;102(5):1116–26.

7. Thalheimer U, Bosch J, Burroughs AK. How to prevent varices from bleeding: shades of grey–the case for nonselective beta blockers. Gastroenterology 2007;133(6):2029–36.

8. Senzolo M, Cholongitas E, Burra P, et al. Beta-Blockers protect against spontaneous bacterial peritonitis in cirrhotic patients: a meta-analysis. Liver Int 2009; 29(8):1189–93.

9. Garcia-Tsao G, Sanyal AJ, Grace ND, et al, Practice Guidelines Committee of the American Association for the Study of Liver Diseases; Practice Parameters Committee of the American College of Gastroenterology. Prevention and management of gastroesophageal varices and variceal hemorrhage in cirrhosis. Hepatology 2007;46(3):922–38.

10. Garcia-Tsao G, Bosch J. Management of varices and variceal hemorrhage in cirrhosis. N Engl J Med 2011;362(9):823–32.

11. Gonzalez R, Zamora J, Gomez-Camarero J, et al. Meta-analysis: combination endoscopic and drug therapy to prevent variceal rebleeding in cirrhosis. Ann Intern Med 2008;149(2):109–22.

12. Thiele M, Krag A, Rohde U, et al. Meta-analysis: banding ligation and medical interventions for the prevention of rebleeding from oesophageal varices. Aliment Pharmacol Ther 2012;35(10):1155–65.

13. Tandon P, Saez R, Berzigotti A, et al. A specialized, nurse-run titration clinic: a feasible option for optimizing beta-blockade in non-clinical trial patients. Am J Gastroenterol 2010;105(9):1917–21.

14. Gluud LL, Langholz E, Krag A. Meta-analysis: isosorbide-mononitrate alone or with either beta-blockers or endoscopic therapy for the management of oesophageal varices. Aliment Pharmacol Ther 2010;32(7):859–71.

15. García-Pagán JC, Villanueva C, Albillos A, et al, Spanish Variceal Bleeding Study Group. Nadolol plus isosorbide mononitrate alone or associated with band ligation in the prevention of recurrent bleeding: a multicentre randomised controlled trial. Gut 2009;58(8):1144–50.

16. Lo GH, Chen WC, Chan HH, et al. A randomized, controlled trial of banding ligation plus drug therapy versus drug therapy alone in the prevention of esophageal variceal rebleeding. J Gastroenterol Hepatol 2009;24(6): 982–7.

17. Ahmad I, Khan AA, Alam A, et al. Propranolol, isosorbide mononitrate and endoscopic band ligation - alone or in varying combinations for the prevention of esophageal variceal rebleeding. J Coll Physicians Surg Pak 2009;19(5): 283–6.

18. Shaheen NJ, Stuart E, Schmitz SM, et al. Pantoprazole reduces the size of post-banding ulcers after variceal band ligation: a randomized, controlled trial. Hepatology 2005;41(3):588–94.

19. Sollano JD, Chan MM, Babaran RP, et al. Propranolol prevents rebleeding after variceal ligation. Gastrointest Endosc 2001;53:AB143.

20. Lo GH, Lai KH, Cheng JS, et al. The effects of endoscopic variceal ligation and propranolol on portal hypertensive gastropathy: a prospective, controlled trial. Gastrointest Endosc 2001;53(6):579–84.

21. Lo GH, Lai KH, Cheng JS, et al. Endoscopic variceal ligation plus nadolol and sucralfate compared with ligation alone for the prevention of variceal rebleeding: a prospective, randomized trial. Hepatology 2000;32(3):461–5.

22. Kumar A, Jha SK, Sharma P, et al. Addition of propranolol and isosorbide mononitrate to endoscopic variceal ligation does not reduce variceal rebleeding incidence. Gastroenterology 2009;137(3):892–901.

23. de la Peña J, Brullet E, Sanchez-Hernández E, et al. Variceal ligation plus nadolol compared with ligation for prophylaxis of variceal rebleeding: a multicenter trial. Hepatology 2005;41(3):572–8.

24. Abdel-Rahim AY, Abdel-Ghany MS, El-Kholy B. Band ligation alone versus band ligation and propranolol in the management of bleeding oesophageal varices. Am J Gastroenterol 2000;95:2442.

25. Villanueva C, Aracil C, Colomo A, et al. Clinical trial: a randomized controlled study on prevention of variceal rebleeding comparing nadolol + ligation vs. hepatic venous pressure gradient-guided pharmacological therapy. Aliment Pharmacol Ther 2009;29(4):397–408.

26. Augustin S, González A, Badia L, et al. Long-term follow-up of hemodynamic responders to pharmacological therapy after variceal bleeding. Hepatology 2012; 56(2):706–14.

27. Bureau C, Péron JM, Alric L, et al. "A La Carte" treatment of portal hypertension: adapting medical therapy to hemodynamic response for the prevention of bleeding. Hepatology 2002;36(6):1361–6.

28. Villanueva C, Miñana J, Ortiz J, et al. Endoscopic ligation compared with combined treatment with nadolol and isosorbide mononitrate to prevent recurrent variceal bleeding. N Engl J Med 2001;345(9):647–55.

29. Abraldes JG, Tarantino I, Turnes J, et al. Hemodynamic response to pharmacological treatment of portal hypertension and long-term prognosis of cirrhosis. Hepatology 2003;37(4):902–8.

30. de Souza AR, La Mura V, Reverter E, et al. Patients whose first episode of bleeding occurs while taking a β-blocker have high long-term risks of rebleeding and death. Clin Gastroenterol Hepatol 2012;10(6):670–6.

31. Ripoll C, Genescà J, Araujo IK, et al. Rebleeding prophylaxis improves outcomes in patients with hepatocellular carcinoma. A multicenter case-control study. Hepatology 2013;58(6):2079–88.

32. Papatheodoridis GV, Goulis J, Leandro G, et al. Transjugular intrahepatic portosystemic shunt compared with endoscopic treatment for prevention of variceal rebleeding: a meta-analysis. Hepatology 1999;30(3):612–22.

33. Khan S, Tudur Smith C, Williamson P, et al. Portosystemic shunts versus endoscopic therapy for variceal rebleeding in patients with cirrhosis. Cochrane Database Syst Rev 2006;(4):CD000553.

34. Escorsell A, Bañares R, García-Pagán JC, et al. TIPS versus drug therapy in preventing variceal rebleeding in advanced cirrhosis: a randomized controlled trial. Hepatology 2002;35(2):385–92.

35. Bureau C, Garcia-Pagan JC, Otal P, et al. Improved clinical outcome using polytetrafluoroethylene-coated stents for TIPS: results of a randomized study. Gastroenterology 2004;126(2):469–75.

36. Albillos A, Bañares R, González M, et al. A meta-analysis of transjugular intrahepatic portosystemic shunt versus paracentesis for refractory ascites. J Hepatol 2005;43(6):990–6.

37. Salerno F, Cammà C, Enea M, et al. Transjugular intrahepatic portosystemic shunt for refractory ascites: a meta-analysis of individual patient data. Gastroenterology 2007;133(3):825–34.

38. Sersté T, Melot C, Francoz C, et al. Deleterious effects of beta-blockers on survival in patients with cirrhosis and refractory ascites. Hepatology 2010;52(3):1017–22.

39. Luca A, Miraglia R, Caruso S, et al. Short- and long-term effects of the transjugular intrahepatic portosystemic shunt on portal vein thrombosis in patients with cirrhosis. Gut 2011;60(6):846–52.

40. Han G, Qi X, Guo W, et al. Transjugular intrahepatic portosystemic shunt for portal vein thrombosis in cirrhosis. Gut 2012;61(2):326–7.

nd Ectopic Varices

Dushant Uppal, MD[a], Wael Saad, MD[b],
MD[a],*

Gastric varices • Duodenal varices • Rectal varices • TIPS
thrombosis • Splenic vein thrombosis

heterogeneity underlying the formation of gastric and ectopic varices;
zation of treatment is difficult.

of gastric and ectopic variceal bleeding should include medical man-
otide or vasopressin analogues and may require temporizing mea-
endoscopically or via balloon tamponade.

gastric and ectopic variceal bleed should involve a combination of
diographic staging to determine the best treatment modality based
ause and vascular anatomy.

tion with cyanoacrylate injection, transjugular intrahepatic portosyste-
on-occluded retrograde transvenous obliteration are potential thera-
ectopic varices whether alone or in combination; but each of these
ique limitations, risks, benefits, and appropriate follow-up measures.

portal vein thrombosis should be considered in both noncirrhotic and
ce the bleeding risk has been controlled; but for isolated splenic vein
tomy, rather than anticoagulation, should be considered in symptom-

LOPMENT OF THE PORTAL VENOUS SYSTEM

enous structure of the portal-collateral pathways, it helps to un-
ologic development. **Fig. 1** shows the changes over time of the
nous system in the embryo and fetus. The portal venous system
vitelline and umbilical veins surrounding the liver bud with both
the sinus venosus. Extensive embryologic remodeling of these

o the portal system and simultaneous remodeling of the paired right and left
eins into the renal/adrenal/gonadal veins (subcardinal) and the azygous/
s veins (supracardinal) lead ultimately to the mature venous system. The
ent of these systems is important when approaching gastric varices (GV)

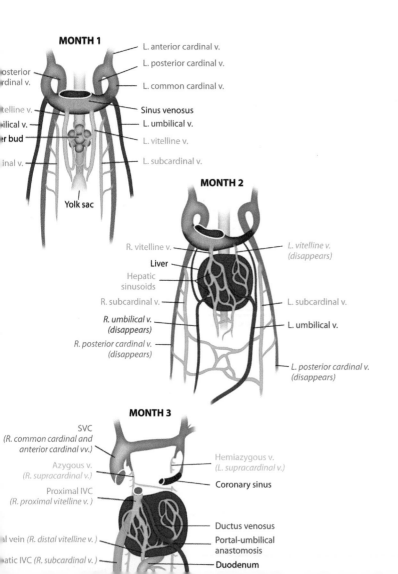

MONTH 1

L. anterior cardinal v.
L. posterior cardinal v.
L. common cardinal v.

osterior
rdinal v.

telline v.
ilical v.
r bud

inal v.

Sinus venosus
L. umbilical v.
L. vitelline v.
L. subcardinal v.

Yolk sac

MONTH 2

R. vitelline v.
Liver
Hepatic
sinusoids
R. subcardinal v.
R. umbilical v.
(disappears)
R. posterior cardinal v.
(disappears)

L. vitelline v.
(disappears)

L. subcardinal v.
L. umbilical v.

L. posterior cardinal v.
(disappears)

MONTH 3

SVC
(R. common cardinal and
anterior cardinal vv.)
Azygous v.
(R. supracardinal v.)
Proximal IVC
(R. proximal vitelline v.)

Hemiazygous v.
(L. supracardinal v.)
Coronary sinus

Ductus venosus
Portal-umbilical
anastomosis
Duodenum

al vein (R. distal vitelline v.)
atic IVC (R. subcardinal v.)

and ectopic varices (ECV) because the connections that arise are often related to their anatomic origins. For example, in patients with splenic vein thrombosis (SVT) and subsequent GV, the hypertensive short gastric veins in the fundus of the stomach, which originate from the vitelline veins, often communicate with the azygous vein, which originates from the supracardinal veins, through small portosystemic collaterals in the distal esophagus.[1] Understanding these anastomoses and the direction of these veins' afferent and efferent flow based on their anatomy can help guide therapeutic interventions, which the authors note in future sections of this review.[2]

GV IN CIRRHOSIS

In patients with cirrhosis and no underlying splanchnic vein thrombosis, studies have found the prevalence of GV to be 17% to 25% compared with a prevalence of esophageal varices (EV) of 50% to 60%.[3,4] GV bleed less frequently than EV but tend to be more severe.[4] Fundal varices tend to bleed more often than varices in the cardia or antrum.[4] The natural history of GV has rarely been reported; but in one study of 132 patients, the bleeding risk was estimated at 16%, 36%, and 44% at 1 year, 3 years, and 5 years, respectively. The presence of a red spot, a varix greater than 5 mm in size, and advanced Child-Pugh class were all found to be predictors of bleeding.[3] The absence of forward flow in the splenic vein has also recently been established as a predictor of GV bleeding, with a 5-year risk of 59% versus 39% when compared with those with forward flow.[5] This finding is consistent with a much earlier study that noted, in comparison with EV, GV are much more likely to have reversed or to-and-fro flow in the splenic vein.[6]

The management of GV in patients with cirrhosis depends greatly on how they are classified because this can provide a guide for the prognosis and treatment approach. The most common system used is the Sarin classification (**Fig. 2**).[4] Using this classification system helped identify gastric fundal varices as higher-risk lesions for bleeding and has guided other studies in evaluating responses to different therapies. For instance, sclerotherapy for GV has not had the same success that it had in the treatment of EV, except in subsets of patients with gastroesophageal varices (GOV) 1. Physiologically, this makes sense because, as the Sarin classification has shown, GOV1 GV are located near the gastroesophageal junction and are often fed from the same venous source as EV. However, with fundal varices, GOV2 and IGV 1, the Sarin classification does not truly describe the underlying vascular heterogeneity,

◄───

Fig. 1. The embryologic development of the portal venous and systemic venous circulation of the abdomen. In gold are the vitelline veins that merge over time to form the intrahepatic portal and hepatic veins as well as the superior portion of the intrahepatic inferior vena cava (IVC). These veins also form the main portal vein and go on to form the splenic and mesenteric veins. In red are the umbilical veins. Over time, the right umbilical vein atrophies and the left umbilical vein maintains a connection to the left portal venous system and forms the ductus venosus with the vitelline veins; the ductus venosus becomes the ligamentum venosum and the umbilical vein atrophies after birth. This vestigial link explains the presence of a recanalized umbilical vein in portal hypertension. Colored teal blue are the paired subcardinal veins, which merge over time to form the abdominal IVC and bilateral renal, adrenal, and gonadal veins. In green are the azygous and hemiazygos veins, which are derived from the supracardinal veins and run inferiorly into the abdomen where the hemiazygos connects into the left adrenal vein. These vestigial connections should atrophy over time but are likely the source of small portosystemic collaterals in portal hypertension[1] and likely play a role in gastrorenal shunt formation.[2] SVC, superior vena cava.

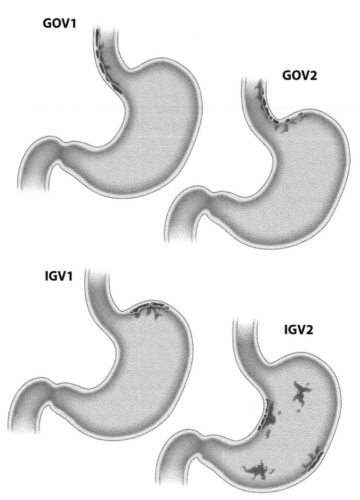

Fig. 2. The Sarin endoscopic classification for GV.[4] GOV, gastroesophageal varices; IGV, isolated GV.

which has made it difficult to use this system alone to standardize an approach to treatment and highlights the need for a better understanding of the vascular anatomy.

Clinical investigators in the 1980s and 1990s, especially in Japan, can be credited with bringing a new appreciation of the architecture of the venous collateral bed underlying cardiofundal varices; these typically involve collaterals arising from the short gastric veins and the posterior gastric veins leading to an outflow trunk that ends in the left renal vein.[6] This study also highlights the difference between a right-sided portal circulation and a left-sided portal circulation in relation to GV. Proposed vascular classifications are based on the afferent veins feeding the varices combined with the venous outflow tract, whether it is through a direct shunt or multiple small collaterals (**Figs. 3** and **4**).[7,8] The vascular classifications can be used in conjunction with the endoscopic classification to determine the best therapy.

The management strategies for bleeding GV have varied over the years but are generally categorized into either endoscopic or radiologic approaches. Appropriate

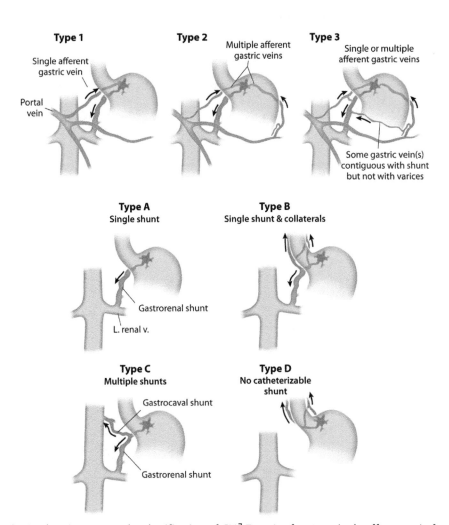

Fig. 3. The Kiyosue vascular classification of GV.[7] Type 1 refers to a single afferent vein for either the right or left portal circulation; type 2 refers to multiple afferent vessels contributing to the varix; type 3 is consistent with type 2 with the addition of small afferent vessels in direct continuity with the outflow track. Type A consists of a gastrorenal shunt (GRS) as the sole outflow; type B describes the presence of a GRS in conjunction with small peridiaphragmatic portosystemic collaterals; type C describes the presence of both a GRS and direct gastro-caval shunt; type D consists of small portosystemic collaterals as the sole outflow track. Types 1, 2, and 3 can be combined with types A, B, C, and D to describe the inflow and outflow of a GV.

medical management of acute GV bleeding is unclear because there are no trials specifically evaluating the use of octreotide or vasopressin analogues; however, the diversion of splanchnic blood flow should decrease bleeding similar to the effect seen in acute esophageal variceal bleeding and should be considered in this population. Balloon tamponade is likely a more effective method to stop bleeding in the acute setting; however, this usually must be followed up by more definitive endoscopic or vascular therapy.

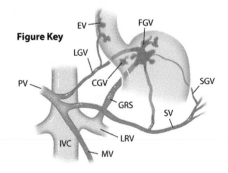

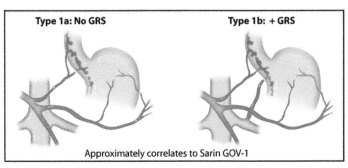

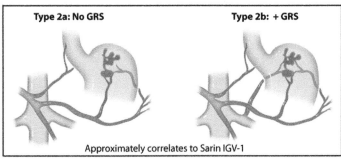

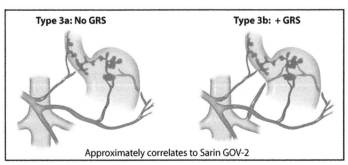

Fig. 4. Saad-Caldwell vascular classification of GV.[8] Type 1a with left-sided (left gastric vein) afferent flow into GV and no gastrorenal shunt (GRS), outflow through small portosystemic collaterals, type 1b with left-sided afferent flow and dominant GRS as outflow; type 2a with right-sided (short gastric vein) afferent flow into GV and outflow through small portosystemic collaterals, type 2b with right-sided afferent flow and dominant GRS as outflow; type 3a with mixed (left and right) afferent flow and outflow through small portosystemic collaterals, type 3b with mixed afferent flow and dominant GRS as outflow. This classification includes a type 4a and 4b, which are the same as 3a and 3b but with the inclusion of portal vein thrombosis. CGV, cardial GV; FGV, fundal GV; IVC, inferior vena cava; LGV, left gastric vein; LRV, left renal vein; MV, mesenteric vein (superior mesenteric vein); PV, portal vein; SGV, short gastric vein; SV, splenic vein.

Endoscopic Treatment of GV

Endoscopic therapies have focused mainly on injection therapy with cyanoacrylate glues, but variceal band ligation has also been evaluated. Cyanoacrylate injection has excellent rates of acute hemostasis, greater than 90%,[9–14] but has variable rates of rebleeding, with an average rate of around 20% within 1 year.[9,10,13,15] When compared directly with band ligation, cyanoacrylate injection is superior at both initial hemostasis as well as long-term rebleeding. In one study, initial hemostasis was 87% with cyanoacrylate versus 45% with band ligation, with rebleeding rates of 31% versus 54%, respectively.[11] A more recent study comparing the two did not show a difference in acute hemostasis (both achieved 93%); however, rebleeding with cyanoacrylate was 23.0% at 1 year compared with 33.5% with the band ligation group.[9] This study also showed a much higher rate of recurrence of GV with band ligation versus cyanoacrylate, 60% versus 23%, respectively. One of the concerns with cyanoacrylate injection is the risk of embolization of the glue thrombus. The risk of severe and potentially fatal embolization with the most commonly used 4-carbon N-butyl-2-cyanoacrylate is estimated to be 0% to 2%.[9,10,13,15] In one of the largest series, the risk of thrombotic complication was only 0.7%; these all occurred in a technique using large volumes of lipiodol, which delays polymerization.[16] The authors' own data comparing the ex vivo polymerization times of various cyanoacrylate mixtures have shown a roughly 2-fold increase in the polymerization time by adding the iodinated plant oil ethiodized oil (Ethiodol) (identical to lipiodol) to N-butyl-2-cyanoacrylate. These results suggest that the use of iodinated contrast oils, although probably decreasing the risk of needle impaction, increases the risk of embolization.[17]

TIPS Treatment of GV

Transjugular intrahepatic portosystemic shunt (TIPS) has been evaluated in the treatment of GV. In comparison with EV, large GV often have lower portal pressures and lower portosystemic gradients before TIPS placement.[6,18] In a study from 1997, results of TIPS procedures in patients with EV and/or GV were compared revealing that EV had a notable reduction in size after TIPS, as would be expected; but 50% of GV did not change in size despite achieving a portosystemic gradient less than 12 mm Hg.[19] These findings were again noted in a study from 2007 comparing cyanoacrylate injection with TIPS for the treatment of GV. Despite a slightly lower rebleeding rate in the TIPS group when follow-up endoscopy was performed, those that underwent glue injection had a much lower rate of persistent GV compared with the TIPS group, 20% versus 57%, respectively.[14] This phenomenon is likely caused by the presence of spontaneous shunts, such as gastrorenal and splenorenal shunts.[6]

In a study from 2003, TIPS had a lower 30-day rate of rebleeding when compared with cyanoacrylate injection, 15% versus 30%, respectively. But there was no mortality difference between the groups, and the cost analysis at 6 months revealed a significant benefit of glue injection over TIPS.[20] In the authors' own data, they found a lower 1-year rebleeding rate in the cyanoacrylate group compared with the TIPS group, 10% and 25% respectively, and also showed no mortality difference.[21] The authors did, however, show an increased morbidity with TIPS caused by hepatic encephalopathy. In an earlier study with this same population, the authors also found a cost benefit to cyanoacrylate treatment when compared with noncyanoacrylate therapy.[22] Although TIPS remains a common and widely accepted means of managing GV bleeding, its application remains problematic in many patients; it is sometimes ineffective.[18,23] This ineffectiveness is especially so in patients with far-left shunts, in whom transhepatic occlusion of the shunt, usually performed by delivering a coil through the TIPS, may be challenging. In addition, TIPS may be less effective in patients with a low transhepatic pressure gradient because of effective decompression through the spontaneous gastrorenal shunt and possibly detrimental in those with marginal hepatic reserve.[18,19,24]

Balloon-Occluded Retrograde Transvenous Obliteration Treatment of GV

Balloon-occluded retrograde transvenous obliteration (BRTO) is a more direct vascular intervention for GV. Access to cardiofundal varices is usually achieved via the femoral vein to the left renal vein and then to the varix outflow tract. The applicability of this procedure depends on the presence and size of the outflow track.[6,25,26]

Success rates for BRTO, as confirmed by endoscopy, have ranged from 75% in earlier studies to 97% more recently.[12,25–27] In one study comparing BRTO with endoscopic cyanoacrylate, the GV obliteration rates were 77% and 43%, respectively.[12] In studies evaluating the success of BRTO alone, the GV rebled rates were 3.2% to 8.7% after successful procedures and 10% to 20% in an intent-to-treat analysis (included failures).[25,28,29] When compared with TIPS, BRTO had a 1-year rebleeding rate of 2% versus 20% in the TIPS group and an improved 1-year survival of 96% versus 81% with TIPS. Encephalopathy was 19% in the TIPS group and 0% in the BRTO group.[30] In contrast to TIPS, which is known to divert blood flow from hepatic parenchyma and may worsen liver function in some patients,[31,32] successful BRTO can augment perfusion of the hepatic parenchyma and may enhance indices of hepatic function, including the Model for End-Stage Liver Disease (MELD) score.[33–35] On the other hand, increasing portal pressure can cause significant aggravation of common problems, including ascites, hepatic hydrothorax, gall bladder edema, intestinal wall edema, and EV.[36,37] In some cases, these problems may require subsequent TIPS placement.[38] Other technical risks include extension of thrombus retrograde into the portal system.[39]

Medical Prophylaxis for GV

Prophylactic therapy for GV has not been evaluated extensively; however, Mishra and colleagues[40] compared cyanoacrylate glue injection with beta-blocker therapy for both primary and secondary prophylaxis of GV bleeding. For secondary prophylaxis, repeat glue injection until obliteration of varices had a much lower rebleeding rate compared with standard beta-blockade therapy titrated to pulse, 15% versus 55%, respectively. As expected, the beta-blocker group had a better reduction in portal pressures; however, this did not affect the results. Also, beta-blockade had a much higher mortality compared with the glue injection group, 25% versus 3%, respectively. In a study comparing glue injection, beta blockade, and no therapy for primary prophylaxis of first GV bleed, the 2-year bleeding rates were 13%, 28%, and 45%, respectively, suggesting that glue injection is superior to beta-blockade, again despite large decreases in portal pressure with beta-blocker therapy.[41]

DUODENAL VARICES

ECV are the cause for bleeding in 1% to 5% of patients with intrahepatic portal hypertension and in 20% to 30% of those with extrahepatic portal hypertension and make up 2% to 5% of all variceal bleeding.[42,43] Duodenal varices (DV) make up 17% of all ECV bleeding.[42] They have a prevalence of 0.2% to 0.4% in all patients undergoing upper endoscopy.[44,45] Because it is rare, there are no controlled trials evaluating DV; however, as with GV, there are varying anatomic considerations to DV. In the largest series of patients with DV, 3 of 14 patients had acute bleeding and underwent endoscopic injection of cyanoacrylate along with one other patient with a red spot on a duodenal varix. All 3 acutely bleeding patients achieved initial hemostasis, and there were no rebleeds among all 4.[46] Two other case reports reveal success with cyanoacrylate injection with no rebleeding out to 1 year, and another investigator reports success in a single case with thrombin injection.[47–49] Most DV have an afferent venous supply from either the portal vein or the superior mesenteric vein with an outflow track directly into the inferior vena cava, making TIPS and BRTO possible.[44,50] In one case of failed endoscopic management, rescue BRTO was performed for DV bleeding with complete obliteration of the varix after 3 months of follow-up and no rebleeding.[51] Another series of 5 patients who underwent BRTO for DV reported 100% technical success and no rebleeding out to 1 year.[50] TIPS has also been successful in one case report of DV in the setting of cirrhosis as a bridge to transplant.[52] Other reports on the general use of TIPS for all kinds of ECV bleeding have shown modest results in the patients with DV.[53] Because of the lack of randomized trials, an exact recommendation for the treatment of DV cannot be made; but the evidence noted here suggests that, similar to GV, there are many viable modalities with similar rates of success.

COLORECTAL VARICES

Rectal varices (RV) are the most prevalent of the ECV, with rates reported as high as 77% of all ECV. Their prevalence in patients with cirrhosis is between 28% and 56%, whereas their prevalence in extrahepatic portal vein obstruction is 63% to 94%.[54–56] Bleeding from RV is rare but can be massive and fatal.[57,58] Most of the data on management are related to TIPS placement in these patients; however, there are a few case reports and case series on endoscopic therapies, BRTO, and even surgical management. Endoscopically there are case reports of cyanoacrylate use as well as band ligation. In contrast to GV, band ligation shows superior results with excellent initial hemostasis and low rebleeding rates compared with glue injection.[58–60] There have been case reports of standard BRTO therapy as well as a transumbilical approach to a BRTO procedure; in both cases, the RV were completely obliterated and there was no rebleeding.[61,62] There have been many retrospective studies evaluating TIPS results in these patients; although initial hemostasis results are quite good, there are rebleeding rates from 10% to 20% despite adequately reduced portal pressure.[53,63–65] This finding is similar to the findings in some patients with GV after TIPS and suggests that, because of the complex vascular outflow pathways seen in these varices, TIPS alone may not be effective. In some cases, BRTO or TIPS with direct embolization of the varix may be necessary.

GV AND ECV IN PORTAL VEIN THROMBOSIS

A discussion of GV and ECV would be incomplete without also addressing the sometimes-important role of portal vein thrombosis (PVT) whether in cirrhotic or noncirrhotic patients.

Cirrhotic PVT and GV/ECV Bleeding

Cirrhotic patients with PVT and variceal bleeding have a much worse prognosis.[66–69] In addition, PVT is much more prevalent in cirrhotic patients when compared with the general population, with an average prevalence around 10% and a range between 2.1% and 23.0%.[70] There are only a few studies that remark on the incidence of PVT, one with a cumulative incidence of 7.4% and another with an annual incidence of 16%.[71,72] The rates of variceal bleeding in cirrhotic patients with PVT range from about 39% to 50% at presentation; however, most of these bleeds are secondary to EV.[73] There are very little data regarding gastric variceal bleeding or ectopic variceal bleeding in cirrhotic patients with PVT; of the data available, there are only case reports or very small case series.

A case report of DV and GV in a patient with cirrhosis and PVT noted hemostasis without rebleeding out to 1 year after endoscopic injection of Histoacryl.[47] TIPS (usually along with postprocedure anticoagulation) is also a viable option in these patients, even with occlusive PVT provided intrahepatic portal branches can be visualized.[74] This approach has the advantage of offering variceal decompression but carries technical challenges and an increased risk of hepatic decompensation with higher MELD scores.[19] There are a few prospective trials that have evaluated the use of anticoagulation in PVT related to cirrhosis and have noted very few bleeding events.[71,74,75] In one of these studies, there was a significantly higher rate of recanalization in patients on anticoagulation; variceal bleeding was worse in patients that did not receive anticoagulation compared with those that did.[74] Certainly, long-term anticoagulation needs to be considered in this population, especially in patients with an underlying thrombophilia.

Noncirrhotic PVT and GV/ECV Bleeding

Although cirrhosis-related portal hypertension may be the most common cause of GV and ECV, PVT and SVT are also known to cause both GV and ECV. Noncirrhotic PVT is the second leading cause of portal hypertension in the Western world, with a prevalence of 5% to 10% in patients with portal hypertension.[76] Within this group of patients, EV are most prevalent at about 78% to 90% in all cases of noncirrhotic PVT, with GV having a reported prevalence from 14% to 50%.[68,77–79] ECV have been reported in 27% to 40% of cases of splanchnic vein thrombosis (PVT alone or with SVT or mesenteric vein thrombosis) and have been noted to be much more common than in cirrhosis.[55,77]

In a study examining 60 patients with splanchnic vein thrombosis, 54 of which had chronic noncirrhotic portal-mesenteric vein thrombosis, Orr and colleagues[78] noted that 91% had EV on initial endoscopy and 50% had GV. Of those 60 patients, 50% presented with gastrointestinal bleeding. Of all bleeding events, the sentinel bleeding episodes were from EV alone; but the secondary bleeding episodes were more commonly GV and ECV, with bleeding rates of 26% and 33%, respectively. Fatal hemorrhage was more often from GV and ECV, suggesting that, although less prevalent, GV and ECV bleeding is more severe. A second study, by Spaander and colleagues,[80] revealed similar results. They found that gastric fundal varices were associated with an increased risk of rebleeding by a factor of 5 (hazard ratio 5.07). Despite rebleeding risks, the overall mortality for these patients is still more closely related to the underlying cause of the PVT.[69,81]

Anticoagulation in the setting of PVT remains a challenging aspect of treatment. Hypercoagulable risks and myeloproliferative disorders (MPD) should be assessed. The prevalence of an inherent clotting disorder, such as factor V Leiden, prothrombin mutation, protein C or S deficiency, or MPD, in these patients is 50% to 60% and can alter long-term management in regard to anticoagulation.[68,82–85] Currently, the Baveno V criteria, and other studies, recommend treating acute PVT for at least 3 to 6 months; however, if there is an underlying coagulopathy or MPD, then lifelong therapy needs to be considered.[86,87] In contrast, the data for anticoagulation in chronic PVT, with cavernoma formation, are less persuasive but still suggest that, in the setting of a hypercoagulable state, lifelong anticoagulation should be considered. The risk of bleeding while on anticoagulation is low, and some series showed that bleeding is less common with anticoagulation than without, likely because of decreased portal pressures secondary to recanalization.[78,88] Amitrano and colleagues[68] evaluated 121 patients with PVT or mesenteric vein thrombosis noting all follow-up bleeding events occurred in the patients that were not on anticoagulation. Despite this low risk of bleeding from varices in this population, experts recommend screening for varices early after diagnosis, performing follow-up endoscopy 6 months later, and then annually from there on, treating the varices as you would in cirrhotic patients.[86,89] Although recanalization decreases the risk of bleeding, not all patients achieve recanalization. In separate studies by Hall and Condat,[88,90] there were recanalization rates of 82% and 90%, respectively.[88,90] However, in most studies, the rates of recanalization on anticoagulation are in the range of 30% to 50%.[87,91] The rates of spontaneous recanalization without anticoagulation range from 0% to 32% in these studies.[86–90] Overall, the mortality risk in these patients is related to the thrombosis itself and/or the underlying disorder causing the thrombosis and not from bleeding risk, suggesting that anticoagulation is beneficial and should be considered in all patients, especially those with an underlying thrombophilic disorder.[69,92]

Noncirrhotic SVT and GV/ECV Bleeding

SVT must also be considered separate from PVT and cirrhosis because the underlying cause is much different. The most common causes of isolated SVT are chronic pancreatitis, acute pancreatitis, pancreatic pseudocyst, and neoplasm, with pancreatitis the most frequent cause.[1,93–97] The overall incidence of SVT ranges from 13% to 45%, with most of these studies evaluating populations of patients with pancreatitis. It is estimated that 60% of cases of SVT are caused by pancreatitis.[94,97–99] The incidence of GV in SVT ranges from 15% to almost 57%, with higher rates in studies that looked specifically at acute and chronic pancreatitis.[1,93,94,98,99] The presenting symptom in patients with SVT is gastrointestinal bleeding in 45% to 72% of cases.[97] Heider and colleagues[93] looked at a large group of patients with pancreatitis over a 10-year period and noted 53 that had SVT. Of these 53 patients, they initially reported that 41 of them were noted to have GV, a prevalence of almost 80%; however, most of these were noted on computed tomography findings. On further analysis, only 36 of these 53 patients underwent esophagogastroduodenoscopy (EGD); of those patients, only 11 had endoscopically notable GV, or about 30%. Another study by Agarwal and colleagues[98] evaluated the incidence and management of SVT in patients with chronic pancreatitis. There was an incidence of SVT of 22% and, within that group, an incidence of all varices of 41%. Of those with GV, 43% experienced a bleeding event.

The definitive treatment of GV bleeding in the setting of SVT is splenectomy; however, performing splenectomy in all patients with SVT is a contentious subject.[93,96,98] Heider and colleagues[93] found that, in their patients with SVT, the overall bleeding risk was only 4%; however, the patients that bled were all patients with GV on EGD. Additionally, Agarwal and colleagues[98] noted a bleeding rate from varices (EV vs GV not specified) of approximately 10% and also noted that, in patients who underwent splenectomy, there was no GV bleeding out to 2 years compared with a 14% GV bleeding rate in those who did not. This finding suggests that splenectomy may prevent GV bleeding.

SUMMARY

In conclusion, GV and ECV have several underlying causes and, therefore, cannot be treated with any one particular intervention. Acute management of both GV and ECV should focus on the stabilization of patients while concurrently attempting to define the underlying cause so that therapy can be tailored to the individual. More randomized controlled trials are needed in the future to better define the subsets of populations that may benefit from one intervention as compared with another. For patients with GV secondary to cirrhosis, the authors recommend the approach shown in (**Fig. 5**). This approach outlines the need for flexibility in treatment options depending on each patient's unique vascular anatomy. A similar algorithm should be used for ectopic variceal bleeding, with an initial focus on stabilization and optimization of coagulation parameters followed by endoscopic assessment and assessment of

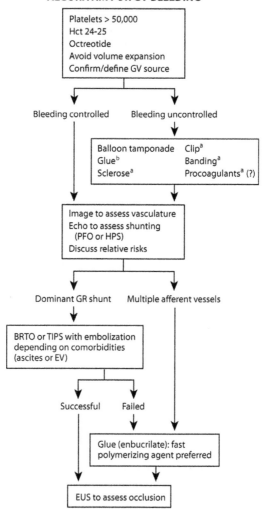

ALGORITHM FOR GV BLEEDING

Platelets > 50,000
Hct 24-25
Octreotide
Avoid volume expansion
Confirm/define GV source

Bleeding controlled   Bleeding uncontrolled

Balloon tamponade   Clip[a]
Glue[b]   Banding[a]
Sclerose[a]   Procoagulants[a] (?)

Image to assess vasculature
Echo to assess shunting
(PFO or HPS)
Discuss relative risks

Dominant GR shunt   Multiple afferent vessels

BRTO or TIPS with embolization
depending on comorbidities
(ascites or EV)

Successful   Failed

Glue (enbucrilate): fast
polymerizing agent preferred

EUS to assess occlusion

Fig. 5. Algorithm for management of gastric variceal bleeding. Enbucrilate (N-2-butyl-cyanoacrylate), procoagulants (recombinant factor VII, aminocaproic acid). Management of ectopic variceal bleeding should follow the same algorithm with the exception that endoscopic management is different depending on varix location. [a] Temporizing measures only. [b] Cyanoacrylate glue injection may not be available at all institutions, and a risk-benefit discussion should be held with patients regarding embolic risk without knowing the underlying vascular anatomy. EUS, endoscopic ultrasound; GR, gastrorenal; Hct, hematocrit; HPS, hepatopulmonary syndrome; PFO, patent foramen ovale.

vascular anatomy. The treatment will vary based on the underlying vascular anatomy and location of the ectopic varices (rectal, duodenal).

In patients whose presenting symptom of SVT is gastric variceal bleeding, then splenectomy, after stabilization, should be the therapy of choice because it can relieve active bleeding and will prevent further bleeding.[95,97–99] In patients with SVT who simply have GV but have not experienced bleeding, the authors would recommend a more measured approach with regular screening endoscopies. If GV seem to be increasing in size or begin showing high-risk marks, then prophylactic splenectomy should be considered.

For all patients with PVT, whether cirrhotic or noncirrhotic, a hypercoagulable workup should be performed. In acute PVT, anticoagulation should be strongly considered for 3 to 6 months with the goal of recanalization of the portal vein once bleeding has been controlled. Patients with acute GV or ECV bleeding should be treated endoscopically before anticoagulation and should undergo variceal surveillance on a regular basis. TIPS after mechanical thrombectomy may be beneficial in some patients; however, long-term anticoagulation may still be needed because of underlying thrombophilia.

REFERENCES

1. Evans GR, Yellin AE, Weaver FA, et al. Sinistral (left-sided) portal hypertension. Am Surg 1990;56(12):758–63.
2. Patten BM, Carlson BM. Patten's foundations of embryology. 6th edition. New York: McGraw-Hill; 1996. p. 752, xii.
3. Kim T, Shijo H, Kokawa H, et al. Risk factors for hemorrhage from gastric fundal varices. Hepatology 1997;25(2):307–12.
4. Sarin SK, Lahoti D, Saxena SP, et al. Prevalence, classification and natural history of gastric varices: a long-term follow-up study in 568 portal hypertension patients. Hepatology 1992;16(6):1343–9.
5. Maruyama H, Ishihara T, Ishii H, et al. Blood flow parameters in the short gastric vein and splenic vein on Doppler ultrasound reflect gastric variceal bleeding. Eur J Radiol 2010;75(1):e41–5.
6. Watanabe K, Kimura K, Matsutani S, et al. Portal hemodynamics in patients with gastric varices. A study in 230 patients with esophageal and/or gastric varices using portal vein catheterization. Gastroenterology 1988;95(2):434–40.
7. Kiyosue H, Mori H, Matsumoto S, et al. Transcatheter obliteration of gastric varices. Part 1. Anatomic classification. Radiographics 2003;23(4):911–20.
8. Saad WE. Vascular anatomy and the morphologic and hemodynamic classifications of gastric varices and spontaneous portosystemic shunts relevant to the BRTO procedure. Tech Vasc Interv Radiol 2013;16(2):60–100.
9. Tan PC, Hou MC, Lin HC, et al. A randomized trial of endoscopic treatment of acute gastric variceal hemorrhage: N-butyl-2-cyanoacrylate injection versus band ligation. Hepatology 2006;43(4):690–7.
10. Rajoriya N, Forrest EH, Gray J, et al. Long-term follow-up of endoscopic Histoacryl glue injection for the management of gastric variceal bleeding. QJM 2011; 104(1):41–7.
11. Lo GH, Lai KH, Cheng JS, et al. A prospective, randomized trial of butyl cyanoacrylate injection versus band ligation in the management of bleeding gastric varices. Hepatology 2001;33(5):1060–4.
12. Hong CH, Kim HJ, Park JH, et al. Treatment of patients with gastric variceal hemorrhage: endoscopic N-butyl-2-cyanoacrylate injection versus

balloon-occluded retrograde transvenous obliteration. J Gastroenterol Hepatol 2009;24(3):372–8.

13. Caldwell SH, Hespenheide EE, Greenwald BD, et al. Enbucrilate for gastric varices: extended experience in 92 patients. Aliment Pharmacol Ther 2007;26(1): 49–59.

14. Lo GH, Liang HL, Chen WC, et al. A prospective, randomized controlled trial of transjugular intrahepatic portosystemic shunt versus cyanoacrylate injection in the prevention of gastric variceal rebleeding. Endoscopy 2007;39(8): 679–85.

15. Kang EJ, Jeong SW, Jang JY, et al. Long-term result of endoscopic Histoacryl (N-butyl-2-cyanoacrylate) injection for treatment of gastric varices. World J Gastroenterol 2011;17(11):1494–500.

16. Cheng LF, Wang ZQ, Li CZ, et al. Low incidence of complications from endoscopic gastric variceal obturation with butyl cyanoacrylate. Clin Gastroenterol Hepatol 2010;8(9):760–6.

17. Caldwell S. Gastric varices: is there a role for endoscopic cyanoacrylates, or are we entering the BRTO era? Am J Gastroenterol 2012;107(12):1784–90.

18. Tripathi D, Therapondos G, Jackson E, et al. The role of the transjugular intrahepatic portosystemic stent shunt (TIPSS) in the management of bleeding gastric varices: clinical and haemodynamic correlations. Gut 2002;51(2):270–4.

19. Sanyal AJ, Freedman AM, Luketic VA, et al. The natural history of portal hypertension after transjugular intrahepatic portosystemic shunts. Gastroenterology 1997;112(3):889–98.

20. Mahadeva S, Bellamy MC, Kessel D, et al. Cost-effectiveness of N-butyl-2-cyanoacrylate (histoacryl) glue injections versus transjugular intrahepatic portosystemic shunt in the management of acute gastric variceal bleeding. Am J Gastroenterol 2003;98(12):2688–93.

21. Procaccini NJ, Al-Osaimi AM, Northup P, et al. Endoscopic cyanoacrylate versus transjugular intrahepatic portosystemic shunt for gastric variceal bleeding: a single-center U.S. analysis. Gastrointest Endosc 2009;70(5):881–7.

22. Greenwald BD, Caldwell SH, Hespenheide EE, et al. N-2-butyl-cyanoacrylate for bleeding gastric varices: a United States pilot study and cost analysis. Am J Gastroenterol 2003;98(9):1982–8.

23. Ryan BM, Stockbrugger RW, Ryan JM. A pathophysiologic, gastroenterologic, and radiologic approach to the management of gastric varices. Gastroenterology 2004;126(4):1175–89.

24. Tripathi D, Jalan R. Transjugular intrahepatic portosystemic stent-shunt in the management of gastric and ectopic varices. Eur J Gastroenterol Hepatol 2006;18(11):1155–60.

25. Akahoshi T, Hashizume M, Tomikawa M, et al. Long-term results of balloon-occluded retrograde transvenous obliteration for gastric variceal bleeding and risky gastric varices: a 10-year experience. J Gastroenterol Hepatol 2008; 23(11):1702–9.

26. Hirota S, Matsumoto S, Tomita M, et al. Retrograde transvenous obliteration of gastric varices. Radiology 1999;211(2):349–56.

27. Hiraga N, Aikata H, Takaki S, et al. The long-term outcome of patients with bleeding gastric varices after balloon-occluded retrograde transvenous obliteration. J Gastroenterol 2007;42(8):663–72.

28. Kitamoto M, Imamura M, Kamada K, et al. Balloon-occluded retrograde transvenous obliteration of gastric fundal varices with hemorrhage. Am J Roentgenol 2002;178(5):1167–74.

29. Kim ES, Kweon YO, Cho CM, et al. The clinical efficacy of the balloon occluded retrograde transvenous obliteration (BRTO) in gastric variceal bleeding. J Hepatol 2003;38:62.

30. Ninoi T, Nakamura K, Kaminou T, et al. TIPS versus transcatheter sclerotherapy for gastric varices. AJR Am J Roentgenol 2004;183(2):369–76.

31. Ferral H, Patel NH. Selection criteria for patients undergoing transjugular intrahepatic portosystemic shunt procedures: current status. J Vasc Interv Radiol 2005;16(4):449–55.

32. Saad WE, Darwish WM, Davies MG, et al. Transjugular intrahepatic portosystemic shunts in liver transplant recipients for management of refractory ascites: clinical outcome. J Vasc Interv Radiol 2010;21(2):218–23.

33. Uehara H, Akahoshi T, Tomikawa M, et al. Prediction of improved liver function after balloon-occluded retrograde transvenous obliteration: relation to hepatic vein pressure gradient. J Gastroenterol Hepatol 2012;27(1):137–41.

34. Kumamoto M, Toyonaga A, Inoue H, et al. Long-term results of balloon-occluded retrograde transvenous obliteration for gastric fundal varices: hepatic deterioration links to portosystemic shunt syndrome. J Gastroenterol Hepatol 2010;25(6): 1129–35.

35. Saad WE, Wagner CC, Al-Osaimi A, et al. The effect of balloon-occluded transvenous obliteration of gastric varices and gastrorenal shunts on the hepatic synthetic function: a comparison between Child-Pugh and model for end-stage liver disease scores. Vasc Endovascular Surg 2013;47(4):281–7.

36. Cho SK, Shin SW, Yoo EY, et al. The short-term effects of balloon-occluded retrograde transvenous obliteration, for treating gastric variceal bleeding, on portal hypertensive changes: a CT evaluation. Korean J Radiol 2007;8(6): 520–30.

37. Tanihata H, Minamiguchi H, Sato M, et al. Changes in portal systemic pressure gradient after balloon-occluded retrograde transvenous obliteration of gastric varices and aggravation of esophageal varices. Cardiovasc Intervent Radiol 2009;32(6):1209–16.

38. Saad WE, Wagner CC, Lippert A, et al. Protective value of TIPS against the development of hydrothorax/ascites and upper gastrointestinal bleeding after balloon-occluded retrograde transvenous obliteration (BRTO). Am J Gastroenterol 2013;108(10):1612–9.

39. Cho SK, Shin SW, Do YS, et al. Development of thrombus in the major systemic and portal veins after balloon-occluded retrograde transvenous obliteration for treating gastric variceal bleeding: its frequency and outcome evaluation with CT. J Vasc Interv Radiol 2008;19(4):529–38.

40. Mishra SR, Chander Sharma B, Kumar A, et al. Endoscopic cyanoacrylate injection versus beta-blocker for secondary prophylaxis of gastric variceal bleed: a randomised controlled trial. Gut 2010;59(6):729–35.

41. Mishra SR, Sharma BC, Kumar A, et al. Primary prophylaxis of gastric variceal bleeding comparing cyanoacrylate injection and beta-blockers: a randomized controlled trial. J Hepatol 2011;54(6):1161–7.

42. Norton ID, Andrews JC, Kamath PS. Management of ectopic varices. Hepatology 1998;28(4):1154–8.

43. Lebrec D, Benhamou JP. Ectopic varices in portal hypertension. Clin Gastroenterol 1985;14(1):105–21.

44. Hashizume M, Tanoue K, Ohta M, et al. Vascular anatomy of duodenal varices: angiographic and histopathological assessments. Am J Gastroenterol 1993; 88(11):1942–5.

45. Al-Mofarreh M, Al-Moagel-Alfarag M, Ashoor T, et al. Duodenal varices. Report of 13 cases. Z Gastroenterol 1986;24(11):673–80.

46. Liu Y, Yang J, Wang J, et al. Clinical characteristics and endoscopic treatment with cyanoacrylate injection in patients with duodenal varices. Scand J Gastroenterol 2009;44(8):1012–6.

47. Bhasin DK, Sharma BC, Sriram PV, et al. Endoscopic management of bleeding ectopic varices with histoacryl. HPB Surg 1999;11(3):171–3.

48. Kim HH, Kim SE. Ruptured duodenal varices successfully managed by endoscopic N-butyl-2-cyanoacrylate injection. J Clin Med Res 2012;4(5): 351–3.

49. Rai R, Panzer SW, Miskovsky E, et al. Thrombin injection for bleeding duodenal varices. Am J Gastroenterol 1994;89(10):1871–3.

50. Zamora CA, Sugimoto K, Tsurusaki M, et al. Endovascular obliteration of bleeding duodenal varices in patients with liver cirrhosis. Eur Radiol 2006; 16(1):73–9.

51. Haruta I, Isobe Y, Ueno E, et al. Balloon-occluded retrograde transvenous obliteration (BRTO), a promising nonsurgical therapy for ectopic varices: a case report of successful treatment of duodenal varices by BRTO. Am J Gastroenterol 1996;91(12):2594–7.

52. Almeida JR, Trevisan L, Guerrazzi F, et al. Bleeding duodenal varices successfully treated with TIPS. Dig Dis Sci 2006;51(10):1738–41.

53. Kochar N, Tripathi D, McAvoy NC, et al. Bleeding ectopic varices in cirrhosis: the role of transjugular intrahepatic portosystemic stent shunts. Aliment Pharmacol Ther 2008;28(3):294–303.

54. Chawla Y, Dilawari JB. Anorectal varices–their frequency in cirrhotic and noncirrhotic portal hypertension. Gut 1991;32(3):309–11.

55. Ganguly S, Sarin SK, Bhatia V, et al. The prevalence and spectrum of colonic lesions in patients with cirrhotic and noncirrhotic portal hypertension. Hepatology 1995;21(5):1226–31.

56. Misra SP, Dwivedi M, Misra V, et al. Colonic changes in patients with cirrhosis and in patients with extrahepatic portal vein obstruction. Endoscopy 2005; 37(5):454–9.

57. Herman BE, Baum S, Denobile J, et al. Massive bleeding from rectal varices. Am J Gastroenterol 1993;88(6):939–42.

58. Chen WC, Hou MC, Lin HC, et al. An endoscopic injection with N-butyl-2-cyanoacrylate used for colonic variceal bleeding: a case report and review of the literature. Am J Gastroenterol 2000;95(2):540–2.

59. Coelho-Prabhu N, Baron TH, Kamath PS. Endoscopic band ligation of rectal varices: a case series. Endoscopy 2010;42(2):173–6.

60. Ryu SH, Moon JS, Kim I, et al. Endoscopic injection sclerotherapy with N-butyl-2-cyanoacrylate in a patient with massive rectal variceal bleeding: a case report. Gastrointest Endosc 2005;62(4):632–5.

61. Anan A, Irie M, Watanabe H, et al. Colonic varices treated by balloon-occluded retrograde transvenous obliteration in a cirrhotic patient with encephalopathy: a case report. Gastrointest Endosc 2006;63(6):880–4.

62. Hashimoto N, Akahoshi T, Kamori M, et al. Treatment of bleeding rectal varices with transumbilical venous obliteration of the inferior mesenteric vein. Surg Laparosc Endosc Percutan Tech 2013;23(3):e134–7.

63. Vangeli M, Patch D, Terreni N, et al. Bleeding ectopic varices–treatment with transjugular intrahepatic porto-systemic shunt (TIPS) and embolisation. J Hepatol 2004;41(4):560–6.

64. Shibata D, Brophy DP, Gordon FD, et al. Transjugular intrahepatic portosystemic shunt for treatment of bleeding ectopic varices with portal hypertension. Dis Colon Rectum 1999;42(12):1581–5.

65. Nayar M, Saravanan R, Rowlands PC, et al. TIPSS in the treatment of ectopic variceal bleeding. Hepatogastroenterology 2006;53(70):584–7.

66. Merkel C, Bolognesi M, Bellon S, et al. Long-term follow-up study of adult patients with non-cirrhotic obstruction of the portal system: comparison with cirrhotic patients. J Hepatol 1992;15(3):299–303.

67. Condat B, Pessione F, Hillaire S, et al. Current outcome of portal vein thrombosis in adults: risk and benefit of anticoagulant therapy. Gastroenterology 2001; 120(2):490–7.

68. Amitrano L, Guardascione MA, Scaglione M, et al. Prognostic factors in noncirrhotic patients with splanchnic vein thromboses. Am J Gastroenterol 2007; 102(11):2464–70.

69. Janssen HL, Wijnhoud A, Haagsma EB, et al. Extrahepatic portal vein thrombosis: aetiology and determinants of survival. Gut 2001;49(5):720–4.

70. Rodriguez-Castro KI, Porte RJ, Nadal E, et al. Management of nonneoplastic portal vein thrombosis in the setting of liver transplantation: a systematic review. Transplantation 2012;94(11):1145–53.

71. Francoz C, Belghiti J, Vilgrain V, et al. Splanchnic vein thrombosis in candidates for liver transplantation: usefulness of screening and anticoagulation. Gut 2005;54(5):691–7.

72. Zocco MA, Di Stasio E, De Cristofaro R, et al. Thrombotic risk factors in patients with liver cirrhosis: correlation with MELD scoring system and portal vein thrombosis development. J Hepatol 2009;51(4):682–9.

73. Amitrano L, Guardascione MA, Brancaccio V, et al. Risk factors and clinical presentation of portal vein thrombosis in patients with liver cirrhosis. J Hepatol 2004;40(5):736–41.

74. Senzolo M, Sartori T, Rossetto V, et al. Prospective evaluation of anticoagulation and transjugular intrahepatic portosystemic shunt for the management of portal vein thrombosis in cirrhosis. Liver Int 2012;32(6):919–27.

75. Amitrano L, Guardascione MA, Menchise A, et al. Safety and efficacy of anticoagulation therapy with low molecular weight heparin for portal vein thrombosis in patients with liver cirrhosis. J Clin Gastroenterol 2010;44(6):448–51.

76. Valla DC, Condat B, Lebrec D. Spectrum of portal vein thrombosis in the West. J Gastroenterol Hepatol 2002;17(Suppl 3):S224–7.

77. Sarin SK, Sollano JD, Chawla YK, et al. Consensus on extra-hepatic portal vein obstruction. Liver Int 2006;26(5):512–9.

78. Orr DW, Harrison PM, Devlin J, et al. Chronic mesenteric venous thrombosis: evaluation and determinants of survival during long-term follow-up. Clin Gastroenterol Hepatol 2007;5(1):80–6.

79. Spaander VM, van Buuren HR, Janssen HL. Review article: the management of non-cirrhotic non-malignant portal vein thrombosis and concurrent portal hypertension in adults. Aliment Pharmacol Ther 2007;26(Suppl 2):203–9.

80. Spaander MC, Darwish Murad S, van Buuren HR, et al. Endoscopic treatment of esophagogastric variceal bleeding in patients with noncirrhotic extrahepatic portal vein thrombosis: a long-term follow-up study. Gastrointest Endosc 2008;67(6):821–7.

81. Primignani M. Portal vein thrombosis, revisited. Dig Liver Dis 2010;42(3):163–70.

82. Primignani M, Martinelli I, Bucciarelli P, et al. Risk factors for thrombophilia in extrahepatic portal vein obstruction. Hepatology 2005;41(3):603–8.

83. Primignani M, Mannucci PM. The role of thrombophilia in splanchnic vein thrombosis. Semin Liver Dis 2008;28(3):293–301.

84. De Stefano V, Teofili L, Leone G, et al. Spontaneous erythroid colony formation as the clue to an underlying myeloproliferative disorder in patients with Budd-Chiari syndrome or portal vein thrombosis. Semin Thromb Hemost 1997;23(5): 411–8.

85. Colaizzo D, Amitrano L, Tiscia GL, et al. The JAK2 V617F mutation frequently occurs in patients with portal and mesenteric venous thrombosis. J Thromb Haemost 2007;5(1):55–61.

86. de Franchis R, Baveno VF. Revising consensus in portal hypertension: report of the Baveno V consensus workshop on methodology of diagnosis and therapy in portal hypertension. J Hepatol 2010;53(4):762–8.

87. Plessier A, Darwish-Murad S, Hernandez-Guerra M, et al. Acute portal vein thrombosis unrelated to cirrhosis: a prospective multicenter follow-up study. Hepatology 2010;51(1):210–8.

88. Hall TC, Garcea G, Metcalfe M, et al. Impact of anticoagulation on outcomes in acute non-cirrhotic and non-malignant portal vein thrombosis: a retrospective observational study. Hepatogastroenterology 2013;60(122):311–7.

89. Garcia-Pagan JC, Hernandez-Guerra M, Bosch J. Extrahepatic portal vein thrombosis. Semin Liver Dis 2008;28(3):282–92.

90. Condat B, Pessione F, Helene Denninger M, et al. Recent portal or mesenteric venous thrombosis: increased recognition and frequent recanalization on anticoagulant therapy. Hepatology 2000;32(3):466–70.

91. Turnes J, Garcia-Pagan JC, Gonzalez M, et al. Portal hypertension-related complications after acute portal vein thrombosis: impact of early anticoagulation. Clin Gastroenterol Hepatol 2008;6(12):1412–7.

92. Donadini MP, Dentali F, Ageno W. Splanchnic vein thrombosis: new risk factors and management. Thromb Res 2012;129(Suppl 1):S93–6.

93. Heider TR, Azeem S, Galanko JA, et al. The natural history of pancreatitis-induced splenic vein thrombosis. Ann Surg 2004;239(6):876–80 [discussion: 880–2].

94. Bernades P, Baetz A, Levy P, et al. Splenic and portal venous obstruction in chronic pancreatitis. A prospective longitudinal study of a medical-surgical series of 266 patients. Dig Dis Sci 1992;37(3):340–6.

95. Bradley EL 3rd. The natural history of splenic vein thrombosis due to chronic pancreatitis: indications for surgery. Int J Pancreatol 1987;2(2):87–92.

96. Butler JR, Eckert GJ, Zyromski NJ, et al. Natural history of pancreatitis-induced splenic vein thrombosis: a systematic review and meta-analysis of its incidence and rate of gastrointestinal bleeding. HPB (Oxford) 2011;13(12):839–45.

97. Weber SM, Rikkers LF. Splenic vein thrombosis and gastrointestinal bleeding in chronic pancreatitis. World J Surg 2003;27(11):1271–4.

98. Agarwal AK, Raj Kumar K, Agarwal S, et al. Significance of splenic vein thrombosis in chronic pancreatitis. Am J Surg 2008;196(2):149–54.

99. Sakorafas GH, Sarr MG, Farley DR, et al. The significance of sinistral portal hypertension complicating chronic pancreatitis. Am J Surg 2000;179(2):129–33.

Portal Hypertensive Gastropathy and Colopathy

Nathalie H. Urrunaga, MD, MS[a], Don C. Rockey, MD[b],*

KEYWORDS

- Cirrhosis • Hemorrhage • Bleeding • Pressure • Portal hypertension

KEY POINTS

- PHG and PHC can cause acute and/or chronic gastrointestinal bleeding.
- Diagnosis for both is endoscopic.
- The specific management of PHG and PHC depends on the clinical presentation.
- For acute bleeding, hemodynamic stabilization with intravenous (IV) fluids, IV antibiotics, and blood transfusion as needed should be begun immediately. This should be followed by IV pharmacologic therapy to decrease portal pressure, and subsequently by nonselective β-blockers.
- In patients with chronic bleeding, therapy with β-blockers and iron replacement is recommended. The role of TIPS is controversial.
- Patients with refractory bleeding should be managed on an individual basis.

INTRODUCTION

The most common cause of portal hypertension is liver cirrhosis, which causes so-called intrahepatic or sinusoidal portal hypertension. Other disorders including presinusoidal and postsinusoidal diseases (ie, portal vein thrombosis, schistosomiasis, veno-occlusive disease, cardiac failure) may also cause increased portal pressure. Portal hypertension likely causes hemodynamic and mucosal changes in the entire gastrointestinal (GI) tract. This article focuses on the pathogenesis, diagnosis, and treatment of portal hypertensive gastropathy (PHG) and colopathy (PHC) (**Table 1**).

The cause of PHG and PHC is incompletely understood. However, available data indicate that portal hypertension is a critical component. It has been recognized

N.H. Urrunaga was supported by the NIH (Research Grant T32 DK 067872).
Disclosure of Conflicts: The authors certify that they have no financial arrangements (eg, consultancies, stock ownership, equity interests, patent-licensing arrangements, research support, major honoraria, and so forth).
[a] Division of Gastroenterology and Hepatology, University of Maryland School of Medicine, 22 S. Greene Street, N3W156, Baltimore, MD 21201, USA; [b] Department of Internal Medicine, Medical University of South Carolina, 96 Jonathan Lucas Street, Suite 803, Charleston, SC 29425, USA
* Corresponding author.
E-mail address: rockey@musc.edu

| Table 1 | | |
| Features of portal hypertensive gastropathy and colopathy | | |
Features	Portal Hypertensive Gastropathy	Portal Hypertensive Colopathy
Endoscopic characteristics	Mosaic pattern and red spots	Mosaic pattern and red spots, sometimes, vascular ectasia appearance
Pathology	Dilated capillaries and venules, no inflammation	Edema and capillary dilatation, lymphocytes and plasma cells, in lamina propria
Treatment	Iron-replacement therapy Transfusions Portal pressure–reducing agents	[a]Iron-replacement therapy Transfusions Portal pressure–reducing agents
Salvage treatment	TIPS/shunt surgery APC Liver transplantation	TIPS/shunt surgery APC Liver transplantation

Current practice is based on case and case series reports.
[a] There are insufficient data for standard recommendations in PHC bleeding.

that mucosal changes in the gastric mucosa of patients with portal hypertension were different pathologically from inflammatory gastritis; this led to the early description "congestive gastropathy."[1] The primary pathologic change was characterized by vascular ectasia. PHG is recognized endoscopically as a mosaic-like pattern called snakeskin mucosa with or without red spots.[2] Additionally, the terms portal hypertensive enteropathy[3,4] and PHC[5,6] were created to describe similar changes in the small bowel and colonic mucosa, respectively. PHC is characterized by erythema of the colonic mucosa, vascular lesions including cherry-red spots, telangiectasias, or angiodysplasia-like lesions.

PHG and PHC are important clinically because they may lead to chronic and/or acute GI bleeding. Both disorders are often confused with other diseases that can present similarly. Careful investigation is essential to accurately delineate the proper diagnostic needs and to start specific treatment.

PORTAL HYPERTENSIVE GASTROPATHY
Epidemiology

The prevalence of PHG in patients with cirrhosis varies from 20% to 98%.[2,7–12] This variation seems to be caused by several factors, including the study of different populations and variable patient selection, different interpretation of endoscopic lesions, and lack of uniform diagnostic criteria and classification.

Some studies have demonstrated a higher prevalence of PHG in patients with advanced liver disease, esophageal varices, or history of sclerotherapy or ligation for esophageal varices.[7,9,10] In general, the available data suggest that PHG is often associated with more severe portal hypertension.[13] It has also been suggested that the prevalence of PHG increases as esophageal varices are obliterated,[2] although this point is controversial.

Clinical Findings

Most patients with PHG are asymptomatic, but a significant number of patients exhibit symptoms related to chronic GI bleeding and chronic blood loss/iron deficiency anemia. A smaller proportion of patients exhibit evidence of active GI bleeding.

Chronic bleeding from PHG has been reported to occur in 3% to 60% of patients.[8,9,14,15] The definition of chronic bleeding most commonly used is decrease of hemoglobin of 2 g/dL within a 6-month time period without evidence of acute bleeding and nonsteroidal anti-inflammatory drug use.[16] Other definitions include the presence of iron deficiency anemia with a positive fecal occult blood test.[15]

Acute GI hemorrhage is less common. The prevalence of acute GI bleeding from PHG in patients with cirrhosis has been reported to be between 2% and 12%.[7–9] Most of these cases are caused by severe PHG (90%–95%).[7,9] The diagnosis of acute hemorrhage from PHG is made when active hemorrhage from PHG lesions or nonremovable clots over these lesions are identified during endoscopy, or if there is evidence of portal hypertension, typical gastric lesions, and no other source of bleeding can be identified after complete evaluation of the GI tract.[17]

Diagnostic Modalities

The diagnosis of PHG is made at the time of endoscopic evaluation. Endoscopic features include a typical snakeskin mosaic pattern, flat or bulging red marks or red spots resembling vascular ectasias,[1] or black-brown spots. The most common location for PHG is the proximal stomach (fundus and body).[18,19]

The simplest way to make the diagnosis is by esophagogastroduodenoscopy. Capsule endoscopy has also been used and was shown to have a sensitivity of 74% and specificity of 83% when compared with esophagogastroduodenoscopy.[20] Another study performed in 119 patients showed that the sensitivity of capsule endoscopy was 69% and specificity 99%.[21] However, the diagnostic yield in the gastric body was significantly greater than in the fundus (100% vs 48%, respectively).[21] These data suggest that its role is more important in the assessment of small bowel enteropathy.[22]

Classification

Classification of PHG is done based on the severity of its appearance. There are several proposed grading systems, but most experts recommend a two-category classification system,[23,24] although a three-category system has also been proposed (**Table 2**).[25] The two-grading classification proposed by Baveno III consensus is similar to older versions.[1] PHG is classified as mild when the only change consists of a snakeskin mosaic pattern, and it is classified as severe when in addition to the mosaic pattern, flat or bulging red or black-brown spots are seen, and/or when there is active hemorrhage (**Fig. 1**).[23]

The two-category classification system has significantly better interobserver and intraobserver reproducibility and agreement.[26] A recent study has shown that the endoscopic criteria for the diagnosis of PHG that were associated with a high rate of interobserver reliability are the mosaic-like pattern, red-point lesions, and cherry-red spots.[27] The clinical importance of this grading system resides in the fact that patients with severe PHG have a higher chance of bleeding or to have chronic anemia than patients with mild PHG.[9,28]

Other Diagnostic Modalities

Nonendoscopic modalities for diagnosis of PHG have been studied. These include magnetic resonance imaging and computed tomography.[29,30] PHG is identified by computed tomography scan as enhancement on the inner layer of the gastric walls, which may reflect gastric congestion. In a study of 32 patients, 10 had PHG and 22 did not.[29] Enhancement of the inner layer of the gastric wall in the delayed phase was observed in nine patients with PHG, and in five without portal hypertension.

Category	Baveno III Consensus	NIEC	McCormack et al,[1] 1985	Tanoue et al,[25] 1992
Table 2 Classification of portal hypertensive gastropathy				
Mild	MLP of mild degree (without redness of the areola)	Mosaic-like pattern Mild: diffusely pink areola Moderate: flat red spot in center of pink areola Severe: diffusely red areola	Fine speckling or scarlatina-type of rash Superficial reddening Snakeskin pattern	Grade 1: Mild reddening Congestive mucosa
Moderate	N/A	N/A	N/A	Grade 2: Severe redness + fine reticular pattern in areas of raised mucosa
Severe	MLP + red signs or if any other red sign or brown-black spot is present	Red marks: red lesions of variable diameter, flat or slightly protruding Discrete or confluent	Cherry-red spots, confluent or not Diffuse hemorrhage	Grade 3: Grade 2 + point bleeding

Abbreviations: MLP, mosaic-like pattern; NIEC, New Italian Endoscopic Club for the Study and Treat of Esophageal Varices.

Magnetic resonance imaging was used to measure the diameter of the left gastric, paraesophageal, and azygos veins in 57 patients with portal hypertension. In patients with PHG, the mean diameters of these veins were not different from those in patients without PHG.[30] These data suggest that imaging is at this time best reserved for experimental purposes.

Pathogenesis

The pathogenesis of PHG is incompletely understood. The presence of portal hypertension seems to be essential. Although studies have failed to demonstrate that there is a linear correlation between the degree of portal hypertension and the severity of PHG,[10,12,31] studies that demonstrate improvement of PHG after shunt surgery or transjugular intrahepatic portosystemic shunt (TIPS) support the connection.[32,33]

The major histologic changes in PHG include dilatation of capillaries and venules in the mucosa and submucosa without significant inflammation.[1] Several studies have shown that abnormalities in the mucosal microcirculation may be related to the congestion seen in PHG.[13] PHG seems to develop secondary to congestion because of blockage of gastric blood drainage.[32,34] A major apparent process in PHG is dysregulation of the mucosal microcirculation, which leads to mucosal hypoxia,[35] altering the epithelial cell integrity by overproduction of oxygen free radicals, nitric oxide, tumor necrosis factor-α, endothelin-1, and prostaglandins.[35–39] In addition, because of the impaired blood flow characteristics, and perhaps dysregulation of local cytokines, and vascular factors, the abnormal mucosa in PHG exhibits impaired healing and mechanisms of defense, which in turn may increase the risk for bleeding.[40,41]

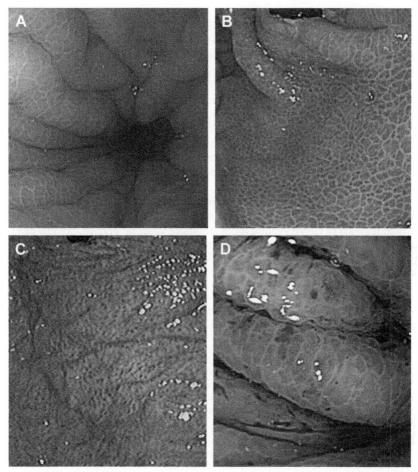

Fig. 1. (*A, B*) Representative images of mild PHG. *A* shows a forward-viewing image of the proximal stomach. *B* shows a retroflex view of the cardia with the classic form of PHG, the typical "mosaic-like pattern" without significant stigmata of bleeding or erythema or edema. (*C, D*) Representative images of severe PHG. Red lesions of variable diameter are evident. There is often irregular mucosa. Cherry spots may be confluent or not. Slow oozing may also be seen as in *D*, an up-close view in the proximal stomach.

Diagnostic Dilemmas

The endoscopic diagnosis of PHG includes several entities. For example, lesions typical of those found in PHG may be seen in patients with irritant injury to the gastric mucosa (ie, caused by nonsteroidal anti-inflammatory drugs or ethanol), although PHG tends to more often be localized to the proximal stomach. One of the main considerations includes gastric antral vascular ectasia (GAVE) or watermelon stomach. GAVE also presents with flat red spots, but usually without the mosaic pattern.[42] GAVE may also appear endoscopically as streaks of erythema, seeming to emanate from the pylorus. GAVE is also usually located in the distal stomach (antrum).[43] Thus, the location of the lesions (PHG, proximal stomach; GAVE, distal stomach) may help distinguish the disorders. On some occasions the red spots can coalesce throughout the entire stomach (proximal and distal) and it is called diffuse gastric vascular ectasia. In situations like this, differentiation from severe PHG is very difficult.

The differentiation between GAVE and PHG may be important because treatment is typically different. Additionally, gastric vascular ectasia, which typically presents with chronic bleeding and iron deficiency, is a relatively uncommon cause of GI hemorrhage in patients with cirrhosis.[44] It is also identified in patients with other diseases including chronic renal failure, bone marrow transplantation, autoimmune and connective tissue diseases including scleroderma, atrophic gastritis, pernicious anemia, and sclerodactyly.[42,45-47] There does not seem to be a direct relationship between the presence of portal hypertension and GAVE,[48] and management of GAVE is different than for PHG. GAVE lesions are usually treated with endoscopic thermoablative methods and respond poorly to β-blockers or TIPS.[33,48]

When the endoscopic diagnosis is unclear, histologic assessment of the mucosa may help (and biopsy in the absence of severe coagulopathy is generally safe). The histologic findings of GAVE include more extensive vascular ectasia, spindle cell proliferation, and fibrin thrombi and fibrohyalinosis.[44]

Treatment Options

Treatment recommendations are targeted according to the presentation and differ depending on the rate of bleeding or whether the patient has specific symptoms (**Fig. 2**).

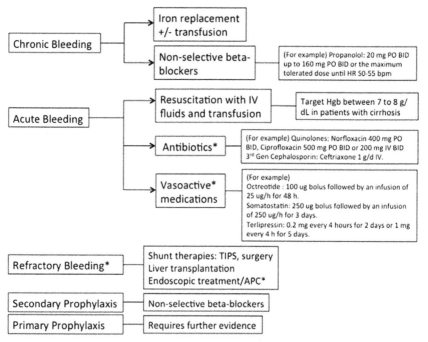

* Based on available studies. Further evidence and research is needed.

Fig. 2. PHG management. Recommended approaches to therapy are shown. It is recommended to manage PHC similarly, although in patients with PHC, management is typically more individualized. APC, argon plasma coagulation.

Primary Prophylaxis

It is not uncommon to identify PHG during endoscopic screening for esophageal varices in patients with cirrhosis. In this scenario, the patient may be asymptomatic without any evidence of bleeding. Primary prophylaxis of GI bleeding in patients with PHG has not been assessed and it is usually not recommended. However, management in these situations needs to be done on an individual basis. The severity of PHG is an important factor to take in consideration. Mild PHG alone usually does not require primary prophylaxis. If the patient has small esophageal varices and mild PHG, the use of nonselective β-blockers may be considered because theoretically it can be of benefit for PHG.[13] In patients with severe PHG and no varices, prophylaxis with nonselective β-blockers should be considered. However, this approach is controversial and more research is needed to clarify if β-blockers should be implemented as primary prophylaxis for bleeding from PHG.

Chronic Bleeding

Patients with PHG may present with iron deficiency anemia, consistent with chronic blood loss. It is important that other causes of iron deficiency anemia be excluded before assigning PHG as the cause. Iron-replacement therapy should be started in all patients with iron deficiency anemia caused by PHG; oral preparations are preferred, but intravenous (IV) iron may be used.[13] The use of nonselective β-blockers seems to reduce chronic bleeding secondary to PHG. In a trial that included 14 patients with PHG who received 24 to 480 mg/day of long acting propanol[49] 13 patients stopped bleeding in 3 days. Propranolol was stopped in seven patients after 2 to 6 months; four of these patients rebled and stopped bleeding when propranolol was restarted. A randomized controlled trial included 54 patients with cirrhosis with acute or chronic bleeding from severe PHG; 26 patients who received propanol daily at a dose to reduce the resting heart rate by 25% or to 55 bpm (from 20–160 mg twice a day) were compared with 28 patients who received placebo.[15] The percentage of patients free from rebleeding was higher in the propranolol group at 12 months (65% vs 38%) and at 30 months (52% vs 7%).

Thus, it is recommended to start iron supplementation and propranolol (up to 160 mg orally twice a day or to the maximum tolerated dose with goal heart rate (HR) of 50–55 bpm). Propanol therapy should be continued as long as the patient continues to have portal hypertension.[17]

Acute Bleeding

The differential diagnosis of acute GI bleeding in patients with cirrhosis includes bleeding varices (which account for approximately two-thirds of the lesions in these patients).[50] Other important causes of bleeding include ulcerative processes, and mucosal lesions, such as PHG. As in all patients with acute GI bleeding, aggressive and early generalized support is essential. It should be emphasized that in the setting of portal hypertension blood transfusion should be performed with goal to maintain hemoglobin level between 7 and 8 g/dL.[17] Oral or IV quinolones (eg, norfloxacin, 400 mg twice a day, or ciprofloxacin, 500 mg orally twice a day or 200 mg IV twice a day) or third-generation cephalosporin (eg, ceftriaxone, 1 g/day) for 7 days are recommended in patients with Child B or C cirrhosis or in patients who are on prophylaxis with quinolones.[51] Initiation of vasoconstrictor therapy with terlipressin, somatostatin, or somatostatin analogues should be started as soon as possible and endoscopy should be performed as early as possible.

Once the diagnosis of PHG is confirmed and bleeding from varices has been ruled out, specific treatment of PHG should be started. Endoscopic treatment of acute bleeding secondary to PHG is generally not effective. In situations where a single or a limited number of lesions is apparent, endoscopic therapy (argon plasma coagulation [APC] or coagulation therapy) might be considered on an individual basis. An attempt to lower portal pressure is reasonable. The use of β-blockers has been evaluated in this setting. In one study that included 14 patients with severe PHG and acute bleeding who were treated with propranolol, bleeding was controlled within 3 days in 13 (93%) of 14 patients.[49] It should be emphasized that β-blockers should be expected to take time to achieve an effective hemodynamic response; thus, in the acute period, the use of IV vasoactive drugs should be considered, even though tachyphylaxis is likely to develop.

In one study of patients with acute GI bleeding caused by PHG, octreotide (100-μg bolus followed by an infusion of 25 μg/h for 48 hours) seemed to be effective.[52] In this randomized controlled trial of 68 patients with acute bleeding from PHG that compared octreotide, vasopressin, and omeprazole, octreotide controlled bleeding in 100% of patients. Of note, omeprazole and vasopressin alone controlled bleeding in 64% and 59% of patients, respectively.[52] Because acid is unlikely to be a primary cause of bleeding, omeprazole probably does not play a major role in treatment of PHG, and the rate of control of bleeding with omeprazole likely mimics placebo. In another study, somatostatin led to cessation of acute bleeding from PHG in 26 patients with cirrhosis, with a rate of relapse of 11.5%.[53]

A double-blind randomized multicenter study of 68 patients with bleeding esophageal varices and PHG evaluated the effect of terlipressin (0.2 mg every 4 hours for 2 days or 1 mg every 4 hours for 5 days) in 68 patients.[54] The study showed a higher proportion of bleeding control and lower recurrence in patients assigned to a higher dose (1 mg every 4 hours),[54] but bleeding caused by PHG versus varices was not clearly differentiated.

Refractory Bleeding

Bleeding refractory to medical treatment may occur in patients with chronic or acute bleeding. In patients who present with chronic GI bleeding, those who become transfusion dependent despite iron therapy and β-blockers are general considered refractory. In patients with acute GI bleeding secondary to PHG, medical treatment failure should be considered when there is recurrent hematemesis (after 2 or more hours of treatment, such as with vasoactive medications), or a 3-g drop in hemoglobin in the absence of transfusion or an inadequate hemoglobin raise after transfusion.[55] In these situations, rescue therapies, such as TIPS or shunt surgery, may be considered.[55] Surgical shunts may be considered in patients with well-preserved liver function or in those with noncirrhotic portal hypertension because they have shown to improve gastric mucosal lesions and decreased the number of transfusions.[56,57] TIPS also seems to be effective in stopping bleeding from severe PHG,[33] having been shown to improve the endoscopic appearance of lesions within 6 to 12 weeks, and also leads to reduced transfusion requirements.[32,58,59]

Although APC is attractive because of its ease of application, and in those with a limited number of lesions, there are insufficient data to currently recommend it.[55] In a small study that evaluated APC in 11 patients with bleeding from PHG, APC of at least 80% of the involved mucosal surface at 30 to 40 W and 1.5 to 2 L/min of AP flow every 2 to 4 weeks led to cessation of bleeding and/or a reduction in transfusion in 81% of patients. These were highly selected patients; its use should be done on an individual basis.

The most effective means of therapy is liver transplantation, but is generally most appropriate for patients with decompensated liver disease.[60]

Secondary Prevention

Secondary prophylaxis of bleeding in PHG should be with a β-blocker.[15,55] In a double-blind placebo controlled cross-over trial that included 22 patients with non-bleeding PHG who received 160 mg of long-acting propranolol per day for 6 weeks, nine patients had improved PHG grading, whereas three had improvement after placebo (40% vs 14%); acute GI bleeding occurred in two patients taking placebo and one patient taking propranolol.[49] Another study assessed the occurrence of PHG after endoscopic variceal ligation in 77 patients who were randomized to band ligation alone (40 patients) or combined with propranolol (37 patients). Patients who received propranolol had a lower occurrence of PHG than patients who had only banding.[61]

PORTAL HYPERTENSIVE COLOPATHY
Introduction and Definition

Portal hypertension produces changes in the colorectal mucosa, likely similar to the upper GI tract. The term PHC was initially described in 1991[62] in a study reporting that colonic vascular ectasias and rectal varices were endoscopic features related to portal hypertension. Endoscopic abnormalities described in patients with portal hypertension range from vascular ectasias, anorectal or colonic varices, hemorrhoids, and nonspecific inflammatory changes.[62,63] PHC is likely common in patients with portal hypertension, although bleeding from this entity seems to be uncommon.

Epidemiology

The prevalence of PHC in patients with cirrhosis varies from 25% to 70%.[62–64] The presence of rectal or colonic varices also varies widely, being reported in from 4% to 40% of patients.[64–66] Bleeding from PHC is estimated to be between 0% and 9%.[65,67–69] Major differences in the reported prevalence and risk of bleeding are likely caused by patient selection, study design, lack of a clear classification system, interobserver variability among endoscopies, or differences in the indication for endoscopy.

In one study, the prevalence of esophageal varices, large esophageal varices, previous history of bleeding from esophageal varices, and rectal varices was significantly higher in patients with purported PHC than in control without colonic PHC.[62] PHC has been reported to be associated with a lower platelet count,[6] an increasing severity of cirrhosis (Child grade),[6] large esophageal varices,[70] gastric varices,[64,69] higher portal pressure,[70,71] and spontaneous bacterial peritonitis.[71] However, some studies have reported no correlation of PHC or colorectal varices with the severity of cirrhosis (Child grade),[65,71,72] portal pressure,[67,73] or gastroesophageal varices.[65,68,69,72]

Clinical Findings

PHC is usually asymptomatic; it may become manifest clinically in some patients as insidious chronic lower GI bleeding causing iron deficiency anemia. It has also been reported to cause massive or acute lower GI hemorrhage.[63] In one study of 35 patients with portal hypertension who underwent colonoscopy, the reported prevalence of PHC was 77%.[70] Among these patients 17% had hemoccult positive stool, and 5% presented with lower GI bleed.

Diagnostic Modalities

The diagnosis of PHC is endoscopic. In 64 patients with cirrhosis[62] who underwent colonoscopy and upper endoscopy, PHC was diagnosed in the setting of flat or slightly raised reddish lesions less than 10 mm in diameter on an otherwise normal-appearing mucosa (**Fig. 3**). Of note, rectal varices were also examined, being defined as prominent submucosal veins, dilated proximal to the pectinate line, which protruded into the rectal lumen. These veins were different from normal rectal veins because of their greater diameter and tortuosity (measuring at least 3–6 mm in diameter). Another early study described vascular-appearing lesions in the colon that resembled gastric cherry spots and spider telangiectasias.[63]

Classification

There is no universally accepted classification system for grading the severity of mucosal abnormalities in patients with PHC. This makes comparisons between studies challenging. Several classifications have been proposed (**Table 3**).[5,6,62,70] Initially, a histologic criteria for the vascular lesions typical of PHC included two types of lesions.[62] A so-called "early lesion" was characterized by moderately dilated, tortuous, thin-walled, and endothelial-lined veins and venules found in the submucosa. A "late-stage lesion" had progressively more dilated submucosal veins and dilated and tortuous venules and capillaries in the mucosa. Another system defined PHC endoscopically when patients had lesions appearing to be vascular ectasias, or diffuse red spots and three or more of the following: vascular irregularity, vascular dilatation, solitary red spots, and hemorrhoid.[70] Vascular ectasia was classified in three types: type 1, a flat, fern-like vascular lesion (spider-like lesion); type 2, flat or slightly elevated red lesion less than 10 mm in diameter or a cherry-red lesion; and type 3, a slightly elevated submucosal tumor-like lesion with a central red color and depression. Vascular irregularity was defined as coil-like appearance of the vessels in the submucosa. Vascular dilatation was defined as numerous prominent veins of greater than 3 to 6 mm in diameter. Solitary red spots were defined as numerous red spots with or without inflammatory changes. Another study proposed that PHC should be classified in three grades: grade 1, characterized by erythema of the colonic mucosa; grade 2, erythema of the colonic mucosa with a mosaic-like pattern; and

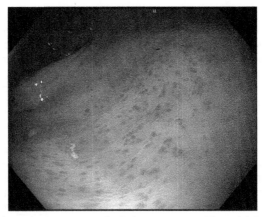

Fig. 3. Image of the colonic mucosa, depicting an area with multiple localized flat red lesions, typical of PHC. (*Courtesy of* A. Brock, MD, Charleston, SC.)

Table 3
Endoscopic classification of portal hypertensive colopathy

	Yamakado et al,[70] 1995	Ito et al,[6] 2005	Bini et al,[5] 2000
Definition of PHC	Vascular ectasia or diffuse red spots + ≥3 of the following: vascular irregularity, vascular dilatation (>3 mm vein), solitary red spots, and hemorrhoid	Vascular ectasia, redness and blue vein	Colitis-like abnormalities and/or vascular lesions
Endoscopic appearance	Type 1: flat, fern-like vascular (spider) lesion	Type 1: solitary vascular ectasia	Grade 1: erythema of colonic mucosa
	Type 2: flat, slightly elevated red lesion of <10 mm in diameter or a cherry-red lesion	Type 2: diffuse vascular ectasia	Grade 2: erythema of the colonic mucosa with mosaic-like pattern
	Type 3: slightly elevated submucosal tumor-like lesion with central red color and depression		Grade 3: vascular lesions including cherry-red spots, telangiectasias or angiodysplasia-like lesions

Abbreviation: PHC, portal hypertensive colopathy.

grade 3, vascular lesions in the colon including cherry-red spots, telangiectasias, or angiodysplasia-like lesions.[5]

Pathology

The pathogenesis of PHC remains poorly understood. Portal hypertension seems to play an important role, and there is an association with a hyperkinetic circulatory state.[70] The main pathologic change in PHC is colonic mucosal capillary ectasia.[62,63] The histomorphometric analysis of colonic samples of cirrhotic patients with PHC and/ or rectal varices had higher mean diameter of vessels and higher mean cross-sectional vascular area than patients with cirrhosis without PHC and/or rectal varices.[62] Another study[63] that included colonic biopsies of 20 patients with cirrhosis who underwent colonoscopy because of history of macroscopic or microscopic rectal bleeding, iron deficiency anemia, or colonic of polyps showed edema and capillary dilation in 50% of patients. The remaining 50% showed a slight increase in number of lymphocytes and plasma cells in the lamina propria; furthermore, four patients with vascular ectasias had diffuse mucosal changes resembling chronic colitis. In a study of colon biopsies of 55 patients with cirrhosis and portal hypertension and 25 control subjects,[64] morphometric analysis showed that the diameter and thickness of the capillary wall was higher in patients with portal hypertension than control subjects. Other features included edema, increased mononuclear cell infiltration, and fibromuscular proliferation in the lamina propria.

In an animal model of portal hypertension,[74] colonic mucosal blood flow and the number of submucosal veins were significantly increased when compared with control rats. Also, there was increased mRNA expression and enzyme activity of the inducible isoform of nitric oxide synthase. It was proposed that excess nitric oxide generated by overexpressed inducible nitric oxide synthase might play a role in the vascular and hemodynamic changes seen in PHC.

Diagnostic Dilemmas

Vascular changes of PHC can sometimes be difficult to differentiate from angiodysplasia of the colon secondary to degenerative changes. The latter is usually reported in patients with chronic renal insufficiency, aortic stenosis, and older patients and these lesions are usually fewer, smaller, and less widely distributed than the lesions seen in PHC.[62,72] Other noninflammatory and inflammatory etiologies of bleeding, such as ischemia, radiation changes, and hereditary hemorrhagic telangiectasia, are also in the differential diagnosis.[69]

For patients with cirrhosis and portal hypertension who present with lower GI bleeding, PHC should be considered. Additionally, colonic varices should be differentiated from hemorrhoids, especially before surgical excision, and angiography may be considered.[75]

Treatment Options

The evidence with which to base treatment strategies in PHC is limited. Indeed, there is no established standard treatment of PHC. Most of the available recommendations are based on case reports or small series reports.

In an animal model comparing saline, octreotide, and propranolol, octreotide and propranolol improved typical changes in the mucosa of rats with PHC (including mucosal edema, hyperemia, and hemorrhage).[76] In patients with chronic lower GI bleeding secondary to PHC, treatment with a β-blocker has been reported to be effective.[77] Another study demonstrated that there was a decreased risk of bleeding from PHC in patients with portal hypertension who were taking β-blockers.[5] In general, if there is evidence of iron deficiency anemia, iron replacement should be started. Treatment with β-blocker therapy as tolerated to achieve a resting heart rate of 50 to 55 bpm is reasonable.

In patients with acute bleeding, vasoactive medications, such as octreotide or terlipressin, could be effective.[77] Nonselective β-blockers are recommended as soon as hemodynamic stability is achieved.[77] A case report of a patient bleeding from PHC demonstrated that octreotide infusion (100-μg bolus followed by continuous infusion at 25 μg/h) decreased hepatic venous pressure gradient and stopped bleeding.[77]

The use of neodymium:yttrium-aluminum-garnet laser photocoagulation therapy was studied in 47 patients with angiodysplasias (20 in the colon, although it was not stated whether they were idiopathic or associated with PHC).[78] A median number of laser sessions (range, 1–8) were necessary to remove the angioectasias. The probability of remaining free of bleeding at 54 months was 61 ± 9%. Bleeding recurred in 15 of the 47 patients.[78] These data further emphasize that angiodyplasias in PHC are usually diffuse, and even after effective therapy (such as with laser) there is a risk of recurrent bleeding from residual vascular lesions.[77]

TIPS has been used as a rescue therapy in patients with refractory GI bleeding that does not respond to vasoactive medications or β-blockers. In one study of persistent bleeding from PHC in a patient with cirrhosis and portal hypertension that did not responded initially to propanol, bleeding was controlled after TIPS placement.[79] The portosystemic gradient was reduced after TIPS placement, and repeat colonoscopy at 9 days showed decrease in size and number of colonic lesions. The patient was followed up for 18 months without recurrence of GI bleeding.[79] Another report demonstrated control of lower GI bleeding from numerous angiodysplastic spots in the right colon after a proximal splenorenal shunt with splenectomy.[75]

Colonic varices may be treated with sclerotherapy or with shunt therapy. A study that included 20 cirrhotic patients, of which 19 were referred for colonoscopy because of iron deficiency anemia or evidence of chronic or acute lower GI bleeding, reported that two patients who had massive rectal bleeding had successful sclerotherapy of bleeding rectal varices and another two patients underwent mesocaval shunt for cecal varices.[63] There are other reports suggesting the use of TIPS to control recurrent bleeding from anorectal and colonic varices.[80,81] There have been reports of the use of surgical ligation,[82] sclerotherapy,[83] and cryosurgery for treatment of anorectal varices.[84]

With lower GI bleeding refractory to medical therapy, endoscopic treatment, and TIPS, surgery may be considered.[85] A 24-year-old patient with portal hypertension from portal vein thrombosis and persistent hematochezia underwent a TIPS procedure and later percutaneous coil embolization of the distal inferior mesenteric vein without control of her hematochezia. Sigmoidoscopy showed edematous, friable mucosa and prominent submucosal vessels in the left colon. Because of her refractory bleeding, a laparotomy with left-sided colectomy and coloanal anastomosis led to control of bleeding.[85]

Prophylaxis

Trials examining the role of β-blockers or other agents for primary or secondary prophylaxis for lower GI bleeding caused by PHC have not been performed. Therefore, the best approach is unknown. In patients with concomitant esophageal varices, nonselective β-blockers are reasonable.

SUMMARY

PHG and PHC can cause acute and/or chronic GI bleeding. Their pathogenesis is still not completely understood, but currently available evidence suggests that their development is related to portal hypertension. Diagnosis for both is endoscopic. The differential diagnosis is sometimes difficult and in these situations biopsy and histologic examination may be helpful. Management of PHG and PHC centers on the clinical presentation; for acute bleeding, hemodynamic stabilization with IV fluids, IV antibiotics, and blood transfusion should be provided as needed. IV pharmacologic therapy to decrease portal pressure followed by nonselective β-blockers as soon as the patient is hemodynamically stable is appropriate. In patients with chronic bleeding, therapy with β-blockers and iron replacement is advised. Patients with refractory bleeding represent difficult clinical challenges and should be managed on an individual basis, typically with the input of specialists. TIPS and shunt procedures may be helpful in some situations. The most effective approach to reduction of portal pressure is liver transplantation, which should be considered in appropriate candidates.

REFERENCES

1. McCormack TT, Sims J, Eyre-Brook I, et al. Gastric lesions in portal hypertension: inflammatory gastritis or congestive gastropathy? Gut 1985;26:1226–32.
2. Thuluvath PJ, Yoo HY. Portal hypertensive gastropathy. Am J Gastroenterol 2002;97:2973–8.
3. Menchén L, Ripoll C, Marín-Jiménez I, et al. Prevalence of portal hypertensive duodenopathy in cirrhosis: clinical and haemodynamic features. Eur J Gastroenterol Hepatol 2006;18:649–53.
4. Higaki N, Matsui H, Imaoka H, et al. Characteristic endoscopic features of portal hypertensive enteropathy. J Gastroenterol 2008;43:327–31.
5. Bini EJ, Lascarides CE, Micale PL, et al. Mucosal abnormalities of the colon in patients with portal hypertension: an endoscopic study. Gastrointest Endosc 2000;52:511–6.

6. Ito K, Shiraki K, Sakai T, et al. Portal hypertensive colopathy in patients with liver cirrhosis. World J Gastroenterol 2005;11:3127–30.

7. D'Amico G, Montalbano L, Traina M, et al. Natural history of congestive gastropathy in cirrhosis. The Liver Study Group of V. Cervello Hospital. Gastroenterology 1990;99:1558–64.

8. Primignani M, Carpinelli L, Preatoni P, et al. Natural history of portal hypertensive gastropathy in patients with liver cirrhosis. The New Italian Endoscopic Club for the study and treatment of esophageal varices (NIEC). Gastroenterology 2000; 119:181–7.

9. Merli M, Nicolini G, Angeloni S, et al. The natural history of portal hypertensive gastropathy in patients with liver cirrhosis and mild portal hypertension. Am J Gastroenterol 2004;99:1959–65.

10. Iwao T, Toyonaga A, Oho K, et al. Portal-hypertensive gastropathy develops less in patients with cirrhosis and fundal varices. J Hepatol 1997;26:1235–41.

11. Fontana RJ, Sanyal AJ, Mehta S, et al. Portal hypertensive gastropathy in chronic hepatitis C patients with bridging fibrosis and compensated cirrhosis: results from the HALT-C trial. Am J Gastroenterol 2006;101:983–92.

12. Sarin SK, Sreenivas DV, Lahoti D, et al. Factors influencing development of portal hypertensive gastropathy in patients with portal hypertension. Gastroenterology 1992;102:994–9.

13. Cubillas R, Rockey DC. Portal hypertensive gastropathy: a review. Liver Int 2010;30:1094–102.

14. Sarin SK, Shahi HM, Jain M, et al. The natural history of portal hypertensive gastropathy: influence of variceal eradication. Am J Gastroenterol 2000;95: 2888–93.

15. Pérez-Ayuso RM, Piqué JM, Bosch J, et al. Propranolol in prevention of recurrent bleeding from severe portal hypertensive gastropathy in cirrhosis. Lancet 1991; 337:1431–4.

16. de Franchis R, editor. Portal Hypertension II. Proceedings of the Second Baveno International Consensus Workshop on Definitions, Methodology and Therapeutic Strategies. Oxford: Blackwell Science; 1996.

17. Ripoll C, Garcia-Tsao G. Management of gastropathy and gastric vascular ectasia in portal hypertension. Clin Liver Dis 2010;14:281–95.

18. Cales P, Pascal JP. Gastroesophageal endoscopic features in cirrhosis: comparison of intracenter and intercenter observer variability. Gastroenterology 1990; 99:1189.

19. Vigneri S, Termini R, Piraino A, et al. The stomach in liver cirrhosis. Endoscopic, morphological, and clinical correlations. Gastroenterology 1991;101:472–8.

20. de Franchis R, Eisen GM, Laine L, et al. Esophageal capsule endoscopy for screening and surveillance of esophageal varices in patients with portal hypertension. Hepatology 2008;47:1595–603.

21. Aoyama T, Oka S, Aikata H, et al. Is small-bowel capsule endoscopy effective for diagnosis of esophagogastric lesions related to portal hypertension? J Gastroenterol Hepatol 2013. [Epub ahead of print].

22. De Palma GD, Rega M, Masone S, et al. Mucosal abnormalities of the small bowel in patients with cirrhosis and portal hypertension: a capsule endoscopy study. Gastrointest Endosc 2005;62:529–34.

23. de Franchis R. Updating consensus in portal hypertension: report of the Baveno III Consensus Workshop on definitions, methodology and therapeutic strategies in portal hypertension. J Hepatol 2000;33:846–52.

24. Spina GP, Arcidiacono R, Bosch J, et al. Gastric endoscopic features in portal hypertension: final report of a consensus conference, Milan, Italy, September 19, 1992. J Hepatol 1994;21:461–7.

25. Tanoue K, Hashizume M, Wada H, et al. Effects of endoscopic injection sclerotherapy on portal hypertensive gastropathy: a prospective study. Gastrointest Endosc 1992;38:582–5.

26. Yoo HY, Eustace JA, Verma S, et al. Accuracy and reliability of the endoscopic classification of portal hypertensive gastropathy. Gastrointest Endosc 2002;56: 675–80.

27. de Macedo GF, Ferreira FG, Ribeiro MA, et al. Reliability in endoscopic diagnosis of portal hypertensive gastropathy. World J Gastrointest Endosc 2013;5: 323–31.

28. Stewart CA, Sanyal AJ. Grading portal gastropathy: validation of a gastropathy scoring system. Am J Gastroenterol 2003;98:1758–65.

29. Ishihara K, Ishida R, Saito T, et al. Computed tomography features of portal hypertensive gastropathy. J Comput Assist Tomogr 2004;28:832–5.

30. Erden A, Idilman R, Erden I, et al. Veins around the esophagus and the stomach: do their calibrations provide a diagnostic clue for portal hypertensive gastropathy? Clin Imaging 2009;33:22–4.

31. Ohta M, Yamaguchi S, Gotoh N, et al. Pathogenesis of portal hypertensive gastropathy: a clinical and experimental review. Surgery 2002;131:S165–70.

32. Mezawa S, Homma H, Ohta H, et al. Effect of transjugular intrahepatic portosystemic shunt formation on portal hypertensive gastropathy and gastric circulation. Am J Gastroenterol 2001;96:1155–9.

33. Kamath PS, Lacerda M, Ahlquist DA, et al. Gastric mucosal responses to intrahepatic portosystemic shunting in patients with cirrhosis. Gastroenterology 2000;118:905–11.

34. Gupta R, Sawant P, Parameshwar RV, et al. Gastric mucosal blood flow and hepatic perfusion index in patients with portal hypertensive gastropathy. J Gastroenterol Hepatol 1998;13:921–6.

35. Albillos A, Colombato LA, Enriquez R, et al. Sequence of morphological and hemodynamic changes of gastric microvessels in portal hypertension. Gastroenterology 1992;102:2066–70.

36. Migoh S, Hashizume M, Tsugawa K, et al. Role of endothelin-1 in congestive gastropathy in portal hypertensive rats. J Gastroenterol Hepatol 2000;15: 142–7.

37. Lopez-Talavera JC, Merrill WW, Groszmann RJ. Tumor necrosis factor alpha: a major contributor to the hyperdynamic circulation in prehepatic portal-hypertensive rats. Gastroenterology 1995;108:761–7.

38. Payen JL, Cales P, Pienkowski P, et al. Weakness of mucosal barrier in portal hypertensive gastropathy of alcoholic cirrhosis. Effects of propranolol and enprostil. J Hepatol 1995;23:689–96.

39. Kawanaka H, Tomikawa M, Jones MK, et al. Defective mitogen-activated protein kinase (ERK2) signaling in gastric mucosa of portal hypertensive rats: potential therapeutic implications. Hepatology 2001;34:990–9.

40. Ferraz JG, Wallace JL. Underlying mechanisms of portal hypertensive gastropathy. J Clin Gastroenterol 1997;25(Suppl 1):S73–8.

41. Perini RF, Camara PR, Ferraz JG. Pathogenesis of portal hypertensive gastropathy: translating basic research into clinical practice. Nat Clin Pract Gastroenterol Hepatol 2009;6:150–8.

42. Gostout CJ, Viggiano TR, Ahlquist DA, et al. The clinical and endoscopic spectrum of the watermelon stomach. J Clin Gastroenterol 1992;15:256–63.

43. Ripoll C, Garcia-Tsao G. The management of portal hypertensive gastropathy and gastric antral vascular ectasia. Dig Liver Dis 2011;43:345–51.

44. Payen JL, Calès P, Voigt JJ, et al. Severe portal hypertensive gastropathy and antral vascular ectasia are distinct entities in patients with cirrhosis. Gastroenterology 1995;108:138–44.

45. Vincent C, Pomier-Layrargues G, Dagenais M, et al. Cure of gastric antral vascular ectasia by liver transplantation despite persistent portal hypertension: a clue for pathogenesis. Liver Transpl 2002;8:717–20.

46. Tobin AB, Budd DC. The anti-apoptotic response of the Gq/11-coupled muscarinic receptor family. Biochem Soc Trans 2003;31:1182–5.

47. Ingraham KM, O'Brien MS, Shenin M, et al. Gastric antral vascular ectasia in systemic sclerosis: demographics and disease predictors. J Rheumatol 2010; 37:603–7.

48. Spahr L, Villeneuve JP, Dufresne MP, et al. Gastric antral vascular ectasia in cirrhotic patients: absence of relation with portal hypertension. Gut 1999;44: 739–42.

49. Hosking SW, Kennedy HJ, Seddon I, et al. The role of propranolol in congestive gastropathy of portal hypertension. Hepatology 1987;7:437–41.

50. Lyles T, Elliott A, Rockey DC. A risk scoring system to predict in-hospital mortality in patients with cirrhosis presenting with upper gastrointestinal bleeding. J Clin Gastroenterol 2013. [Epub ahead of print].

51. Fernández J, Ruiz del Arbol L, Gómez C, et al. Norfloxacin vs ceftriaxone in the prophylaxis of infections in patients with advanced cirrhosis and hemorrhage. Gastroenterology 2006;131:1049–56 [quiz: 1285].

52. Zhou Y, Qiao L, Wu J, et al. Comparison of the efficacy of octreotide, vasopressin, and omeprazole in the control of acute bleeding in patients with portal hypertensive gastropathy: a controlled study. J Gastroenterol Hepatol 2002;17: 973–9.

53. Kouroumalis EA, Koutroubakis IE, Manousos ON. Somatostatin for acute severe bleeding from portal hypertensive gastropathy. Eur J Gastroenterol Hepatol 1998;10:509–12.

54. Bruha R, Marecek Z, Spicak J, et al. Double-blind randomized, comparative multicenter study of the effect of terlipressin in the treatment of acute esophageal variceal and/or hypertensive gastropathy bleeding. Hepatogastroenterology 2002;49:1161–6.

55. de Franchis R, Faculty BV. Revising consensus in portal hypertension: report of the Baveno V consensus workshop on methodology of diagnosis and therapy in portal hypertension. J Hepatol 2010;53:762–8.

56. Soin AS, Acharya SK, Mathur M, et al. Portal hypertensive gastropathy in non-cirrhotic patients. The effect of lienorenal shunts. J Clin Gastroenterol 1998; 26:64–7 [discussion: 68].

57. Orloff MJ, Orloff MS, Orloff SL, et al. Treatment of bleeding from portal hypertensive gastropathy by portacaval shunt. Hepatology 1995;21:1011–7.

58. Urata J, Yamashita Y, Tsuchigame T, et al. The effects of transjugular intrahepatic portosystemic shunt on portal hypertensive gastropathy. J Gastroenterol Hepatol 1998;13:1061–7.

59. Vignali C, Bargellini I, Grosso M, et al. TIPS with expanded polytetrafluoroethylene-covered stent: results of an Italian multicenter study. AJR Am J Roentgenol 2005; 185:472–80.

60. DeWeert TM, Gostout CJ, Wiesner RH. Congestive gastropathy and other upper endoscopic findings in 81 consecutive patients undergoing orthotopic liver transplantation. Am J Gastroenterol 1990;85:573–6.
61. Lo GH, Lai KH, Cheng JS, et al. The effects of endoscopic variceal ligation and propranolol on portal hypertensive gastropathy: a prospective, controlled trial. Gastrointest Endosc 2001;53:579–84.
62. Naveau S, Bedossa P, Poynard T, et al. Portal hypertensive colopathy. A new entity. Dig Dis Sci 1991;36:1774–81.
63. Kozarek RA, Botoman VA, Bredfeldt JE, et al. Portal colopathy: prospective study of colonoscopy in patients with portal hypertension. Gastroenterology 1991;101:1192–7.
64. Misra SP, Dwivedi M, Misra V. Prevalence and factors influencing hemorrhoids, anorectal varices, and colopathy in patients with portal hypertension. Endoscopy 1996;28:340–5.
65. Bresci G, Parisi G, Capria A. Clinical relevance of colonic lesions in cirrhotic patients with portal hypertension. Endoscopy 2006;38:830–5.
66. Rabinovitz M, Schade RR, Dindzans VJ, et al. Colonic disease in cirrhosis. An endoscopic evaluation in 412 patients. Gastroenterology 1990;99:195–9.
67. Chen LS, Lin HC, Lee FY, et al. Portal hypertensive colopathy in patients with cirrhosis. Scand J Gastroenterol 1996;31:490–4.
68. Ganguly S, Sarin SK, Bhatia V, et al. The prevalence and spectrum of colonic lesions in patients with cirrhotic and noncirrhotic portal hypertension. Hepatology 1995;21:1226–31.
69. Misra V, Misra SP, Dwivedi M, et al. Colonic mucosa in patients with portal hypertension. J Gastroenterol Hepatol 2003;18:302–8.
70. Yamakado S, Kanazawa H, Kobayashi M. Portal hypertensive colopathy: endoscopic findings and the relation to portal pressure. Intern Med 1995;34:153–7.
71. Diaz-Sanchez A, Nuñez-Martinez O, Gonzalez-Asanza C, et al. Portal hypertensive colopathy is associated with portal hypertension severity in cirrhotic patients. World J Gastroenterol 2009;15:4781–7.
72. Misra SP, Dwivedi M, Misra V, et al. Colonic changes in patients with cirrhosis and in patients with extrahepatic portal vein obstruction. Endoscopy 2005;37:454–9.
73. Wang TF, Lee FY, Tsai YT, et al. Relationship of portal pressure, anorectal varices and hemorrhoids in cirrhotic patients. J Hepatol 1992;15:170–3.
74. Ohta M, Kaviani A, Tarnawski AS, et al. Portal hypertension triggers local activation of inducible nitric oxide synthase gene in colonic mucosa. J Gastrointest Surg 1997;1:229–35.
75. Leone N, Debernardi-Venon W, Marzano A, et al. Portal hypertensive colopathy and hemorrhoids in cirrhotic patients. J Hepatol 2000;33:1026–7.
76. Aydede H, Sakarya A, Erhan Y, et al. Effects of octreotide and propranolol on colonic mucosa in rats with portal hypertensive colopathy. Hepatogastroenterology 2003;50:1352–5.
77. Yoshie K, Fujita Y, Moriya A, et al. Octreotide for severe acute bleeding from portal hypertensive colopathy: a case report. Eur J Gastroenterol Hepatol 2001;13:1111–3.
78. Naveau S, Aubert A, Poynard T, et al. Long-term results of treatment of vascular malformations of the gastrointestinal tract by neodymium YAG laser photocoagulation. Dig Dis Sci 1990;35:821–6.
79. Balzer C, Lotterer E, Kleber G, et al. Transjugular intrahepatic portosystemic shunt for bleeding angiodysplasia-like lesions in portal-hypertensive colopathy. Gastroenterology 1998;115:167–72.

80. Katz JA, Rubin RA, Cope C, et al. Recurrent bleeding from anorectal varices: successful treatment with a transjugular intrahepatic portosystemic shunt. Am J Gastroenterol 1993;88:1104–7.

81. Fantin AC, Zala G, Risti B, et al. Bleeding anorectal varices: successful treatment with transjugular intrahepatic portosystemic shunting (TIPS). Gut 1996; 38:932–5.

82. Johansen K, Bardin J, Orloff MJ. Massive bleeding from hemorrhoidal varices in portal hypertension. JAMA 1980;244:2084–5.

83. Richon J, Berclaz R, Schneider PA, et al. Sclerotherapy of rectal varices. Int J Colorectal Dis 1988;3:132–4.

84. Mashiah A. Massive bleeding from hemorrhoidal varices in portal hypertension. JAMA 1981;246:2323–4.

85. Ozgediz D, Devine P, Garcia-Aguilar J, et al. Refractory lower gastrointestinal bleeding from portal hypertensive colopathy. J Am Coll Surg 2008;207:613.

Hepatopulmonary Syndrome

David G. Koch, MD, MSCR[a],*, Michael B. Fallon, MD[b]

KEYWORDS

- Hepatopulmonary syndrome • Intrapulmonary vasodilatation • Hypoxemia
- Portal hypertension • Contrast echocardiography • Liver transplantation

KEY POINTS

- The hepatopulmonary syndrome (HPS) is a pulmonary complication of cirrhosis and/or portal hypertension that occurs in up to 30% of patients and results in arterial hypoxemia.
- The degree of hypoxemia does not correlate with the severity of liver disease, but patients with cirrhosis with HPS have a higher mortality than do patients with cirrhosis without HPS.
- There are no therapeutic options for HPS aside from liver transplantation.

HISTORICAL PERSPECTIVE

The coexistence between chronic liver disease and alterations in lung function has long been recognized by physicians, with the first report of cyanosis and finger clubbing in patients with cirrhosis appearing in the medical literature in 1884.[1] This clinical association was followed by confirmation that some patients with cirrhosis develop arterial hypoxemia.[2–6] However, the vascular changes that can occur in the lung with liver cirrhosis was not recognized until 1966 when physicians from the Royal Free and Brompton Hospitals in London performed a postmortem examination of the lungs from 13 patients with cirrhosis and described widespread vasodilatation of the precapillary pulmonary arterioles, even commenting on the appearance of "lung spider nevi" along the pleural surface.[7] A few relevant findings from the arteriography and histologic analyses were that (1) there was an increase in the number of vessels along the alveolar wall compared with patients without cirrhosis, especially in vessels measuring less than 35 μm, caused by widespread precapillary arteriole vasodilation; and (2) the primary lung structures (alveoli and connective tissues) were normal. However, a direct correlation with the degree of vasodilatation and severity

Financial Disclosures: None.
[a] Division of Gastroenterology and Hepatology, Department of Internal Medicine, Medical University of South Carolina, 25 Courtenay Drive ART 7100A, MSC 290, Charleston, SC 29425, USA; [b] Division of Gastroenterology, Hepatology and Nutrition, Department of Internal Medicine, The University of Texas Medical School at Houston, 6431 Fannin Street, MSB 4234, Houston, TX 77030, USA
* Corresponding author.
E-mail address: kochd@musc.edu

Clin Liver Dis 18 (2014) 407–420
http://dx.doi.org/10.1016/j.cld.2014.01.003
1089-3261/14/$ – see front matter © 2014 Elsevier Inc. All rights reserved.

of hypoxemia could not be established. The recognition of the hepatopulmonary syndrome (HPS) as a pathologic entity in cirrhosis came 12 years later when the concept that intrapulmonary vasodilatation (IPVD) could cause hypoxemia was accepted.[8]

PATHOPHYSIOLOGY
Animal Model of HPS

Understanding of the pathogenesis of HPS is limited, and derives almost entirely from a rat common bile duct ligation (CBDL) model that uniquely recreates the features of human HPS.[9–16] In this model, proliferating cholangiocytes in the liver produce and secrete endothelin-1 (ET-1),[9–13] whereas other animal models of portal hypertension that do not result in bile duct proliferation and subsequent biliary cirrhosis do not develop HPS (**Fig. 1**).[14] Sheer stress results in upregulation of the endothelin B receptor (ET$_B$R) in the pulmonary vasculature that subsequently binds the increased circulating ET-1 and augments pulmonary nitrous oxide (NO) production via endothelial nitrous oxide synthase (eNOS).[9,12,16–21] In addition, CBDL rats with HPS also have increased pulmonary intravascular monocytes caused by increased pulmonary NO levels and bacterial translocation resulting in increased blood levels of tumor necrosis factor alpha (TNF-α).[22–28] These pulmonary monocytes then contribute to IPVD by increasing levels of NO (via inducible nitric oxide synthase [iNOS])[11,29,30] and carbon monoxide (via heme oxygenase-1 [HO-1]).[11,31] Blood levels of vascular endothelial growth factor (VEGF)[30,32–34] are also increased. The complimentary effects of ET-1, pulmonary monocytes, and VEGF on the pulmonary vasculature not only contribute to IPVD but also to pulmonary angiogenesis, which in turn contributes to the underlying oxygen impairment.[11,30,32–34] The role of angiogenesis in HPS is supported by the presence of neovascularization in the lungs of CBDL rats with HPS[30,34] and the improvement in oxygenation with the antiangiogenesis therapy, sorafenib.[32,33] The CBDL model has provided a possible mechanism for IPVD and HPS (**Fig. 2**), but these pulmonary vascular abnormalities in humans are not exclusive to cholestatic liver disease and biliary cirrhosis because IPVD and HPS occur in cirrhosis of any cause.

Human Disease

Understanding of the pathophysiology of HPS in humans is limited. Nitric oxide has been implicated as a mediator of IPVD in cirrhotic patients with HPS because they have higher exhaled levels of NO compared with patients without HPS, and exhaled NO levels normalize after liver transplantation (LT).[35–37] However, attempts to inhibit NO production pharmacologically have given discrepant results.[38–44] Pulmonary angiogenesis has also been implicated in humans because single nucleotide polymorphisms that regulate angiogenesis are associated with the presence of HPS in patients with cirrhosis.[45] Adding to the angiogenesis hypothesis is the observation that resolution of hypoxemia from HPS after LT is not immediate and may take up to 1 year,

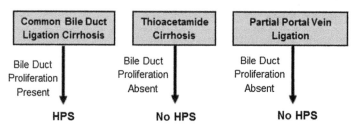

Fig. 1. Outcomes in 3 animal models of portal hypertension. Only the rat CBDL model with accompanying bile duct proliferation and portal hypertension develops hypoxemia.

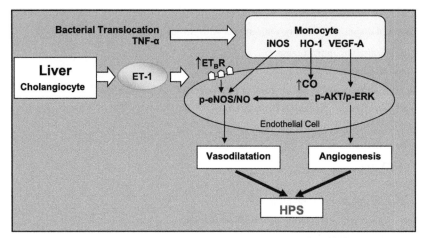

Fig. 2. Conceptual model of the pathogenesis of HPS in the rat CBDL model. CO, carbon monoxide; ET-1, endothelin-1; $ET_{\beta}R$, endothelin β receptor; HO-1, heme oxygenase-1; HPS, hepatopulmonary syndrome; iNOS, inducible nitric oxide synthase; NO, nitric oxide; p-eNOS, phosphorylated endothelial nitric oxide synthase; TNF-α tumor necrosis factor alpha; VEGF-A vascular endothelial growth factor A.

suggesting that there is remodeling of the pulmonary vasculature in addition to IPVD. The potential role of ET-1 in human disease was also shown in a single study in which blood levels of ET-1 in the hepatic vein were higher in patients with cirrhosis with IPVD and HPS compared with those without IPVD, and blood ET-1 levels correlated with the degree of bile duct proliferation in the corresponding liver biopsy specimens.[46] However, whether cholangiocytes in human cirrhosis develop an endocrine capability to produce ET-1 resulting in higher blood levels is still not known. A causal relationship between ET-1 and impairment in oxygenation in HPS has also never been established.

Although the humoral and genetic mediators in HPS are not clearly defined in humans, the underlying vascular pathobiology is better understood. Patients with HPS have dilatation of the capillary and precapillary vessels up to 100 μm in diameter as well as an increase in the number of these dilated vessels.[7] The vessels may also have impaired hypoxic-induced pulmonary vascular vasoconstriction.[47] As a result, mixed venous blood passes rapidly to the pulmonary veins, thereby increasing flow in the setting of preserved alveolar ventilation. This condition results in a ventilation-perfusion (V/Q) mismatch that is the predominant mechanism of hypoxemia, and also oxygen diffusion impairment. The latter results from the room air concentration of oxygen in the alveolus being insufficient to effectively oxygenate blood near the center of the dilated alveolar capillaries and can be overcome by increasing the amount of oxygen inspired, distinguishing HPS as a physiologic shunt rather than an anatomic (right-to-left) shunt.

CLINICAL MANIFESTATIONS

The features of HPS in patients with cirrhosis are nonspecific and typically involve respiratory symptoms, particularly dyspnea. However, dyspnea is a common complaint in patients with cirrhosis, being reported in up to 70% of patients.[48] The symptom may result from many causes aside from HPS, including complications of advanced liver disease and portal hypertension (such as ascites and hepatic hydrothorax), intrinsic lung disease, volume overload, or anemia (**Box 1**). These comorbid conditions

---

Box 1
Differential diagnosis of dyspnea in patients with cirrhosis

Intrinsic cardiopulmonary disease

  Congestive heart failure

  Chronic Obstructive Pulmonary Disease/asthma/restrictive lung disease

Complications of cirrhosis/portal hypertension

  Ascites

  Hepatic hydrothorax

  Muscle wasting

  Anemia

Cause-specific pulmonary complications

  Alpha1-antitrypsin deficiency: panacinar emphysema

  Cystic fibrosis: bronchiectasis

  Primary biliary cirrhosis: fibrosing alveolitis, pulmonary hemorrhage, pulmonary granulomas

  Sarcoidosis: interstitial lung disease, pulmonary hypertension

Pulmonary vascular complications of cirrhosis

  Hepatopulmonary syndrome

  Portopulmonary hypertension

---

are prevalent in patients with cirrhosis. In addition, HPS can coexist with them and still contribute to the hypoxemia. Because changes in position can alter pulmonary blood flow distribution by preferentially perfusing dilated vessels in the lung bases, hypoxemia in HPS may worsen in the upright position (orthodeoxia),[49] with patients reporting increased shortness of breath while sitting as opposed to lying (platypnea). However, these classically described manifestations of HPS are not sensitive indicators of the disease.[50] Spider nevi may be a marker of IPVD and an indicator of more severe hypoxemia, but this cutaneous manifestation is also common in patients with cirrhosis without HPS.[47] Although patients may report shortness of breath, cough is not a common symptom. In addition, patients with significant hypoxemia may also have clubbing in the fingers and toes as well as distal cyanosis if the hypoxemia is severe.[51]

DIAGNOSIS

Formal diagnostic criteria for HPS are now accepted and include documentation of impaired oxygenation in the setting of IPVD and liver disease or portal hypertension (**Table 1**).[52] It is not necessary that patients be hypoxemic because milder forms of HPS are associated solely with a reduction in the partial pressure of carbon dioxide ($Paco_2$) caused by hyperventilation. Therefore, the alteration in oxygenation in patients with HPS is determined by calculating the alveolar-arterial oxygen gradient ($Aapo_2$) from an arterial blood gas (ABG); a threshold of greater than 15 mm Hg is used except for patients older than 64 years, in whom 20 mm Hg is appropriate. Using this threshold of the $Aapo_2$, the severity of HPS is then determined by the degree of hypoxemia, providing a classification scheme with 4 stages from mild to very severe disease (**Table 2**).[52] Although the hypoxemia may be severe while breathing ambient air, the partial pressure of oxygen (Pao_2) usually increases to greater than 300 mm Hg by breathing 100% oxygen.[47] As was also mentioned, the syndrome may occur in

Table 1
Diagnostic criteria for the hepatopulmonary syndrome

	Defining Criteria
Impaired oxygenation	Pao_2 <80 mm Hg Or Increased age-corrected $Aapo_2{}^a$ (>15 mm Hg or >20 mm Hg if age >64 y) while breathing ambient air
Intrapulmonary vasodilatation	Confirmed by contrast-enhanced echocardiography or lung perfusion scanning (brain shunt fraction >6%)
Liver disease	Cirrhosis and/or portal hypertension

Abbreviation: $Aapo_2$, alveolar-arterial oxygen gradient.
a $Aapo_2 = (Fio_2 [P_{atm}-P_{H_2O}]-[Pco_2/0.8])-Pao_2$, where Pao_2 represents partial pressure of arterial oxygen; Fio_2, fraction of inspired oxygen; P_{atm}, atmospheric pressure; P_{H_2O}, partial pressure of water vapor at body temperature; and $Paco_2$, partial pressure of arterial carbon dioxide (0.8 corresponds with the standard gas-exchange respiratory ratio at rest).

patients with comorbid primary lung diseases,[53,54] and having cirrhosis is not imperative because HPS has been described in cases of acute and chronic hepatitis without cirrhosis or portal hypertension[55,56] as well as in noncirrhotic portal hypertension without chronic liver disease.[57–59]

Several radiographic modalities exist to evaluate for the presence of IPVD.[53,60,61] The most sensitive is a contrast-enhanced transthoracic echocardiogram (CEE), in which saline is agitated (creating microbubbles >10 μm in size) and infused into a peripheral vein, opacifying the right atrium and ventricle of the heart within seconds.[60] Under normal circumstances, the bubbles are absorbed in the lung vasculature. Early visualization of bubbles in the left heart in fewer than 3 cardiac cycles after being seen on the right side is a result of intracardiac shunting, whereas delayed appearance (>3 cardiac cycles) is caused by IPVD. Up to 60% of patients with cirrhosis referred for liver transplant have a positive CEE, but only half of them have HPS.[50,60,62] The clinical significance of subclinical IPVD, namely IPVD with a normal $Aapo_2$, is not known. Contrasted echocardiography is a qualitative test designed to determine the absence or presence of IPVD. A semiquantitative measurement of shunting has been developed, but a correlation between the degree of shunting and severity of hypoxemia has not been established.[61]

Another diagnostic modality that is less sensitive than CEE is a nuclear medicine lung perfusion scan, in which technetium-labeled macroaggregates of albumin (99mTcMAA) up to 20 μm are injected in a peripheral vein. The aggregates are trapped in the normal pulmonary vasculature but gain access to the systemic circulation in patients with IPVD or any other form of intracardiac or pulmonary venous-arterial shunting, allowing the aggregates to be detected and measured by scintigraphy. The shunt fraction is the ratio of brain to total-body 99mTcMAA; a positive result is greater than

Table 2
Staging severity of the hepatopulmonary syndrome

Stage	Partial Pressure of Oxygen Thresholds (mm Hg)
Mild	≥80
Moderate	≥60 to <80
Severe	≥50 to <60
Very severe	<50 (or <300 while breathing 100% oxygen)

6%.[53] The lung perfusion scan is less sensitive that CEE in detecting IPVD and is most useful in trying to determine the contribution of HPS to hypoxemia in patients with co-morbid lung diseases. In addition, pulmonary arteriography can be done, but is not routinely recommended unless there is poor responsiveness to 100% inspired oxygen or if there is a suggestion of direct arteriovenous communications that might be amenable to coil embolization because this diagnostic modality is expensive, invasive, and insensitive in detecting IPVD.

Screening for HPS

Because the diagnosis of HPS requires an ABG, it is not practical to screen all patients with cirrhosis using this modality. Pulse oximetry to measure arterial oxygen saturation (SaO_2) can be readily obtained in the clinical setting and has been validated as a means of screening for arterial hypoxemia in patients with cirrhosis.[63,64] Pulse oximetry over-estimates SaO_2. Therefore, an SaO_2 threshold of less than or equal to 97% is able to detect patients with HPS with a PaO_2 less than 70 mm Hg with good sensitivity and specificity (100% and 65% respectively), whereas an SaO_2 threshold of less than or equal to 94% can be used to identify patients with HPS with more severe hypoxemia (ie, PaO_2 <60 mm Hg; sensitivity 100% and specificity 93%).[63] Screening with pulse oximetry is cost-effective, restricting the need for CEE and ABG testing to those patients with cirrhosis with significant hypoxemia (see **Fig. 3** for an overview of the evaluation of hypoxemia in patients with chronic liver disease).[64]

THERAPEUTIC OPTIONS
Pharmacologic Treatment

There are no therapeutic options that reliably improve oxygenation in patients with HPS aside from LT. Several uncontrolled therapeutic trials have been reported, but

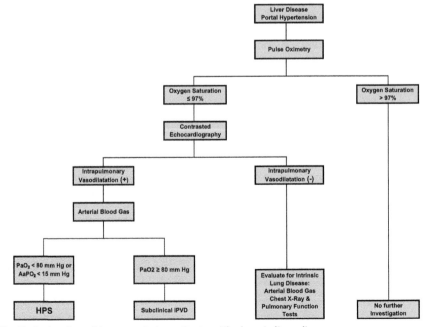

Fig. 3. Evaluation of hypoxemia in patients with chronic liver disease.

none have been sufficiently powered to show a durable improvement in oxygenation. These trials have included agents that manipulate the NO pathway, such as intravenous methylene blue (inhibits the effect of NO on guanylate cyclase)[39–42] and N(G)-nitro-L-arginine methyl ester (L-NAME; reduces NO production by inhibiting eNOS),[43,44] somatostatin,[65] almitrine (pulmonary vasoconstrictor),[66,67] cyclooxygenase inhibitors,[68,69] propranolol (ameliorate portal hypertension),[70,71] antibiotics (selective gut decontamination),[22,72] pentoxifylline (TNF-α inhibitor),[27] and garlic.[73] In addition, patients with HPS are offered oxygen for severe hypoxemia, particularly with significant exercise-induced desaturation. However, supplemental oxygen has never been shown to reliably help dyspnea or improve quality of life in patients with HPS. Nonetheless, it is inexpensive and without significant side effects, so it is routinely used in clinical practice.

Transjugular Intrahepatic Portosystemic Shunt

There have been 7 case reports studying the effect of transjugular intrahepatic shunt (TIPS) in patients with HPS.[74–83] Similar to the pharmacologic therapies discussed, TIPS has not been a consistently beneficial treatment option for HPS. Although some patients did have an improvement in oxygenation after the TIPS was placed,[75–79] the short duration of follow-up[83] and comorbid complications of cirrhosis such as hepatic hydrothorax that are improved by TIPS placement[83] make it difficult to know whether the TIPS provides a lasting benefit. Adding doubt to the therapeutic potential of TIPS, there was no improvement in the pulmonary vasodilatation on the lung perfusion scan in 1 case report,[75] and there are reported cases of HPS developing de novo after TIPS placemen.[74] Given the potential risk for hepatic decompensation and encephalopathy after TIPS placement, its use is not recommended to treat HPS. However, TIPS does not seem to exacerbate the oxygen impairment in HPS, so it can be used to manage the complications of portal hypertension for which it is indicated (such as refractory ascites and variceal bleeding) in patients with concurrent HPS.

LT

LT is the only therapeutic option that can dependably improve oxygenation and survival in patients with HPS.[84–86] However, several reports suggest that patients with more significant hypoxemia (Pao_2 <50 mm Hg while breathing ambient air) had high post-LT mortality,[87] resulting in patients with severe HPS being excluded from their only potential therapeutic option. In addition, the severity of HPS does not correlate with the degree of liver disease, so patients with HPS might not otherwise need an LT for the underlying cirrhosis. Although LT is an effective treatment of HPS, the hypoxemia is usually slow to resolve, with most patients requiring 6 to 12 months for oxygenation to normalize.[84,85,87,88] There are also reports of recovery times of longer than 12 months,[89] especially for patients with more severe pre-LT hypoxemia.[84,89]

Because HPS is progressive and is associated with high pre-LT mortality, patients with significant hypoxemia are eligible for Model for End-stage Liver Disease (MELD) exception points.[90] Post-LT survival may have improved in patients with HPS since introducing the MELD exception policy,[86] but this has not been rigorously studied across the transplant centers. An analysis of the data from the Scientific Registry of Transplant Recipients (SRTR) from 2002 to 2005 compared post-LT survival between patients with HPS listed with a MELD exception with patients with cirrhosis transplanted without an HPS exception. Applying MELD exception points for HPS favored these patients in terms of overall survival.[91] However, the SRTR database does not collect data to allow confirmation of the diagnosis of HPS or determination of the severity of hypoxemia.

Aside from this analysis of the SRTR database, the published outcomes after LT in patients with HPS have largely been confined to single-center studies with small numbers of patients being analyzed. To date, there have been 16 retrospective case series that included at least 5 patients with HPS in the report[84,86–89,92–102] and 1 prospective cohort study published.[103] There is significant heterogeneity among the series with regard to the criteria used to diagnose HPS, making comparisons between them difficult. The 30-day mortality in these publications ranged from 0% to 44%. As mentioned, some reports raised concern that mortality was higher in those patients with more severe pre-LT hypoxemia,[87,96,98] but others did not find this relationship.[84,86,88,89,102] The largest of these studies was a recent, retrospective, single-center study representing patients with severe HPS (defined as a Pao_2 $\leq$70 mm Hg) over 25 years.[86] The investigators determined that severity of hypoxemia did not predict early post-LT mortality and that outcomes may have improved over time as a result of the MELD exception policy for HPS (although this time-sensitive analysis did not reach statistical significance),[86] supporting the existing HPS exception policy for LT.

SUMMARY

HPS is a common complication of cirrhosis that results from alterations in the intrapulmonary vasculature. The pathophysiology of HPS is not clearly defined in humans, and this has limited the discovery of pharmacologic agents that could reverse the underlying process and improve oxygenation. The disorder is associated with increased mortality compared with patients with cirrhosis without HPS, and LT is the only available treatment option. However, severity of hypoxemia does not necessarily parallel the degree of liver dysfunction, so patients are currently eligible for MELD exception points to permit transplantation.

REFERENCES

1. Fluckiger M. Vorkommen von trommelschagel formigen fingerendphalangen ohne chronische veranderungen an der lungen oder am herzen. Wien Med Wochenschr 1884;34:1457.
2. Rodman T, Hurwitz JK, Pastor BH, et al. Cyanosis, clubbing and arterial oxygen unsaturation associated with Laennec's cirrhosis. Am J Med Sci 1959;238: 534–41.
3. Evans PR. Biliary cirrhosis with cyanosis and finger-clubbing. Proc R Soc Med 1937;30:406–9.
4. Keys A, Snell AM. Respiratory properties of the arterial blood in normal man and in patients with disease of the liver: position of the oxygen dissociation curve. J Clin Invest 1938;17:59–67.
5. Heinemann HO, Emirgil C, Mijnssen JP. Hyperventilation and arterial hypoxemia in cirrhosis of the liver. Am J Med 1960;28:239–46.
6. Abelmann WH, Kramer GE, Verstraeten JM, et al. Cirrhosis of the liver and decreased arterial oxygen saturation. Arch Intern Med 1961;108:34–40.
7. Berthelot P, Walker JG, Sherlock S, et al. Arterial changes in the lungs in cirrhosis of the liver–lung spider nevi. N Engl J Med 1966;274:291–8.
8. Kennedy TC, Knudson RJ. Exercise-aggravated hypoxemia and orthodeoxia in cirrhosis. Chest 1977;72:305–9.
9. Fallon MB, Abrams GA, Luo B, et al. The role of endothelial nitric oxide synthase in the pathogenesis of a rat model of hepatopulmonary syndrome. Gastroenterology 1997;113:606–14.

10. Fallon MB, Abrams GA, McGrath JW, et al. Common bile duct ligation in the rat: a model of intrapulmonary vasodilatation and hepatopulmonary syndrome. Am J Phys 1997;272:G779–84.

11. Zhang J, Ling Y, Luo B, et al. Analysis of pulmonary heme oxygenase-1 and nitric oxide synthase alterations in experimental hepatopulmonary syndrome. Gastroenterology 2003;125:1441–51.

12. Zhang M, Luo B, Chen SJ, et al. Endothelin-1 stimulation of endothelial nitric oxide synthase in the pathogenesis of hepatopulmonary syndrome. Am J Phys 1999;277:G944–52.

13. Zhang XJ, Katsuta Y, Akimoto T, et al. Intrapulmonary vascular dilatation and nitric oxide in hypoxemic rats with chronic bile duct ligation. J Hepatol 2003;39: 724–30.

14. Katsuta Y, Zhang XJ, Ohsuga M, et al. Arterial hypoxemia and intrapulmonary vasodilatation in rat models of portal hypertension. J Gastroenterol 2005;40: 811–9.

15. Lee KN, Yoon SK, Lee JW, et al. Hepatopulmonary syndrome induced by common bile duct ligation in a rabbit model: correlation between pulmonary vascular dilatation on thin-section CT and angiography and serum nitrite concentration or endothelial nitric oxide synthase (eNOS)1 expression. Korean J Radiol 2004;5: 149–56.

16. Liu M, Tian D, Wang T, et al. Correlation between pulmonary endothelin receptors and alveolar-arterial oxygen gradient in rats with hepatopulmonary syndrome. J Huazhong Univ Sci Technolog Med Sci 2005;25: 494–6.

17. Ling Y, Zhang J, Luo B, et al. The role of endothelin-1 and the endothelin B receptor in the pathogenesis of hepatopulmonary syndrome in the rat. Hepatology 2004;39:1593–602.

18. Luo B, Abrams GA, Fallon MB. Endothelin-1 in the rat bile duct ligation model of hepatopulmonary syndrome: correlation with pulmonary dysfunction. J Hepatol 1998;29:571–8.

19. Luo B, Liu L, Tang L, et al. Increased pulmonary vascular endothelin B receptor expression and responsiveness to endothelin-1 in cirrhotic and portal hypertensive rats: a potential mechanism in experimental hepatopulmonary syndrome. J Hepatol 2003;38:556–63.

20. Luo B, Tang L, Wang Z, et al. Cholangiocyte endothelin 1 and transforming growth factor beta1 production in rat experimental hepatopulmonary syndrome. Gastroenterology 2005;129:682–95.

21. Luo B, Tang L, Zhang J, et al. Biliary epithelium derived endothelin-1: an endocrine mediator of experimental hepatopulmonary syndrome. Hepatology 2004; 40:214A.

22. Rabiller A, Nunes H, Lebrec D, et al. Prevention of gram-negative translocation reduces the severity of hepatopulmonary syndrome. Am J Respir Crit Care Med 2002;166:514–7.

23. Sztrymf B, Libert JM, Mougeot C, et al. Cirrhotic rats with bacterial translocation have higher incidence and severity of hepatopulmonary syndrome. J Gastroenterol Hepatol 2005;20:1538–44.

24. Liu L, Liu N, Zhao Z, et al. TNF-alpha neutralization improves experimental hepatopulmonary syndrome in rats. Liver Int 2012;32:1018–26.

25. Luo B, Liu L, Tang L, et al. ET-1 and TNF-alpha in HPS: analysis in prehepatic portal hypertension and biliary and nonbiliary cirrhosis in rats. Am J Physiol Gastrointest Liver Physiol 2004;286:G294–303.

26. Sztrymf B, Rabiller A, Nunes H, et al. Prevention of hepatopulmonary syndrome and hyperdynamic state by pentoxifylline in cirrhotic rats. Eur Respir J 2004;23: 752–8.

27. Tanikella R, Philips GM, Faulk DK, et al. Pilot study of pentoxifylline in hepatopulmonary syndrome. Liver Transpl 2008;14:1199–203.

28. Zhang J, Ling Y, Tang L, et al. Pentoxifylline attenuation of experimental hepatopulmonary syndrome. J Appl Phys 2007;102:949–55.

29. Thenappan T, Goel A, Marsboom G, et al. A central role for CD68(+) macrophages in hepatopulmonary syndrome. Reversal by macrophage depletion. Am J Respir Crit Care Med 2011;183:1080–91.

30. Zhang J, Yang W, Luo B, et al. The role of CX(3)CL1/CX(3)CR1 in pulmonary angiogenesis and intravascular monocyte accumulation in rat experimental hepatopulmonary syndrome. J Hepatol 2012;57:752–8.

31. Carter EP, Hartsfield CL, Miyazono M, et al. Regulation of heme oxygenase-1 by nitric oxide during hepatopulmonary syndrome. Am J Physiol Lung Cell Mol Physiol 2002;283:L346–53.

32. Mejias M, Garcia-Pras E, Tiani C, et al. Beneficial effects of sorafenib on splanchnic, intrahepatic, and portocollateral circulations in portal hypertensive and cirrhotic rats. Hepatology 2009;49:1245–56.

33. Chang CC, Chuang CL, Lee FY, et al. Sorafenib treatment improves hepatopulmonary syndrome in rats with biliary cirrhosis. Clin Sci (Lond) 2013;124: 457–66.

34. Zhang J, Luo B, Tang L, et al. Pulmonary angiogenesis in a rat model of hepatopulmonary syndrome. Gastroenterology 2009;136:1070–80.

35. Cremona G, Higenbottam TW, Mayoral V, et al. Elevated exhaled nitric oxide in patients with hepatopulmonary syndrome. Eur Respir J 1995;8:1883–5.

36. Rolla G, Brussino L, Colagrande P, et al. Exhaled nitric oxide and oxygenation abnormalities in hepatic cirrhosis. Hepatology 1997;26:842–7.

37. Rolla G, Brussino L, Colagrande P, et al. Exhaled nitric oxide and impaired oxygenation in cirrhotic patients before and after liver transplantation. Ann Intern Med 1998;129:375–8.

38. Fallon MB. Methylene blue and cirrhosis: pathophysiologic insights, therapeutic dilemmas. Ann Intern Med 2000;133:738–40.

39. Groneberg DA, Fischer A. Methylene blue improves the hepatopulmonary syndrome. Ann Intern Med 2001;135:380–1.

40. Jounieaux V, Leleu O, Mayeux I. Cardiopulmonary effects of nitric oxide inhalation and methylene blue injection in hepatopulmonary syndrome. Intensive Care Med 2001;27:1103–4.

41. Rolla G, Bucca C, Brussino L. Methylene blue in the hepatopulmonary syndrome. N Engl J Med 1994;331:1098.

42. Schenk P, Madl C, Rezaie-Majd S, et al. Methylene blue improves the hepatopulmonary syndrome. Ann Intern Med 2000;133:701–6.

43. Brussino L, Bucca C, Morello M, et al. Effect on dyspnoea and hypoxaemia of inhaled N(G)-nitro-L-arginine methyl ester in hepatopulmonary syndrome. Lancet 2003;362:43–4.

44. Gomez FP, Barbera JA, Roca J, et al. Effects of nebulized N(G)-nitro-L-arginine methyl ester in patients with hepatopulmonary syndrome. Hepatology 2006;43: 1084–91.

45. Roberts KE, Kawut SM, Krowka MJ, et al. Genetic risk factors for hepatopulmonary syndrome in patients with advanced liver disease. Gastroenterology 2010; 139:130–9.e24.

46. Koch DG, Bogatkevich G, Ramshesh V, et al. Elevated levels of endothelin-1 in hepatic venous blood are associated with intrapulmonary vasodilatation in humans. Dig Dis Sci 2012;57(2):516–23.
47. Rodriguez-Roisin R, Roca J, Agusti AG, et al. Gas exchange and pulmonary vascular reactivity in patients with liver cirrhosis. Am Rev Respir Dis 1987;135:1085–92.
48. Sood G, Fallon MB, Niwas S, et al. Utility of dyspnea-fatigue index for screening liver transplant candidates for hepatopulmonary syndrome. Hepatology 1998;28:2319 [abstract].
49. Gomez FP, Martinez-Palli G, Barbera JA, et al. Gas exchange mechanism of orthodeoxia in hepatopulmonary syndrome. Hepatology 2004;40:660–6.
50. Martinez GP, Barbera JA, Visa J, et al. Hepatopulmonary syndrome in candidates for liver transplantation. J Hepatol 2001;34:651–7.
51. Fallon M, Abrams G. Pulmonary dysfunction in chronic liver disease. Hepatology 2000;32:859–65.
52. Rodriguez-Roisin R, Krowka MJ, Herve P, et al. Pulmonary-hepatic vascular disorders (PHD). Eur Respir J 2004;24:861–80.
53. Abrams GA, Nanda NC, Dubovsky EV, et al. Use of macroaggregated albumin lung perfusion scan to diagnose hepatopulmonary syndrome: a new approach. Gastroenterology 1998;114:305–10.
54. Martinez G, Barbera JA, Navasa M, et al. Hepatopulmonary syndrome associated with cardiorespiratory disease. J Hepatol 1999;30:882–9.
55. Regev A, Yeshurun M, Rodriguez M, et al. Transient hepatopulmonary syndrome in a patient with acute hepatitis A. J Viral Hepat 2001;8:83–6.
56. Teuber G, Teupe C, Dietrich CF, et al. Pulmonary dysfunction in non-cirrhotic patients with chronic viral hepatitis. Eur J Intern Med 2002;13:311–8.
57. Gupta D, Vijaya DR, Gupta R, et al. Prevalence of hepatopulmonary syndrome in cirrhosis and extrahepatic portal venous obstruction. Am J Gastroenterol 2001;96:3395–9.
58. De BK, Sen S, Biswas PK, et al. Occurrence of hepatopulmonary syndrome in Budd-Chiari syndrome and the role of venous decompression. Gastroenterology 2002;122:897–903.
59. Krowka MJ. Hepatopulmonary syndrome and extrahepatic vascular abnormalities. Liver Transpl 2001;7:656–7.
60. Abrams GA, Jaffe CC, Hoffer PB, et al. Diagnostic utility of contrast echocardiography and lung perfusion scan in patients with hepatopulmonary syndrome. Gastroenterology 1995;109:1283–8.
61. Vedrinne JM, Duperret S, Bizollon T, et al. Comparison of transesophageal and transthoracic contrast echocardiography for detection of an intrapulmonary shunt in liver disease. Chest 1997;111:1236–40.
62. Schenk P, Fuhrmann V, Madl C, et al. Hepatopulmonary syndrome: prevalence and predictive value of various cut offs for arterial oxygenation and their clinical consequences. Gut 2002;51:853–9.
63. Arguedas MR, Singh H, Faulk DK, et al. Utility of pulse oximetry screening for hepatopulmonary syndrome. Clin Gastroenterol Hepatol 2007;5:749–54.
64. Roberts DN, Arguedas MR, Fallon MB. Cost-effectiveness of screening for hepatopulmonary syndrome in liver transplant candidates. Liver Transpl 2007;13:206–14.
65. Krowka MJ, Dickson ER, Cortese DA. Hepatopulmonary syndrome. Clinical observations and lack of therapeutic response to somatostatin analogue. Chest 1993;104:515–21.

66. Krowka MJ, Cortese DA. Severe hypoxemia associated with liver disease: Mayo Clinic experience and the experimental use of almitrine bismesylate. Mayo Clin Proc 1987;62:164–73.

67. Nakos G, Evrenoglou D, Vassilakis N, et al. Haemodynamics and gas exchange in liver cirrhosis: the effect of orally administered almitrine bismesylate. Respir Med 1993;87:93–8.

68. Shijo H, Sasaki H, Yuh K, et al. Effects of indomethacin on hepatogenic pulmonary angiodysplasia. Chest 1991;99:1027–9.

69. Song JY, Choi JY, Ko JT, et al. Long-term aspirin therapy for hepatopulmonary syndrome. Pediatrics 1996;97:917–20.

70. Agusti AG, Roca J, Bosch J, et al. Effects of propranolol on arterial oxygenation and oxygen transport to tissues in patients with cirrhosis. Am Rev Respir Dis 1990;142:306–10.

71. Lambrecht GL, Malbrain ML, Coremans P, et al. Orthodeoxia and platypnea in liver cirrhosis: effects of propranolol. Acta Clin Belg 1994;49: 26–30.

72. Anel RM, Sheagren JN. Novel presentation and approach to management of hepatopulmonary syndrome with use of antimicrobial agents. Clin Infect Dis 2001;32:E131–6.

73. Abrams GA, Fallon MB. Treatment of hepatopulmonary syndrome with *Allium sativum* L. (garlic): a pilot trial. J Clin Gastroenterol 1998;27:232–5.

74. Corley DA, Scharschmidt B, Bass N, et al. Lack of efficacy of TIPS for hepatopulmonary syndrome. Gastroenterology 1997;113:728–30.

75. Allgaier HP, Haag K, Ochs A, et al. Hepato-pulmonary syndrome: successful treatment by transjugular intrahepatic portosystemic stent-shunt (TIPS). J Hepatol 1995;23:102.

76. Benitez C, Arrese M, Jorquera J, et al. Successful treatment of severe hepatopulmonary syndrome with a sequential use of TIPS placement and liver transplantation. Ann Hepatol 2009;8:71–4.

77. Chevallier P, Novelli L, Motamedi JP, et al. Hepatopulmonary syndrome successfully treated with transjugular intrahepatic portosystemic shunt: a three-year follow-up. J Vasc Interv Radiol 2004;15:647–8.

78. Nistal MW, Pace A, Klose H, et al. Hepatopulmonary syndrome caused by sarcoidosis of the liver treated with transjugular intrahepatic portosystemic shunt. Thorax 2013;68:889–90.

79. Paramesh AS, Husain SZ, Shneider B, et al. Improvement of hepatopulmonary syndrome after transjugular intrahepatic portasystemic shunting: case report and review of literature. Pediatr Transplant 2003;7:157–62.

80. Lasch HM, Fried MW, Zacks SL, et al. Use of transjugular intrahepatic portosystemic shunt as a bridge to liver transplantation in a patient with severe hepatopulmonary syndrome. Liver Transpl 2001;7:147–9.

81. Martinez-Palli G, Drake BB, Garcia-Pagan JC, et al. Effect of transjugular intrahepatic portosystemic shunt on pulmonary gas exchange in patients with portal hypertension and hepatopulmonary syndrome. World J Gastroenterol 2005;11: 6858–62.

82. Riegler JL, Lang KA, Johnson SP, et al. Transjugular intrahepatic portosystemic shunt improves oxygenation in hepatopulmonary syndrome. Gastroenterology 1995;109:978–83.

83. Selim KM, Akriviadis EA, Zuckerman E, et al. Transjugular intrahepatic portosystemic shunt: a successful treatment for hepatopulmonary syndrome. Am J Gastroenterol 1998;93:455–8.

84. Gupta S, Castel H, Rao RV, et al. Improved survival after liver transplantation in patients with hepatopulmonary syndrome. Am J Transplant 2010;10: 354–63.
85. Swanson KL, Wiesner RH, Krowka MJ. Natural history of hepatopulmonary syndrome: impact of liver transplantation. Hepatology 2005;41:1122–9.
86. Iyer VN, Swanson KL, Cartin-Ceba R, et al. Hepatopulmonary syndrome: favorable outcomes in the MELD exception era. Hepatology 2013;57:2427–35.
87. Arguedas MR, Abrams GA, Krowka MJ, et al. Prospective evaluation of outcomes and predictors of mortality in patients with hepatopulmonary syndrome undergoing liver transplantation. Hepatology 2003;37:192–7.
88. Collisson EA, Nourmand H, Fraiman MH, et al. Retrospective analysis of the results of liver transplantation for adults with severe hepatopulmonary syndrome. Liver Transpl 2002;8:925–31.
89. Taille C, Cadranel J, Bellocq A, et al. Liver transplantation for hepatopulmonary syndrome: a ten-year experience in Paris, France. Transplantation 2003;75: 1482–9 [discussion: 46–7].
90. Fallon MB, Mulligan DC, Gish RG, et al. Model for end-stage liver disease (MELD) exception for hepatopulmonary syndrome. Liver Transpl 2006; 12(Suppl 3):S105–7.
91. Sulieman BM, Hunsicker LG, Katz DA, et al. OPTN policy regarding prioritization of patients with hepatopulmonary syndrome: does it provide equitable organ allocation? Am J Transplant 2008;8:954–64.
92. Barbe T, Losay J, Grimon G, et al. Pulmonary arteriovenous shunting in children with liver disease. J Pediatr 1995;126:571–9.
93. Deberaldini M, Arcanjo AB, Melo E, et al. Hepatopulmonary syndrome: morbidity and survival after liver transplantation. Transplant Proc 2008;40: 3512–6.
94. Egawa H, Kasahara M, Inomata Y, et al. Long-term outcome of living related liver transplantation for patients with intrapulmonary shunting and strategy for complications. Transplantation 1999;67:712–7.
95. Fewtrell MS, Noble-Jamieson G, Revell S, et al. Intrapulmonary shunting in the biliary atresia/polysplenia syndrome: reversal after liver transplantation. Arch Dis Child 1994;70:501–4.
96. Hobeika J, Houssin D, Bernard O, et al. Orthotopic liver transplantation in children with chronic liver disease and severe hypoxemia. Transplantation 1994;57: 224–8.
97. Kim HY, Choi MS, Lee SC, et al. Outcomes in patients with hepatopulmonary syndrome undergoing liver transplantation. Transplant Proc 2004;36: 2762–3.
98. Krowka MJ, Mandell MS, Ramsay MA, et al. Hepatopulmonary syndrome and portopulmonary hypertension: a report of the multicenter liver transplant database. Liver Transpl 2004;10:174–82.
99. Schenk P, Schoniger-Hekele M, Fuhrmann V, et al. Prognostic significance of the hepatopulmonary syndrome in patients with cirrhosis. Gastroenterology 2003; 125:1042–52.
100. Schiffer E, Majno P, Mentha G, et al. Hepatopulmonary syndrome increases the postoperative mortality rate following liver transplantation: a prospective study in 90 patients. Am J Transplant 2006;6:1430–7.
101. Saigal S, Choudhary N, Saraf N, et al. Excellent outcome of living donor liver transplantation in patients with hepatopulmonary syndrome: a single centre experience. Clin Transplant 2013;27:530–4.

102. Scott V, Miro A, Kang Y, et al. Reversibility of the hepatopulmonary syndrome by orthotopic liver transplantation. Transplant Proc 1993;25:1787–8.
103. Fallon MB, Krowka MJ, Brown RS, et al. Impact of hepatopulmonary syndrome on quality of life and survival in liver transplant candidates. Gastroenterology 2008;135(4):1168–75.

Portopulmonary Hypertension

Rodrigo Cartin-Ceba, MD*, Michael J. Krowka, MD

KEYWORDS

- Portopulmonary hypertension • Cirrhosis • Liver transplant • Portal hypertension
- Pulmonary hypertension

KEY POINTS

- Pulmonary arterial hypertension (PAH) is a serious pulmonary vascular disease. When PAH occurs in the setting of portal hypertension, it is known as portopulmonary hypertension (POPH).
- Pulmonary hypertension in patients with liver disease or portal hypertension can be caused by multiple mechanisms, including hyperdynamic (high-flow) state, increased pulmonary venous congestion (pulmonary venous hypertension), and vascular constriction or obstruction of the pulmonary arterial bed (POPH).
- POPH is an uncommon and serious yet treatable pulmonary vascular consequence of cirrhotic and noncirrhotic portal hypertension; its pathophysiology remains unclear with no clear relationship to the cause of the liver disease or the severity of the portal hypertension. Its main presenting symptom is exertional dyspnea, and POPH may lead to right heart failure and death if untreated.
- Because of the spectrum of pulmonary hemodynamic changes associated with hepatic dysfunction, screening by transthoracic echocardiography and confirmation by right heart catheterization is necessary for accurate diagnosis and therapeutic considerations.
- Despite the lack of controlled studies, PAH-specific therapy in POPH can significantly improve pulmonary hemodynamics and right ventricular function. The potential to cure POPH, at least hemodynamically, with a combination of PAH-specific therapy and liver transplant seems to be an attainable goal in a cohort of patients with POPH yet to be optimally characterized.

INTRODUCTION

Portopulmonary hypertension (POPH) is a well-known serious complication of portal hypertension from cirrhotic and noncirrhotic causes. POPH is defined as the presence of pulmonary artery hypertension (PAH) that evolves as a consequence of portal hypertension[1] and is included in group I of the 2008 Dana Point classification of PAH.[1]

The authors have no disclosures.
Division of Pulmonary and Critical Care Medicine, Mayo Clinic, 200 1st Street Southwest, Rochester, MN 55905, USA
* Corresponding author.
E-mail address: cartinceba.rodrigo@mayo.edu

In epidemiologic studies, POPH has been documented in approximately 4.5% to 8.5% of liver transplant (LT) candidates.[2,3] Historically, the first description of POPH was provided by Mantz and Craige[4] in 1951 after describing the necropsy results of a 53-year-old woman with spontaneous portacaval shunt (caused by a probable congenital portal vein narrowing) that originated at the confluence of the portal, splenic, and mesenteric veins and coursed through to the mediastinum. The shunt was lined by varying amounts of thrombus thought to have embolized via the innominate vein into the right heart and pulmonary arteries. In addition to embolized small pulmonary arteries, an extreme endothelial proliferation and recanalization process was documented.[4] For POPH, specific screening recommendations and diagnostic criteria are now clearly defined, including the management of POPH in the setting of LT candidacy. Despite the lack of POPH-specific randomized controlled trials for PAH-specific therapy, extrapolation of the therapeutic advances in treating PAH with beneficial effects in POPH has stimulated ongoing interest and importance in this syndrome. This review article recapitulates the evolving knowledge in the diagnosis, management, and treatment of POPH.

POPH DEFINITION AND GENERAL CHARACTERISTICS

POPH should be clearly defined and recognized based on an accurate interpretation of hemodynamics obtained by right heart catheterization (RHC). All the following criteria should be met for the diagnosis of POPH:

- Portal hypertension: clinical diagnosis (ascites, varices, splenomegaly)
- Mean pulmonary artery pressure (MPAP): 25 mm Hg or greater
- Pulmonary vascular resistance (PVR): greater than 240 dyne/s/cm^{-5}
- Pulmonary capillary wedge pressure (PCWP): 15 mm Hg or less
- Transpulmonary gradient (TPG): greater than 12 mm Hg

In addition, the severity of POPH is defined based on the MPAP as follows: mild ($\geq$25 MPAP, <35 mm Hg), moderate ($\geq$35 MPAP, <45 mm Hg), and severe (>45 mm Hg MPAP). There are different pulmonary hemodynamic patterns that complicate advanced liver disease and are important to recognize during RHC (**Table 1**).[5,6] Distinguishing these 3 patterns is extremely important in the management of portal hypertension because therapies and outcomes clearly differ:

1. Hyperdynamic circulatory state induced by liver dysfunction
2. Excess pulmonary venous volume caused by diastolic dysfunction and/or renal insufficiency (pulmonary venous hypertension)
3. PAH caused by vascular obstruction (POPH)[7]

Furthermore, POPH should be distinguished from hepatopulmonary syndrome (HPS),[5,8] which is another major pulmonary vascular consequence of liver disease. In HPS, arterial hypoxemia is caused by intrapulmonary vascular dilatations (exactly opposite to the vascular obstructions documented in POPH) that form as a remodeling process caused by factors yet to be identified. In addition, the pulmonary hemodynamics associated with HPS reflect a normal PVR and usually a high-flow state characterized by an increased cardiac output (CO). The distinction between these two syndromes is very important, especially if LT is to be considered, because of the differences in risk, treatment options, and outcomes between these two syndromes.[8]

Mainly affecting adults, POPH has also been reported in the pediatric age group.[9] Autoimmune liver disorders (primary biliary cirrhosis and cirrhosis from autoimmune hepatitis) and female sex are more frequently associated with POPH according to

Table 1
Pulmonary hemodynamic patterns documented by RHC in advanced liver disease

	MPAP	PVR	Cardiac Output	PCWP
Vasoconstriction with vasoproliferation (POPH)	Elevated	Elevated	Low or normal	Normal
Fluid overload (excess volume)	Elevated	Normal or elevated	Elevated	Elevated
Hyperdynamic circulatory state (high flow)	Elevated	Normal	Elevated	Normal

a recent study.[10] The presence of spontaneous portacaval shunts is more frequent in those with POPH; patients with previous surgical portacaval shunts have a high frequency of POPH years after that surgery.[11–13] Splenectomy accomplished during portacaval shunt surgery may also be a risk factor for POPH.[14] There seems to be no relationship to the existence or severity of POPH with the severity of liver dysfunction as characterized by the Child-Turcotte-Pugh or Model for End-Stage Liver Disease (MELD) scores.[9,15]

Important similarities and differences between POPH and other phenotypes of PAH exist. Compared with idiopathic PAH (IPAH), POPH is characterized by higher CO and generally less degrees of severity as measured by MPAP and PVR.[16,17] In addition, patients with POPH not infrequently have a history of splenectomy, which may be an independent factor to develop PAH.[14] Finally, it is not uncommon for patients with an initial diagnosis of IPAH to later determine, because of thrombocytopenia and other imaging (even in the setting of normal liver function tests), that portal hypertension exists and POPH is the correct diagnosis.

PATHOPHYSIOLOGY

Genetic predisposition may play a role because not all patients with portal hypertension caused by cirrhosis develop POPH.[18] Furthermore, the histopathologic changes from POPH are indistinguishable from the changes observed in other PAH phenotypes.[7,19] Based on autopsy and lung explant studies, POPH is characterized by a spectrum of obstructive and remodeling changes in the pulmonary arterial bed. Initially, medial hypertrophy with smooth muscle proliferation and a transition to myofibroblasts has been documented. As this proliferative pathologic process advances, platelet aggregates, in situ thrombosis, intimal fibrosis, and finally, weblike shape lesions develop involving the entire pulmonary arterial wall with recanalization for the passage of pulmonary arterial blood.[7,19] This weblike lesion is termed *plexogenic arteriopathy*, and it is unknown whether such structures are irreversible.[19] The factors leading to such pulmonary vascular obstruction in the setting of liver disease are complex but originate from the development of portal hypertension. The pulmonary vascular changes occurs within the context of a hyperdynamic state caused by extrahepatic (splanchnic) vasodilation.[9] It is unknown if this persistent high flow state initiates (by shear stress) or exacerbates (in combination with circulating mediators) the pulmonary vascular proliferative process. It has been demonstrated that the pulmonary endothelial cells lack prostacyclin synthase in patients with POPH (hence a lack of prostacyclin-vasodilation)[20]; the pulmonary vascular bed is exposed to increased levels of circulating endothlin-1 in the setting of cirrhosis (a potent vasoconstrictor and facilitator of smooth muscle proliferation)[21,22] and may be deficient in local nitric oxide effect (for vasodilation).[23] The role of other circulating and receptor factors that may affect the pulmonary endothelium is speculative. These factors include vasoconstrictive/proliferative mediators, such as serotonin, thromboxane, vasoactive intestinal peptide, and vascular endothelial growth factor, as well as the possible imbalance of endothelin receptors (Endothelin receptor A [mediating vasoconstriction] and Endothelin receptor B [mediating vasodilation]) in the pulmonary arterial bed.[23] The mechanistic link between estrogen signaling, serum estradiol levels, circulating endothelial progenitor cells, and the development of POPH is a current research hypothesis of interest.[24,25]

Another hypothesis states that the intrahepatic injury leads to an intrahepatic increased resistance to flow-evoking mediators that cause splanchnic vasodilation via enhanced local nitric oxide effect and presumed angiogenesis effect.[9,26] The splanchnic bed becomes hyporesponsive to vasoconstrictors; excess volume occurs because of renal retention, and a hyperdynamic state is generated. This high flow exacerbates the existing portal hypertension because of increased intrahepatic resistance to flow, leading to the creation of alternative flow pathways: portacaval shunts and esophagogastric varices. Presumably, such aberrant pathways allow other mediators to reach the pulmonary arterial bed and, in the setting of high flow, trigger the pulmonary arterial proliferative process.

The resulting pulmonary hemodynamics have been well described: increased MPAP, high CO, and normal PCWP but an increased calculated PVR caused by the proliferative, obstructive process in the pulmonary arterial bed. Note that if the pulmonary vascular pathologic proliferative process does not occur, only a high-flow state exists with no obstruction to flow with resultant normal calculated PVR. Marked excess volume caused by fluid retention may occur and be reflected by increased PCWP. Depending on the existence of proliferation and the degree of such fluid retention, an increase in both PVR and PCWP can confuse the interpretation of pulmonary hemodynamics.[6] In that scenario, which may occur in up to 25% of patients with POPH,[9] the existence of obstruction to pulmonary arterial flow is manifest by an increased TPG (MPAP-PCWP >12 mm Hg). These patients should not be excluded from the diagnosis of POPH because of high PCWP alone. As the pulmonary vasoproliferative process progresses, the increasing resistance to flow will at some point begin to restrict the degree of CO flowing through the pulmonary vascular bed. Strain on the right ventricle (RV) will be seen with dilation of the RV and reduction in systolic function (as measured by reduced longitudinal contractility).[27] Progressive reduction in CO will then evolve with right heart failure leading to hepatic venous engorgement and worsening portal hypertension. Death of either right heart failure or portal hypertension complications will occur if no PAH-specific therapeutic intervention is attempted.[9]

EPIDEMIOLOGY AND MAIN OUTCOMES

The term POPH seems to have been initially used by Yoshida and colleagues[28] in 1993 as they described the first case of POPH to undergo successful LT (39-year-old man with long-standing chronic active hepatitis). Subsequently, several small series and case reports with autopsy results have described pulmonary arterial obstruction and pulmonary plexogenic arteriopathy with and without thromboemboli.[19,29–32] Large series have confirmed the coexistence of these portal and pulmonary vascular abnormalities and have shown that the association is not coincidental. An unselected series of 17,901 autopsies revealed that PAH was 5 times more likely in cirrhotic patients than those without liver disease.[33] Within the 1981–1987 National Institutes of Health's national registry of primary pulmonary hypertension from 32 centers reported by Rich and colleagues,[34] additional analyses by Groves and colleagues[35] concluded that

8.3% likely had POPH (17 of 204; 187 had primary pulmonary hypertension). The largest prospective study of patients with portal hypertension (n = 507) concluded that 2% had POPH.[15]

More recently, in the French pulmonary hypertension registry experience over a 12-month period (2002–2003), POPH was identified in 10.4% of the cases (70 of 674) from 17 university hospitals.[36] The Registry to Evaluate Early And Long-term Pulmonary Arterial Hypertension Disease Management (REVEAL registry) documented a 5.3% POPH frequency (174 of 3525) in the United States.[16] The largest POPH-LT center experiences reported to date are as follows: 8.5% (Baylor 102 of 1205; PVR >120 dyne/s/cm^{-5}), 6.1% (Clichy, France 10 of 165; PVR >120 dyne/s/cm^{-5}), and 5.3% (Mayo Clinic 66 of 1235; PVR >240 dyne/s/cm^{-5}).[6,37,38]

Outcomes of POPH have been confounded by small series from eras in which none of the current PAH-specific therapies were available or the experience with LT was not fully developed. Previous to the availability of continuous intravenous (IV) prostacyclin infusion, Robalino and Moodie[39] reported only a dismal 5-year 4% survival (n = 78). From the Mayo Clinic, Swanson and colleagues[40] reported a 14% 5-year survival in patients with POPH (n = 19) whereby LT was denied and patients were not treated with any of the current PAH-specific therapy. From the French National Center for PAH (n = 154 over a 20-year span until 2004, only one-third had been treated with PAH-specific therapy), Le Pavec and colleagues[2] described 1-, 3-, and 5-year survivals of 88%, 75%, and 68%, respectively, for patients with POPH (but mainly Child A and alcoholic cirrhosis). The causes of death in all series mentioned herein were equally distributed between right heart failure caused by POPH and direct complications of liver disease (bleeding, sepsis, hepatocellular carcinoma).

The REVEAL registry also presented 2 important observations related to POPH treatment and outcomes.[16] First, POPH treatment patterns demonstrated that the use of any PAH-specific therapy for POPH was delayed compared with patients diagnosed with IPAH. Specifically, at the time of entry into the registry only 25% were on PAH-specific therapy; by the end of the 12-month follow-up, 74% of those alive were on treatment. Second, although the baseline hemodynamics in POPH (MPAP and PVR) were significantly better than those with IPAH, the 1- and 3-year survivals were worse (**Fig. 1**); the 5-year survival for all patients with POPH was 40% versus 64% for IPAH. The causes of liver disease and causes of death were not determined in the registry, and survival was not analyzed by the type of PAH-specific therapy.

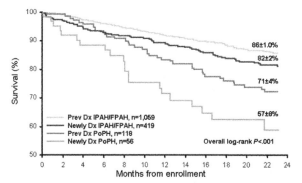

Fig. 1. REVEAL 2-year survival patterns for POPH and IPAH categorized by previous versus newly diagnosed (Dx) at the time of entry into the registry. FPAH, familial PAH. (*From* Krowka MJ, Miller DP, Barst RJ, et al. Portopulmonary hypertension: a report from the US-based REVEAL Registry. Chest 2012;141:909; with permission.)

Up until the publication of the Pulmonary Arterial Hypertension Soluble Guanylate Cyclase–Stimulator Trial (PATENT-1), which evaluated the use of riociguat in PAH and included 13 patients with POPH,[41] every controlled randomized study of PAH has excluded patients with POPH. This universal exclusion of POPH cases from clinical trials complicated the understanding of POPH outcomes compared with other PAH disorders. It is also important to mention that beginning in 2002, a higher priority for LT was an option for highly selected patients with POPH in the United States.[42] Only patients with moderate to severe POPH (MPAP >35 mm Hg) who attained significant hemodynamic improvement with PV therapy (MPAP <35 mm Hg and PVR <400 dyne/s/cm^{-5}) were granted higher priority for LT. From 2002 through 2010, 155 patients with POPH were granted such priority and underwent transplant by regional review boards.[43]

SCREENING FOR POPH

The most used and practical screening method to detect POPH has been transthoracic echocardiography (TTE).[44–46] By assessing the tricuspid regurgitant peak velocity (TR), estimating the right atrial pressure by inferior vena cava changes with inspiration, and using the modified Bernoulli equation, an estimate of RV systolic pressure (RVSP) can be determined in approximately 80% of patients with portal hypertension.[44] Determining the RVSP allows the clinician to decide which patients should proceed to RHC for the definitive diagnosis. At the authors' institution, the presence of RVSP greater than 50 mm Hg has been the cutoff criteria to proceed to RHC in a clinical algorithm followed since 1996.[6] Rarely, immeasurable TR with abnormal qualitative RV size or function results in RHC. TTE has been noted to have a 97% sensitivity and 77% specificity to detect moderate to severe PAH before LT.[44] A recent study reported that using a threshold of RVSP greater than 38 mm Hg by TTE, the sensitivity and specificity for the diagnosis of POPH was 100% and 82%, respectively.[3]

The American Association for the Study of Liver disease recommends TTE screening to detect pulmonary hypertension in every patient considered for LT in the United States.[47] LT candidates on no PAH-specific therapy and MPAP of 35 mm Hg or greater had significant elevated mortality.[48] Additional studies[49–51] reported first diagnosing POPH in the operating room after anesthesia induction (in the era before current PAH-specific therapy), noting that patients with mild to moderate POPH (MPAP <35 mm Hg) do quite well without pre-LT PAH-specific therapy. The goal of screening is to identify and treat those who have the highest risk of cardiopulmonary adversity during and after LT. Pulmonary hemodynamics in LT candidates may change over time; therefore, repetitive screening (every 12 months) is recommended.[37] Recent data also suggest that pretransplant echocardiographic findings, such as severity of tricuspid regurgitation, are associated with increased mortality and graft failure.[52]

CLINICAL MANIFESTATIONS

Dyspnea at rest or with exertion is by far the most common presenting symptom of POPH. Other causes of dyspnea that are common in patients with portal hypertension need to be excluded: ascites, anemia, fluid retention, and muscle wasting. Symptoms such as chest pain or syncope are usually markers of severe POPH.[9] Physical findings in POPH are usually absent, subtle, and nonspecific; however, some important findings may be noted, such as the presence of hyperdynamic precordium, an accentuated second heart sound (best heard at the apex) reflecting forceful closure of the pulmonic valve caused by high pulmonary artery pressures, and a systolic murmur during RV systolic function caused by tricuspid valve regurgitation. With severe POPH, there may be marked distension of the jugular veins, peripheral edema, ascites, and a RV third heart sound (S3). The lung examination is usually normal, and it is quite uncommon to have clubbing or cyanosis (as seen in HPS). Mild hypoxemia is common and often associated with abnormal overnight pulse oximetry. Rarely is severe hypoxemia documented, as opposed to being commonly seen in HPS.[9]

The chest radiograph usually demonstrates cardiomegaly and enlargement of the central pulmonary arteries as the duration and severity of POPH progresses (usually over many months).[9] The electrocardiogram may show a rightward electrical axis, right bundle branch block pattern; when POPH is severe, the presence of inverted T waves in the precordial V1-V4 leads can be seen, which suggests a severe effect on the RV. Although rare, it is important to rule out chronic pulmonary emboli as a cause of PAH even in the setting of liver disease, especially in the setting of portal vein and hepatic vein thromboses. Pulmonary function tests are usually not helpful in the diagnosis or management because a common abnormality seen in PAH, a reduced single breath diffusing capacity, is frequently seen in most patients with advanced liver disease.

MANAGEMENT AND MEDICAL TREATMENT OF POPH

The main initial questions that the clinician needs to answer in regard to the management of POPH are

1. Does the patient unequivocally have POPH?
2. What is the severity of POPH?
3. Does the patient need PAH-specific therapy?
4. What are the risks and what is the right timing for potential LT?

Patients with POPH with MPAP greater than 35 mm Hg are particularly vulnerable to poor outcomes with attempted LT, especially if there is no attempt to treat the POPH with current PAH-specific medications. With current treatments, POPH outcomes are variable; yet in highly selected patients with POPH, with aggressive treatment and successful LT, pulmonary hemodynamics may completely normalize. RV size and function normalizes, and liberation from PAH-specific medications may be allowed. In **Fig. 2**, the authors summarize the clinical algorithm followed at their institution based on RHC results.

The immediate goal in the management and treatment of POPH is to improve pulmonary hemodynamics by reducing the obstruction to pulmonary arterial flow. This goal can be accomplished by medications that result in vasodilation, antiplatelet aggregation, and antiproliferative effects.[9] This goal may be achieved by augmenting the lack of pulmonary endothelial prostacyclin synthase deficiency (prostacyclin infusion), blocking circulating endothelin-1 effects (endothelin receptor antagonists), and enhancing local nitric oxide vasodilatation effects (phosphodiesterase inhibitors and soluble guanylate cyclase stimulators).[9,53] The ultimate goal, in addition to favorably affecting pulmonary hemodynamics ($\downarrow$MPAP, $\downarrow$PVR, and $\uparrow$CO), is to stabilize, improve, and/or normalize RV function. It is very important to stress that improvements in both MPAP and PVR are the ideal goals in treating POPH. However, MPAP may not decrease as much as desired because increases in CO associated with reduced obstruction to flow (measured by decreased PVR) will result in higher flow (and increased pressure).

Uncontrolled small series and recent case reports have demonstrated that PAH-specific therapies used for other types of PAH could be beneficial for patients with

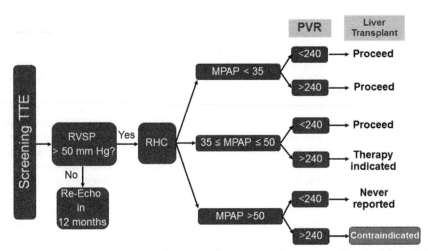

Fig. 2. Current POPH screening evaluation and treatment algorithm used at the Mayo Clinic. *Contraindicated* indicates high risk of intraoperative event at graft reperfusion; MPAP (normal <25 mm Hg); PVR (normal <240 dyne/s/cm^{-5} [or 3 Wood units]); RVSP estimated by TTE. NR, never reported.

POPH (**Table 2**).[54–71] The only randomized controlled trial that included patients with POPH was recently published (PATENT-1) and included a total of 13 patients with POPH, 11 of which received the study drug riociguat. The study showed that riociguat significantly improved exercise capacity and secondary end points; however, the small group of patients with POPH preclude definitive conclusions regarding the efficacy of this drug in this particular group of patients with PAH.[41]

Prostanoids

Continuous prostacyclin infusion via a central catheter in combination with oral endothelin receptor antagonists has shown the most dramatic PAH-specific therapy effect in individuals with POPH. In a summary of 48 patients treated with IV epoprostenol from 5 studies, MPAP decreased by 25% (48 → 36 mm Hg), PVR decreased by 52% (550 → 262 dyne/s/cm^{-5}), and CO increased by 38% (6.3 → 8.7 L/min, all $P<.01$).[30,55–59] Other prostacyclins (IV treprostinil and inhaled iloprost) have resulted in significant pulmonary hemodynamic improvement in POPH.[63,67,69]

Endothelin Receptor Antagonists

Hoeper and colleagues[62] documented 1- and 3-year survival of 94% and 89% in 18 patients with POPH and Child A liver disease using the nonselective endothelin antagonist bosentan. No liver toxicity was noted. However, Eriksson and colleagues[56] have correctly warned about potential liver toxicity with the use of bosentan, occurring in up to 10% of patients without documented POPH. Although Kahler and colleagues[64] have reported success in POPH with the use of a selective endothelin receptor antagonist (ET$_A$) sitaxsentan, this medication has not been approved in the United States, has been associated with fatal hepatic failure, and has now been removed from the market by its manufacturer. Cartin-Ceba and colleagues[55] reported 13 patients with POPH using the ET$_A$ receptor antagonist ambrisentan (10 mg daily) and documented at 1-year an improvement in each of 8 patients with POPH (MPAP 58 → 41 mm Hg and PVR 445 → 174 dyne/s/cm^{-5}; $P = .004$). Of note, 5 of the 8 patients normalized

Table 2
PAH-specific therapy use in POPH

PAH-Specific Therapy Group	Drug	Study's First Author and Reference	Number of Subjects Included	Study Main Outcomes
Endothelin receptor antagonist	Bosentan	Hoeper[62]	18	1- and 3-y survivals 94% and 89%, respectively
	Bosentan	Savale[72]	34	Event-free survival estimates were 82%, 63%, and 47% at 1, 2, and 3 y, respectively
	Ambrisentan	Cartin-Ceba[55]	13	At 1 y, MPAP and PVR improved in 8 of 8; PVR normalized in 5
Phosphodiesterase inhibitors	Sildenafil	Reichenberger[68]	12	Improvement at 3 mo; not sustained at 1 y
	Sildenafil	Gough[58]	11	PVR decreased in all at first RHC follow-up
	Sildenafil	Hemnes[60]	10	At 1-y MPAP and PVR decreased in 3 of 5 patients
Prostanoids	Epoprostenol	Kuo[66]	4	MPAP and PVR improved
	Epoprostenol	Krowka[65]	15	15 MPAP and PVR improved
	Epoprostenol	Ashfaq[54]	16	Successful LT in 11 patients; 5-y survival 67%
	Epoprostenol	Fix[57]	19	PVR improved in 14 of 14; MPAP improved in 11 of 14
	Epoprostenol	Sussman[70]	8	MPAP and PVR improved in 7 of 8
	Treprostinil	Sakai[69]	3	Successful LT in 2 patients (moderate POPH)
	Inhaled iloprost	Hoeper[62]	13	1- and 3-y survivals 77% and 46%, respectively
	Inhaled iloprost	Melgosa[67]	21	Acute, but no long-term hemodynamic improvement
	Epoprostenol	Awdish[88]	21	Clearance for transplant in 52% of patients within 1 y
Combination therapy	Sildenafil alone or combined with prostacyclins in 9 patients	Hollatz[63]	11	MPAP and PVR improved in all patients, all underwent LT, and 7 of 11 are off PAH-specific therapy
	Sildenafil and bosentan combined in 6 patients, 1 patient only on prostacyclins	Raevens[71]	7	MPAP and PVR improved in the 5 of 6 patients treated with combination of sildenafil and bosentan, 2 underwent LT

their PVR. In further support of ambrisentan in POPH, Halank and colleagues[59] described significant improvement in both exercise capacity and symptoms in 14 patients with POPH. Importantly, neither of the uncontrolled ambrisentan studies was associated with hepatic toxicity. This finding may be caused by the differences in chemical structure (ambrisentan-propionic acid; bosentan and sitaxsentan-sulfa base) and distinct hepatic metabolic pathways.[61] More recently, Savale and colleagues[72] described 34 patients with POPH (Child A or B severity of liver disease) treated with bosentan documenting significant hemodynamic improvement (more so in the Child B subgroup), and event-free survival estimates were 82%, 63%, and 47% at 1, 2, and 3 years, respectively. Two clinical trials specifically designed for patients with POPH are evaluating the role of ambrisentan in this population; both studies are currently recruiting patients (ClinicalTrials.gov numbers NCT01733095 and NCT01224210).

Phosphodiesterase-5 Inhibitors

Phosphodiesterase-5 inhibitors prevent the breakdown of cyclic guanosine monophosphate, the mediator of nitric oxide–induced vasodilation. The use of phosphodiesterase inhibition (sildenafil) to enhance the nitric oxide vasodilating effect, either alone or in combination with other PAH-specific therapies, has successfully improved POPH pulmonary hemodynamics and facilitated successful LT. Most of the published experiences have been in patients with less severe POPH.[58,60,68]

Other Therapies

Imatinib (a tyrosine kinase inhibitor) was reported in a single case report and could suggest a different pathway of PAH-specific therapy. A dramatic hemodynamic improvement was observed with the 6-week addition of imatinib 400 mg daily to pre-LT IV epoprostenol and post-LT bosentan therapy, resulting in liberation of all PAH-specific medications and normalization of RV function 1 year after LT.[73]

Beta-blockers are generally used in patients with portal hypertension to prevent gastrointestinal bleeding; however, its use may impair RV function. In moderate to severe POPH (n = 10; mean MPAP = 52 mm Hg), withdrawal of beta-blockade increased CO by 28%, decreased PVR by 19% with no change in MPAP, and increased the 6-minute walk by 79 m.[74]

Transjugular intrahepatic portosystemic shunting (TIPS) is used as a treatment of uncontrollable gastrointestinal bleeding or refractory ascites or hydrothorax. TIPS can temporarily increase MPAP, CO, and PVR. In a study of 16 patients with cirrhosis without pulmonary hypertension, the increase in MPAP was greater than that noted in CO, suggesting an increase in the PVR after TIPS.[75] Such changes remained for at least 30 days after TIPS and reflected neurohumoral effects as opposed to increased preload. A significant increase in RV work was documented, and the potential effect on RV function could be deleterious in patients with preexisting POPH.[76] RVSP greater than 50 mm Hg along with abnormal RV size and function is a relative contraindication to elective TIPS at the authors' institution.

LT

LT is a potentially curative intervention for patients with underlying cirrhosis, which is the most common cause of portal hypertension. In the United States, a total of 6256 LTs were performed in 2012. As of September 2013, there were approximately 15,831 patients on the wait list in more than 120 US LT centers.[77] Assuming up to 8.5% of LT candidates have POPH, at any point in time there may be approximately 1300

POPH-LT candidates.[2] A summary of outcomes related to POPH following LT is presented in **Table 3**. Unfortunately, the outcomes of LT in patients with POPH remain unpredictable despite adequate screening, careful patient selection, higher priority for LT, and advances in single and combination PAH-specific therapies.[49-51,78-84] Effective PAH-specific therapy has resulted in successful LT and subsequent liberation from pre-LT PAH-specific therapy (see **Table 3**). Importantly, reperfusion during the LT procedure represents a critical time when preload can increase, cytokines may be released, thrombi may migrate into the pulmonary circulation, and intraoperative death follows from acute right heart failure.[85] Despite limited supporting data, LT programs in the United States now allow higher priority to conduct LT if pulmonary hemodynamics can be significantly improved and meet standardized MELD exception guidelines. Current treatment targets for POPH MELD exception in the United States are detailed next:

1. Moderate to severe POPH diagnosis confirmed by RHC
   a. MPAP 35 mm Hg or greater
   b. PVR 240 dyne/s/cm^{-5} or greater
   c. PCWP 15 mm Hg or less
2. PAH-specific therapy initiated; improvement documented
   a. MPAP less than 35 mm Hg
   b. PVR less than 400 dyne/s/cm^{-5} regardless of MPAP and
   c. Satisfactory RV function by TTE
3. MELD exception updated (additional 10% MELD points) every 3 months
   a. Give additional MELD exception if RHC data satisfy criteria 2

Failure to reduce MPAP to less than 50 mm Hg is considered by most centers to be a contraindication to LT or, if discovered at the time of the operation, grounds to cancel the LT procedure before the abdominal incision. Despite limited experience, at this time it seems logical that similar pulmonary hemodynamic guidelines should be followed when living-donor-POPH transplants are considered.[79,86] Although the role of LT in the setting of POPH is evolving with experience, the recognition that severe POPH (measured hemodynamically and qualitatively by echocardiography) can resolve after LT with aggressive pre-LT PAH therapy is quite remarkable. Although preliminary observations are encouraging, the normalization of pulmonary hemodynamics after LT does not necessarily equate to pulmonary vascular histopathology changes resolution or long-term stability. Finally, it should be noted that clinically significant PAH could develop de novo following LT (ie, normal pulmonary hemodynamics are noted at the time of LT) for reasons that are clearly not understood.[87]

An important pressing issue regarding MELD exception deserves further comment. MELD exception is generally not granted under current US policy if the MPAP remains greater than 35 mm Hg despite normalization of PVR and RV function with pre-LT therapy. In such patients, the elevation in MPAP reflects a change in physiology and is the result of pulmonary vasoactive therapy increasing the existing high-flow state and decreasing the PVR to flow. The authors consider that in those patients with normalization of RV function and PVR, MELD exception should be granted despite the abnormal MPAP. Based on observational data, it is hypothesized that for those individuals, cure of POPH after LT can be obtained. Indeed, it is unknown whether pulmonary hemodynamic normalization after LT reflects a pathologic pulmonary vascular cure. In addition, in most post-LT patients that have clinical improvement and echocardiographic normalization of RV function, size, and RVSP, RHC is not routinely performed to corroborate the normalization of the hemodynamics.

Table 3
LT outcomes in the setting of POPH

Outcomes	Study's First Author and Reference
POPH wait-list mortality	Colle[37]
	Fix[57]
	Gough[58]
	Sussman[70]
POPH MELD exception pre-LT	Sussman[70]
	Krowka[43]
Case canceled in operating room	Fukazawa[80]
	Krowka[48]
	Kuo[66]
	Ramsay[38]
Intraoperative death	Krowka[82]
	Krowka[48]
	Le Pavec[2]
	Ramsay[38]
	Swanson[40]
	Krowka[43]
Transplant hospitalization death	Taura[84]
	Ramsay[38]
	Krowka[48]
	Starkel[50]
	Krowka[82]
	Kawut[81]
	Saner[51]
	Ashfaq[54]
	Krowka[43]
	Raevens[71]
Late death not caused by POPH	Ramsay[38]
	Ashfaq[54]
	Swanson[40]
Late death caused by POPH	Ramsay[38]
	Le Pavec[2]
Multiorgan (H-Lu-Lv; Lu-Lv transplant)[a]	Scouras[83]
De novo PAH post-LT[b]	Koch[87]
Post-LV outcomes	
Resolved (PAH-specific therapy discontinued)	Sussman[70]
	Ashfaq[54]
	Fix[57]
	Gough[58]
	Sakai[69]
	Tapper[73]
	Bandara[79]
	Cartin-Ceba[55]
	Hollatz[63]
	Krowka[43,c]
Resolved/stable without PAH-specific therapy	Yoshida[28]
	Castro[49]
	Starkel[50]
	Colle[37]
	Ashfaq[54]

(continued on next page)

Table 3 (continued)	
Outcomes	**Study's First Author and Reference**
Improved/stabilized PAH-specific therapy continued	Reichenberger[68]
	Sussman[70]
	Fix[57]
	Austin[78]
	Hemnes[60]
	Sakai[69]
	Hollatz[63]
	Krowka[43]
	Raevens[71,d]
Progressive despite PAH-specific therapy	Ramsay[38]

Abbreviation: H-Lu-Lv, heart, double lung, liver transplants; Lu-Lv, double lung, liver transplants.

[a] It is noted that multiorgan transplants have been reported in the literature for cystic fibrosis, alpha-1 antitrypsin deficiency, and sarcoidosis; but these entities also affect lung parenchyma, and many cases were accomplished in the era before current PAH-specific medications and, therefore, were not included herein.

[b] A literature review of 13 such cases.

[c] Living donor LT (3 patients).

[d] Combined PAH-specific therapy use.

PRACTICE GUIDELINES

In addition to the POPH screening guidelines espoused by the American Association for the Study of Liver Diseases[47] and evolving MELD exception,[43] the International Liver Transplant Society will publish POPH diagnostic and management guidelines in 2014.

SUMMARY

POPH is a serious pulmonary vascular complication of cirrhotic and noncirrhotic portal hypertension; its pathophysiology remains unclear, with no clear relationship to the cause of the liver disease or the severity of the portal hypertension. POPH can lead to right heart failure and death if untreated. Because of the different spectrum of pulmonary hemodynamic changes associated with hepatic dysfunction, screening by TTE and confirmation by RHC is necessary for accurate diagnosis and therapeutic considerations. Despite the lack of controlled studies, PAH-specific therapies in POPH can significantly improve pulmonary hemodynamics and RV function. The potential to cure POPH, at least hemodynamically, with a combination of PAH-specific therapy and LT seems to be an attainable goal in a cohort of patients with POPH yet to be optimally characterized.

REFERENCES

1. Simonneau G, Robbins IM, Beghetti M, et al. Updated clinical classification of pulmonary hypertension. J Am Coll Cardiol 2009;54:S43–54.
2. Le Pavec J, Souza R, Herve P, et al. Portopulmonary hypertension: survival and prognostic factors. Am J Respir Crit Care Med 2008;178:637–43.
3. Raevens S, Colle I, Reyntjens K, et al. Echocardiography for the detection of portopulmonary hypertension in liver transplant candidates: an analysis of cutoff values. Liver Transpl 2013;19:602–10.

4. Mantz FA Jr, Craige E. Portal axis thrombosis with spontaneous portacaval shunt and resultant cor pulmonale. AMA Arch Pathol 1951;52:91–7.

5. Rodriguez-Roisin R, Krowka MJ, Herve P, et al. Pulmonary-hepatic vascular disorders (PHD). Eur Respir J 2004;24:861–80.

6. Krowka MJ, Swanson KL, Frantz RP, et al. Portopulmonary hypertension: results from a 10-year screening algorithm. Hepatology 2006;44:1502–10.

7. Krowka MJ, Edwards WD. A spectrum of pulmonary vascular pathology in portopulmonary hypertension. Liver Transpl 2000;6:241–2.

8. Rodriguez-Roisin R, Krowka MJ. Hepatopulmonary syndrome–a liver-induced lung vascular disorder. N Engl J Med 2008;358:2378–87.

9. Krowka MJ. Portopulmonary hypertension. Semin Respir Crit Care Med 2012; 33:17–25.

10. Kawut SM, Krowka MJ, Trotter JF, et al. Clinical risk factors for portopulmonary hypertension. Hepatology 2008;48:196–203.

11. Lockhart A. Pulmonary arterial hypertension in portal hypertension. Clin Gastroenterol 1985;14:123–38.

12. Senior RM, Britton RC, Turino GM, et al. Pulmonary hypertension associated with cirrhosis of the liver and with portacaval shunts. Circulation 1968;37:88–96.

13. Talwalkar JA, Swanson KL, Krowka MJ, et al. Prevalence of spontaneous portosystemic shunts in patients with portopulmonary hypertension and effect on treatment. Gastroenterology 2011;141:1673–9.

14. Peacock AJ. Pulmonary hypertension after splenectomy: a consequence of loss of the splenic filter or is there something more? Thorax 2005;60:983–4.

15. Hadengue A, Benhayoun MK, Lebrec D, et al. Pulmonary hypertension complicating portal hypertension: prevalence and relation to splanchnic hemodynamics. Gastroenterology 1991;100:520–8.

16. Krowka MJ, Miller DP, Barst RJ, et al. Portopulmonary hypertension: a report from the US-based REVEAL Registry. Chest 2012;141:906–15.

17. Kuo PC, Plotkin JS, Johnson LB, et al. Distinctive clinical features of portopulmonary hypertension. Chest 1997;112:980–6.

18. Roberts KE, Fallon MB, Krowka MJ, et al. Genetic risk factors for portopulmonary hypertension in patients with advanced liver disease. Am J Respir Crit Care Med 2009;179:835–42.

19. Edwards BS, Weir EK, Edwards WD, et al. Coexistent pulmonary and portal hypertension: morphologic and clinical features. J Am Coll Cardiol 1987;10: 1233–8.

20. Tuder RM, Cool CD, Geraci MW, et al. Prostacyclin synthase expression is decreased in lungs from patients with severe pulmonary hypertension. Am J Respir Crit Care Med 1999;159:1925–32.

21. Kamath PS, Carpenter HA, Lloyd RV, et al. Hepatic localization of endothelin-1 in patients with idiopathic portal hypertension and cirrhosis of the liver. Liver Transpl 2000;6:596–602.

22. Benjaminov FS, Prentice M, Sniderman KW, et al. Portopulmonary hypertension in decompensated cirrhosis with refractory ascites. Gut 2003;52:1355–62.

23. Pellicelli AM, Barbaro G, Puoti C, et al. Plasma cytokines and portopulmonary hypertension in patients with cirrhosis waiting for orthotopic liver transplantation. Angiology 2010;61:802–6.

24. Yeager ME, Frid MG, Stenmark KR. Progenitor cells in pulmonary vascular remodeling. Pulm Circ 2011;1:3–16.

25. Arnal JF, Fontaine C, Billon-Gales A, et al. Estrogen receptors and endothelium. Arterioscler Thromb Vasc Biol 2010;30:1506–12.

26. Iwakiri Y, Groszmann RJ. The hyperdynamic circulation of chronic liver diseases: from the patient to the molecule. Hepatology 2006;43:S121–31.
27. Bogaard HJ, Abe K, Vonk Noordegraaf A, et al. The right ventricle under pressure: cellular and molecular mechanisms of right-heart failure in pulmonary hypertension. Chest 2009;135:794–804.
28. Yoshida EM, Erb SR, Pflugfelder PW, et al. Single-lung versus liver transplantation for the treatment of portopulmonary hypertension–a comparison of two patients. Transplantation 1993;55:688–90.
29. Lebrec D, Capron JP, Dhumeaux D, et al. Pulmonary hypertension complicating portal hypertension. Am Rev Respir Dis 1979;120:849–56.
30. Matsubara O, Nakamura T, Uehara T, et al. Histometrical investigation of the pulmonary artery in severe hepatic disease. J Pathol 1984;143:31–7.
31. Naeye RL. "Primary" pulmonary hypertension with coexisting portal hypertension. A retrospective study of six cases. Circulation 1960;22:376–84.
32. Sankey EA, Crow J, Mallett SV, et al. Pulmonary platelet aggregates: possible cause of sudden peroperative death in adults undergoing liver transplantation. J Clin Pathol 1993;46:222–7.
33. McDonnell PJ, Toye PA, Hutchins GM. Primary pulmonary hypertension and cirrhosis: are they related? Am Rev Respir Dis 1983;127:437–41.
34. Rich S, Dantzker DR, Ayres SM, et al. Primary pulmonary hypertension. A national prospective study. Ann Intern Med 1987;107:216–23.
35. Groves BM, Brundage BH, Elliott CG, et al. Pulmonary hypertension associated with cirrhosis. Philadelphia: University of Pennsylvania Press; 1990.
36. Humbert M, Sitbon O, Chaouat A, et al. Pulmonary arterial hypertension in France: results from a national registry. Am J Respir Crit Care Med 2006;173:1023–30.
37. Colle IO, Moreau R, Godinho E, et al. Diagnosis of portopulmonary hypertension in candidates for liver transplantation: a prospective study. Hepatology 2003;37:401–9.
38. Ramsay MA, Simpson BR, Nguyen AT, et al. Severe pulmonary hypertension in liver transplant candidates. Liver Transpl Surg 1997;3:494–500.
39. Robalino BD, Moodie DS. Association between primary pulmonary hypertension and portal hypertension: analysis of its pathophysiology and clinical, laboratory and hemodynamic manifestations. J Am Coll Cardiol 1991;17:492–8.
40. Swanson KL, Wiesner RH, Nyberg SL, et al. Survival in portopulmonary hypertension: Mayo Clinic experience categorized by treatment subgroups. Am J Transplant 2008;8:2445–53.
41. Ghofrani HA, Galie N, Grimminger F, et al. Riociguat for the treatment of pulmonary arterial hypertension. N Engl J Med 2013;369:330–40.
42. Krowka MJ, Fallon MB, Mulligan DC, et al. Model for end-stage liver disease (MELD) exception for portopulmonary hypertension. Liver Transpl 2006;12:S114–6.
43. Krowka MJ, Wiesner RH, Rosen CB, et al. Portopulmonary hypertension outcomes in the era of MELD exception. Liver Transpl 2012;18:S259.
44. Kim WR, Krowka MJ, Plevak DJ, et al. Accuracy of Doppler echocardiography in the assessment of pulmonary hypertension in liver transplant candidates. Liver Transpl 2000;6:453–8.
45. Donovan CL, Marcovitz PA, Punch JD, et al. Two-dimensional and dobutamine stress echocardiography in the preoperative assessment of patients with end-stage liver disease prior to orthotopic liver transplantation. Transplantation 1996;61:1180–8.

46. Cotton CL, Gandhi S, Vaitkus PT, et al. Role of echocardiography in detecting portopulmonary hypertension in liver transplant candidates. Liver Transpl 2002;8:1051–4.

47. Murray KF, Carithers RL Jr. AASLD practice guidelines: evaluation of the patient for liver transplantation. Hepatology 2005;41:1407–32.

48. Krowka MJ, Plevak DJ, Findlay JY, et al. Pulmonary hemodynamics and perioperative cardiopulmonary-related mortality in patients with portopulmonary hypertension undergoing liver transplantation. Liver Transpl 2000;6:443–50.

49. Castro M, Krowka MJ, Schroeder DR, et al. Frequency and clinical implications of increased pulmonary artery pressures in liver transplant patients. Mayo Clin Proc 1996;71:543–51.

50. Starkel P, Vera A, Gunson B, et al. Outcome of liver transplantation for patients with pulmonary hypertension. Liver Transpl 2002;8:382–8.

51. Saner FH, Nadalin S, Pavlakovic G, et al. Portopulmonary hypertension in the early phase following liver transplantation. Transplantation 2006;82:887–91.

52. Kia L, Shah SJ, Wang E, et al. Role of pretransplant echocardiographic evaluation in predicting outcomes following liver transplantation. Am J Transplant 2013;13:2395–401.

53. Stasch JP, Pacher P, Evgenov OV. Soluble guanylate cyclase as an emerging therapeutic target in cardiopulmonary disease. Circulation 2011;123:2263–73.

54. Ashfaq M, Chinnakotla S, Rogers L, et al. The impact of treatment of portopulmonary hypertension on survival following liver transplantation. Am J Transplant 2007;7:1258–64.

55. Cartin-Ceba R, Swanson K, Iyer V, et al. Safety and efficacy of ambrisentan for the treatment of portopulmonary hypertension. Chest 2011;139:109–14.

56. Eriksson C, Gustavsson A, Kronvall T, et al. Hepatotoxicity by bosentan in a patient with portopulmonary hypertension: a case-report and review of the literature. J Gastrointestin Liver Dis 2011;20:77–80.

57. Fix OK, Bass NM, De Marco T, et al. Long-term follow-up of portopulmonary hypertension: effect of treatment with epoprostenol. Liver Transpl 2007;13:875–85.

58. Gough MS, White RJ. Sildenafil therapy is associated with improved hemodynamics in liver transplantation candidates with pulmonary arterial hypertension. Liver Transpl 2009;15:30–6.

59. Halank M, Knudsen L, Seyfarth HJ, et al. Ambrisentan improves exercise capacity and symptoms in patients with portopulmonary hypertension. Z Gastroenterol 2011;49:1258–62.

60. Hemnes AR, Robbins IM. Sildenafil monotherapy in portopulmonary hypertension can facilitate liver transplantation. Liver Transpl 2009;15:15–9.

61. Hoeper MM. Liver toxicity: the Achilles' heel of endothelin receptor antagonist therapy? Eur Respir J 2009;34:529–30.

62. Hoeper MM, Seyfarth HJ, Hoeffken G, et al. Experience with inhaled iloprost and bosentan in portopulmonary hypertension. Eur Respir J 2007;30:1096–102.

63. Hollatz TJ, Musat A, Westphal S, et al. Treatment with sildenafil and treprostinil allows successful liver transplantation of patients with moderate to severe portopulmonary hypertension. Liver Transpl 2012;18:686–95.

64. Kahler CM, Graziadei I, Vogelsinger H, et al. Successful treatment of portopulmonary hypertension with the selective endothelin receptor antagonist sitaxentan. Wien Klin Wochenschr 2011;123:248–52.

65. Krowka MJ, Frantz RP, McGoon MD, et al. Improvement in pulmonary hemodynamics during intravenous epoprostenol (prostacyclin): a study of 15 patients

with moderate to severe portopulmonary hypertension. Hepatology 1999;30: 641–8.

66. Kuo PC, Johnson LB, Plotkin JS, et al. Continuous intravenous infusion of epoprostenol for the treatment of portopulmonary hypertension. Transplantation 1997;63:604–6.

67. Melgosa MT, Ricci GL, Garcia-Pagan JC, et al. Acute and long-term effects of inhaled iloprost in portopulmonary hypertension. Liver Transpl 2010;16:348–56.

68. Reichenberger F, Voswinckel R, Steveling E, et al. Sildenafil treatment for portopulmonary hypertension. Eur Respir J 2006;28:563–7.

69. Sakai T, Planinsic RM, Mathier MA, et al. Initial experience using continuous intravenous treprostinil to manage pulmonary arterial hypertension in patients with end-stage liver disease. Transpl Int 2009;22:554–61.

70. Sussman N, Kaza V, Barshes N, et al. Successful liver transplantation following medical management of portopulmonary hypertension: a single-center series. Am J Transplant 2006;6:2177–82.

71. Raevens S, De Pauw M, Reyntjens K, et al. Oral vasodilator therapy in patients with moderate to severe portopulmonary hypertension as a bridge to liver transplantation. Eur J Gastroenterol Hepatol 2013;25:495–502.

72. Savale L, Magnier R, Le Pavec J, et al. Efficacy, safety, and pharmacokinetics of bosentan in portopulmonary hypertension. Eur Respir J 2013;41(1):96–103.

73. Tapper EB, Knowles D, Heffron T, et al. Portopulmonary hypertension: imatinib as a novel treatment and the Emory experience with this condition. Transplant Proc 2009;41:1969–71.

74. Provencher S, Herve P, Jais X, et al. Deleterious effects of beta-blockers on exercise capacity and hemodynamics in patients with portopulmonary hypertension. Gastroenterology 2006;130:120–6.

75. Van der Linden P, Le Moine O, Ghysels M, et al. Pulmonary hypertension after transjugular intrahepatic portosystemic shunt: effects on right ventricular function. Hepatology 1996;23:982–7.

76. van der Heijde RM, Lameris JS, van den Berg B, et al. Pulmonary hypertension after transjugular intrahepatic portosystemic shunt (TIPS). Eur Respir J 1996;9: 1562–4.

77. 2013. Available at: http://optn.transplant.hrsa.gov. Accessed September 25, 2013.

78. Austin MJ, McDougall NI, Wendon JA, et al. Safety and efficacy of combined use of sildenafil, bosentan, and iloprost before and after liver transplantation in severe portopulmonary hypertension. Liver Transpl 2008;14:287–91.

79. Bandara M, Gordon FD, Sarwar A, et al. Successful outcomes following living donor liver transplantation for portopulmonary hypertension. Liver Transpl 2010;16:983–9.

80. Fukazawa K, Pretto EA Jr. Poor outcome following aborted orthotopic liver transplantation due to severe porto-pulmonary hypertension. J Hepatobiliary Pancreat Sci 2010;17:505–8.

81. Kawut SM, Taichman DB, Ahya VN, et al. Hemodynamics and survival of patients with portopulmonary hypertension. Liver Transpl 2005;11:1107–11.

82. Krowka MJ, Mandell MS, Ramsay MA, et al. Hepatopulmonary syndrome and portopulmonary hypertension: a report of the multicenter liver transplant database. Liver Transpl 2004;10:174–82.

83. Scouras NE, Matsusaki T, Boucek CD, et al. Portopulmonary hypertension as an indication for combined heart, lung, and liver or lung and liver transplantation: literature review and case presentation. Liver Transpl 2011;17:137–43.

84. Taura P, Garcia-Valdecasas JC, Beltran J, et al. Moderate primary pulmonary hypertension in patients undergoing liver transplantation. Anesth Analg 1996;83: 675–80.

85. Ramsay M. Portopulmonary hypertension and right heart failure in patients with cirrhosis. Curr Opin Anaesthesiol 2010;23:145–50.

86. Ogawa E, Hori T, Doi H, et al. Living-donor liver transplantation for moderate or severe porto-pulmonary hypertension accompanied by pulmonary arterial hypertension: a single-centre experience over 2 decades in Japan. J Hepatobiliary Pancreat Sci 2012;19:638–49.

87. Koch DG, Caplan M, Reuben A. Pulmonary hypertension after liver transplantation: case presentation and review of the literature. Liver Transpl 2009;15: 407–12.

88. Awdish RL, Cajigas HR. Early initiation of prostacyclin in portopulmonary hypertension: 10 years of a transplant center's experience. Lung 2013;191(6): 593–600.

Hepatic Hydrothorax

John Paul Norvell, MD*, James R. Spivey, MD

KEYWORDS

- Hepatic hydrothorax • Thoracentesis
- Transjugular intrahepatic portosystemic shunt • Cirrhosis
- Spontaneous bacterial empyema

KEY POINTS

- Hepatic hydrothorax is an uncommon complication of portal hypertension defined as a transudative pleural effusion in absence of cardiopulmonary pathology and is usually left-sided.
- Early diagnosis via pleural fluid sampling is essential to rule out other causes, which are found in up to 30% of suspected hepatic hydrothorax cases, and to diagnosis spontaneous bacterial empyema.
- Spontaneous bacterial empyema is under-recognized, present in up to 16% of patients with hepatic hydrothorax, and it is associated with a mortality rate of over 20%.
- In diuretic-refractory cases, thoracentesis is a main stay of treatment but is associated with complications. Both transjugular intrahepatic portosystemic shunt and other surgical procedures are considered bridging measures to liver transplantation in select patients, although management remains challenging and are frequently associated with poor outcomes.

INTRODUCTION: HEPATIC HYDROTHORAX

Hepatic hydrothorax (HH) is a relatively uncommon complication in patients with end-stage liver disease, and it is defined as a transudative pleural effusion usually greater than 500 mL in a patient with portal hypertension without any other underlying primary cardiopulmonary source.[1–3] Although approximately 50% of patients with end-stage liver disease will develop ascites, only 5% to 10% develop hepatic hydrothorax, which may result in dyspnea, hypoxia, and infection, and portends a poor prognosis. The most likely explanation for development is passage of fluid from the peritoneal space to the pleural space due to small diaphragmatic defects. Initial management consists of diuretics with dietary sodium restriction and thoracentesis, and a transjugular intrahepatic portosystemic shunt (TIPS) may ultimately be required. Despite its relative

Financial Disclosure: Neither of the authors have any financial relationships in the subject matter or materials discussed in this article.
Division of Digestive Diseases, Department of Digestive Diseases, Department of Medicine, Emory Transplant Center, Emory University, 1365 Clifton Road, NE, Clinic B, Suite 1200, Atlanta, GA 30322, USA
* Corresponding author.
E-mail address: jpnorvell@emory.edu

infrequency, afflicted patients can be quite symptomatic, develop morbid and fatal complications, pose management dilemmas, and should warrant evaluation for liver transplantation.

CLINICAL FEATURES
Epidemiology

The largest case series have described the incidence of hepatic hydrothorax to be approximately 5% to 10% of cirrhotic patients.[4–6] It is presumably more common in later stages of cirrhosis and has been estimated to be present in 4% to 6% of all patients with cirrhosis and in up to 10% of decompensated patients.[7] The estimation of the incidence is also affected by the sensitivity of detection as illustrated by a study of 862 cirrhotic patients requiring hospital admission that were evaluated with radiography, ultrasound, and computed tomography (CT), which found 15% had pleural effusions, although only 6.5% of patients had enough fluid to perform a thoracentesis.[8] Additionally, persistent massive ascites and HH have been reported in 2% of liver transplant recipients, all of whom had hepatitis C virus.[9]

Clinical Manifestations and Complications

Presentation

HH should always be suspected when a cirrhotic patient develops a pleural effusion. Most patients will first present with clinical signs and symptoms of cirrhosis and portal hypertension, although in other patients, pulmonary symptoms may dominate the clinical presentation. Although 5 to 8 L of ascites can accumulate in the abdominal cavity with only mild symptoms, relatively small amounts of fluid in the thoracic cavity (1–2 L) can cause severe symptoms such as shortness of breath, nonproductive cough, chest discomfort or tightness, and hypoxia. Because the development of HH is thought to be related to ascites, most patients will have concurrent ascites; however, it may not be detectable in 21% of patients.[1] Multiple clinical factors such as volume, rapidity of accumulation, and presence of associated pulmonary disease determine the severity of symptoms, ranging from a lack of symptoms to life-threatening respiratory failure.[1] In addition to dyspnea and hypoxia, patients with HH may develop further complications such as acute tension hydrothorax and infection, called spontaneous bacterial empyema.

A rarely reported presentation of HH is acute tension hydrothorax, which is associated with severe dyspnea and hypotension. It has been reported to occur acutely over the course of an hour and may be secondary to a sudden pleuroperitoneal bleb.[10]

Spontaneous bacterial empyema

Spontaneous bacterial empyema (SBEM) is an important and under-recognized distinct complication of HH and is defined as a spontaneous infection of a pre-existing HH. The name is somewhat misleading, as there is usually no pus or abscess in the thoracic cavity, and the pathogenesis, course, and treatment are very different from empyema secondary to pneumonia. Although SBEM and spontaneous bacterial peritonitis (SBP) are closely related, SBEM is rarely described, and there are only a handful of dedicated studies describing the condition. Two studies from Taiwan found the overall incidence of SBEM to be 2% of all cirrhotic patients and 13% to 16% among cirrhotic patients with HH, which is similar to the prevalence of SBP in patients with ascites.[2,3] SBEM can easily be confused with a pleural empyema, as there is usually no evidence of pus or abscess formation in the thoracic cavity. The pathogenesis of SBEM remains unclear; one hypothesis postulates that pleural infection is caused by flow of infected ascites from the peritoneal to the pleural cavity via defects in the diaphragm. However, two studies found that 40% to 50% of episodes of SBEM were not associated with SBP.[2,11] Thus SBP is not a prerequisite for SBEM, prompting another hypothesis for pathogenesis involving spontaneous bacteremia as the cause. Identified risk factors for the development of SBEM include the severity of the underlying liver disease, decreased serum albumin, lower pleural fluid levels of total protein and C3, and associated SBP.[2,12]

Given the observed mortality rate of 20% to 38%,[2] rapid diagnosis of SBEM is essential for timely initiation of treatment. Although affected patients may present with dyspnea, pleuritic pain, fever, or symptoms from associated SBP such as abdominal pain, SBEM is often associated with minimal clinical signs; thus the clinician must have a low threshold to perform a thoracentesis for pleural fluid analysis (**Box 1**) to make the diagnosis per proposed criteria.[13] The diagnosis of SBEM is established if the pleural fluid cultures are positive, and a polymorphonuclear (PMN) count is greater than 250 cells/mm^3. In cases with negative cultures, the diagnosis is made with a pleural fluid PMN count greater than 500 cells/mm^3 and by excluding a parapneumonic infection.[13] As with ascitic fluid cultures, immediate inoculation of blood culture bottles at the bedside is recommended to increase culture yields, a technique that increased the yield of positive cultures from 33% to 75% in one study.[11] The presence of pleural neutrophilia can suggest an early diagnosis of SBEM while awaiting culture results.[14] The pleural fluid total protein, lactate dehydrogenase, and glucose have been found to not differ significantly between patients with SBEM and noninfected HH.[15] Given its close relationship with SBP, it is not surprising that *Enterobacteriaceae* are among the most commonly isolated causative pathogens: *Escherichia coli*, *Klebsiella pneumonia*, *Enterococcus* subspecies, and *Pseudomonas aeruginosa* (in decreasing frequency).[2]

Prompt initiation of appropriate treatment is essential because of the high mortality associated with SBEM. Given the association with SBP, the initial antibiotic regimen is similar, and appropriate third-generation cephalosporins are recommended for 7 to 10 days.[11] However, there has been evidence of cephalosporin resistance due to extended-spectrum β-lactamase organisms in up to 41% of nosocomially acquired episodes of SBP,[16] in which case carbapenems should be used. Although albumin has been shown to reduce the risk of renal failure in SBP,[17] and some centers administer albumin similarly in patients with SBEM, the use of albumin has not been studied in treatment of SBEM. The only indication for placement of a chest tube for drainage is pus in the pleural space, and it is not necessary for SBEM without pus, even in culture-positive cases. Placement of a chest tube is in general contraindicated in cirrhotic patients due to poor outcomes from fluid depletion, protein loss, infection due to poor wound healing, and renal failure.[11,18] Even with appropriate treatment, the mortality is significant, and independent

---

Box 1
Diagnostic criteria for SBEM

- Positive pleural fluid culture and PMN count >250 cells/mm^3 or

- Negative pleural fluid culture and PMN count >500 cells/mm^3

- No evidence of pneumonia/parapneumonic effusion on chest radiograph or CT

Data from Xiol X, Castellote J, Baliellas C, et al. Spontaneous bacterial empyema in cirrhotic patients: analysis of eleven cases. Hepatology 1990;11(3):365–70; and Tu CY, Chen CH. Spontaneous bacterial empyema. Curr Opin Pulm Med 2012;18(4):355–8.

predictors for death are high Model for End-stage Liver Disease (MELD)-Na score, initial intensive care unit (ICU) admission, and initial antibiotic treatment failure.[2]

PATHOPHYSIOLOGY

The early literature postulated several mechanisms to explain the development of hepatic hydrothoraces in cirrhotic patients with portal hypertension: direct passage of peritoneal fluid via diaphragmatic defects,[19] azygous vein hypertension with leakage of plasma, passage of peritoneal fluid via lymphatics, thoracic duct lymphatic leakage, and hypoalbuminemia with decreased colloid osmotic pressure.[20]

The most commonly accepted theory is the direct passage of peritoneal ascites via diaphragmatic defects. This hypothesis was first proposed following the observation that in patients with pre-existing hepatic hydrothoraces, a right-sided pneumothorax would develop within 24 to 48 hours after 500 to 1000 mL of air were infused in the peritoneal cavity.[19]

A pressure gradient between the peritoneal and pleural space favors the unidirectional passage of ascitic fluid into the chest, possibly with a valvular mechanism. It is interesting to note that despite the prevalence of these congenital defects, a pneumothorax is only rarely observed after abdominal laparoscopic procedures.[21] Ascitic fluid that collects in the abdomen raises the peritoneal pressure and may stretch the diaphragm and alter the pressure gradient between the intra-abdominal and intrathoracic compartments. It is proposed that in patients with cirrhosis and ascites, the increased abdominal pressure and thinning of the diaphragm due to malnutrition may increase gaps between diaphragmatic muscle fibers and lead to small herniations of the peritoneum into the pleural space called pleuroperitoneal blebs. These blebs may rupture and facilitate passage of fluid, which is one-way given the negative intrathoracic pressure,[4,19,22,23] and may explain the observation that 20% of patients with HH do not have clinically significant ascites.[1] Diaphragmatic defects are thought to occur in up to 20% of the population and occur more frequently on the right side for poorly understood reasons. It is proposed that because of embryonic development, the left hemidiaphragm is more muscular and the right side is more tendinous because of the close anatomic relationship of the bare areas of the liver with the diaphragm. This may explain why hepatic hydrothoraces are right-sided in 85% of patients, left-sided in 13% of patients, and bilateral in 2% of patients.[22,23]

The direct passage of fluid across the diaphragm via a valvular mechanism theory can be demonstrated by various imaging methods. Intraperitoneal injection of methylene blue can be used intraoperatively to demonstrate and localize defects, and contrast-enhanced ultrasonography has been used to detect flow across the diaphragm in real time.[24] Additionally, scintigraphic studies using intraperitoneal instillation of ^{99m}Tc-human serum albumin or ^{99m}Tc-sulphor-colloid can be used to demonstrate the unidirectional passage of these markers from the abdominal to the pleural cavity within minutes to hours after administration.[25] The movement of the radioisotope is unidirectional, caused by the negative intrathoracic pressure associated with normal respiration. These radioactive isotope scans have confirmed communication between the peritoneal cavity and the pleural space even in the absence of ascites (**Fig. 1**).[26] Ascites is present in patients with HH only if the formation of ascitic fluid exceeds its absorption by peritoneal lymphatics and transfer into the pleural space.[22]

DIAGNOSIS

The diagnosis of HH is commonly made on clinical grounds in a cirrhotic patient with portal hypertension and a right-sided pleural effusion without known cardiopulmonary

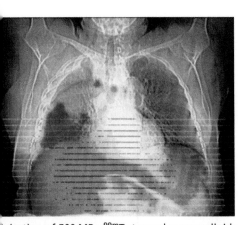

injection of 500 MBq ^{99m}Tc-tagged nannocolloids, followed by scinti-
and 24 hours after injection, demonstrating a transdiaphragmatic
ght pleural cavity. (*From* Truninger K, Frey LD. Hepatic hydrothorax
iz Med Wochenschr 2000;130:1706.)

horacentesis should be performed to confirm the diagnosis and
ses. A prospective study of 60 cirrhotic patients admitted with
underwent diagnostic thoracentesis found that 30% were the
her than HH including SBEM (15%), pleural tuberculosis, adeno-
monic effusions, and undiagnosed exudates.[1] When the effusion
5% of cases were uncomplicated HH.[1]
hould routinely be sent for the following diagnostic tests: cell
d culture in blood culture bottles, serum and fluid protein, albu-
drogenase (LDH). Other tests that maybe useful depending on
lude triglyceride level, pleural pH, adenosine deaminase, and
action (PCR) for mycobacterium, amylase, and cytology to rule
yema, tuberculosis, pancreatitis, and malignancy, respectively.[4]
e proposed pathophysiology, the composition of HH is always
e and similar to ascitic fluid. However, analysis of ascitic and
only slightly different because of the greater efficacy of water
ural surface. In general, the total protein, albumin, cholesterol,
may be marginally higher in pleural fluid.[19,22] Although diuresis
rted to increase the pleural total protein levels, one study found
dant exudate in only 1 of 34 patients on diuretics.[15]
of pleural fluid in HH are described in **Box 2**. In addition to
of transudative fluid, uncomplicated HH has a polymorphonu-
than 500 cells/mm^3, and the total protein concentration is less
tion to pleural fluid analysis, other tests can be helpful to eluci-
ch as CT of the chest and echocardiogram to exclude malig-

d laboratory features of HH

d (85%)

(13%)

2%)

id analysis[4,50]

onuclear cell count <500 cells/mm^3 and negative culture

ein concentration <2.5 g/dL

ein pleural fluid to serum total protein ratio <0.5

al fluid to serum ratio <0.6

pleural fluid albumin gradient >1.1 g/dL

7.4–7.55

id amylase concentration < serum amylase concentration

cose level similar to serum level

T OPTIONS/MANAGEMENT/OUTCOMES
anagement

anagement of HH, like that of abdominal ascites, includes dietary sodium diuretic therapy, and when required based on symptoms or complications, sis or other invasive means. Patients presenting with either ascites and/or be educated regarding restricting dietary sources of sodium to less than aily. When symptomatic volume overload develops, treatment with a com-loop diuretics (furosemide) and aldosterone receptor antagonist (spirono-often effective. Doses may be escalated to include 160 mg of furosemide g of spironolactone daily, although aggressive diuresis is often challenging, f these patients have concurrent renal dysfunction and electrolyte imbal-ding hyponatremia. When these doses are insufficient for therapeutic effect, t may be consuming excessive dietary sodium. In obese patients with nd either ascites or HH, emphasis on carbohydrate restriction often results fective diuresis, but the effect may simply be due to more effective sodium . Care must be taken not to induce more severe malnutrition. For a more nsive discussion of the conservative treatment of ascites, the reader is sources such as the review by Runyon.[29]

esis

etics result in renal dysfunction in the setting of insufficient therapeutic

Transjugular Intrahepatic Portosystemic Shunt

Given the underlying contribution of portal hypertension to the development of hepatic hydrothorax, it stands to reason that portal decompression may be effective in relieving HH, as it is frequently used to reduce ascites formation. Several studies have demonstrated the effectiveness of TIPS in controlling HH.[30–34] A review of 73 patients treated at Emory University Hospital showed favorable clinical responses of 79% and 75% at 1 and 6 months, respectively, following TIPS insertion.[33] The 30-day mortality rate in this group of patients was 19%, which correlated with pre-TIPS creatinine values. Complications in this group of patients included hepatic encephalopathy (15%), a predictable complication from portaprival flow with all central shunts, as well as infection (8.2%), bleeding related to the procedure (6.8%), acute renal failure, and acute respiratory distress syndrome (2.7%). It is worthwhile to remember that the MELD score was originally devised to predict outcomes after TIPS and not to stratify risk for cirrhosis patients per se.[35] Dhanaskaran and colleagues[33] confirmed that the clinical response and longer survival after TIPS in their patients were associated with pre-TIPS MELD scores less than 15. Given the risk of further decompensation of liver function after TIPS placement, the authors' group typically completes the transplant evaluation prior to TIPS insertion in these patients.

Liver Transplantation

Liver transplantation should be considered in patients who develop refractory HH; however some symptomatic patients may still have relatively low MELD scores that will not lead to timely transplantation. Although HH may require perioperative thoracentesis, outcomes in these transplanted patients are not inferior to those in patients transplanted without HH.[36] The authors have found that perioperative use of indwelling pleural catheters on a short-term basis is better tolerated after liver transplantation, and these catheters can often be removed within days without significant reaccumulation of pleural fluid.

Other Surgical Interventions

Local surgical therapy for hepatic hydrothorax is often either ineffective or impractical. Chest tube placement with or without pleurodesis often fails, primarily because of the relentless reaccumulation of fluid in the pleural space. Additionally, complications such as pain, fever, pneumothorax, renal failure, and empyema make this approach unappealing. Repeat application of talc or other sclerosant is often required.[37] One abstract, however, found that indwelling tunneled pleural catheters led to diminishing hydrothorax drainage and ultimate pleurodesis in 8 of 14 patients, 2 of whom developed empyema.[38] Surgical repair of diaphragmatic defects may be considered via a thoracoscopic approach, as more invasive surgical intervention would likely prove too morbid. These procedures require concomitant pleurodesis and carry essentially the same risks as pleurodesis delivered by chest tube. Nevertheless, some success has been described in small case series.[39,40] Finally, peritoneovenous shunts have been used for years to treat refractory ascites, which were devised in a time when few other nonsurgical options existed. The technical challenges and complications, along with the frequent failure of the devises to function properly, have led to their obsolescence in a time when other, better options exist. Despite this history, thoracovenous shunts are occasionally mentioned as a possible treatment option for refractory HH. The experience with these shunts is limited, including rare reports of success and complications.[41–43]

Future Directions

HH drainage and pleurodesis are appealing as a treatment option, but as mentioned previously, the failure and complication rates are formidable. More effective use of video-assisted thorascopic surgical techniques (VATS) to repair diaphragmatic defects, followed by pleurodesis, may be more effective when the culprit defects can be identified.[40] Reducing the pressure differential between peritoneal and pleural spaces using continuous positive airway pressure (CPAP) has been utilized to treat HH, either alone or in conjunction with VATS. The experience is limited, and the contribution of the CPAP in cases where pleurodesis was used remains poorly defined.[44,45] One case using CPAP during sleep saw HH diminish significantly, only to return when the CPAP was stopped and respond again when CPAP was resumed.[46] More experience with this relatively simple and easily administered modality is needed. Finally, other agents such as somatostatin and terlipressin may have a role in the treatment of HH, but their true efficacy remains unproven.[47–49]

SUMMARY

HH is an uncommon but vexing complication of portal hypertension, made more challenging by its location and pathophysiology. The importance of making a correct diagnosis to exclude other causes is essential. The recognition of spontaneous bacterial empyema is of the upmost importance in order to initiate potentially life-saving therapy in a timely manner. An understanding of the pathophysiology of HH is important to avoid the pitfalls of therapeutic misadventures such as chest tube placement. All patients with refractory HH should be considered for liver transplantation, but in the MELD era, transplantation may not be available in a timely manner. Thus effective management is needed but difficult to achieve. Thoracentesis is the initial treatment of choice in diuretic-refractory cases, although attempts to treat HH with any invasive means may result in a myriad of complications including pneumothorax, infection, bleeding, renal failure, and pain. Local therapies such as talc pleurodesis often fail when even a relatively dry field is difficult to obtain. In carefully selected patients, insertion of a transjugular intrahepatic portosystemic shunt may be effective when medical treatment has failed.

REFERENCES

1. Xiol X, Castellote J, Cortes-Beut R, et al. Usefulness and complications of thoracentesis in cirrhotic patients. Am J Med 2001;111(1):67–9.
2. Chen CH, Shih CM, Chou JW, et al. Outcome predictors of cirrhotic patients with spontaneous bacterial empyema. Liver Int 2011;31(3):417–24.
3. Chen TA, Lo GH, Lai KH. Risk factors for spontaneous bacterial empyema in cirrhotic patients with hydrothorax. J Chin Med Assoc 2003;66(10):579–86.
4. Krok KL, Cardenas A. Hepatic hydrothorax. Semin Respir Crit Care Med 2012; 33(1):3–10.
5. Cardenas A, Kelleher T, Chopra S. Review article: hepatic hydrothorax. Aliment Pharmacol Ther 2004;20(3):271–9.
6. Baikati K, Le DL, Jabbour II, et al. Hepatic hydrothorax. Am J Ther 2014;21(1): 43–51.
7. Gur C, Ilan Y, Shibolet O. Hepatic hydrothorax—pathophysiology, diagnosis and treatment—review of the literature. Liver Int 2004;24(4):281–4.
8. Chen CY, Chen JS, Huang LM, et al. Favorable outcome of parapneumonic empyema in children managed by primary video-assisted thoracoscopic debridement. J Formos Med Assoc 2003;102(12):845–50.

9. Urbani L, Catalano G, Cioni R, et al. Management of massive and persistent ascites and/or hydrothorax after liver transplantation. Transplant Proc 2003;35(4): 1473–5.
10. Castellote J, Gornals J, Lopez C, et al. Acute tension hydrothorax: a life-threatening complication of cirrhosis. J Clin Gastroenterol 2002;34(5):588–9.
11. Xiol X, Castellvi JM, Guardiola J, et al. Spontaneous bacterial empyema in cirrhotic patients: a prospective study. Hepatology 1996;23(4):719–23.
12. Sese E, Xiol X, Castellote J, et al. Low complement levels and opsonic activity in hepatic hydrothorax: its relationship with spontaneous bacterial empyema. J Clin Gastroenterol 2003;36(1):75–7.
13. Xiol X, Castellote J, Baliellas C, et al. Spontaneous bacterial empyema in cirrhotic patients: analysis of eleven cases. Hepatology 1990;11(3):365–70.
14. Tu CY, Chen CH. Spontaneous bacterial empyema. Curr Opin Pulm Med 2012; 18(4):355–8.
15. Gurung P, Goldblatt M, Huggins JT, et al. Pleural fluid analysis and radiographic, sonographic, and echocardiographic characteristics of hepatic hydrothorax. Chest 2011;140(2):448–53.
16. Ariza X, Castellote J, Lora-Tamayo J, et al. Risk factors for resistance to ceftriaxone and its impact on mortality in community, healthcare and nosocomial spontaneous bacterial peritonitis. J Hepatol 2012;56(4):825–32.
17. Sort P, Navasa M, Arroyo V, et al. Effect of intravenous albumin on renal impairment and mortality in patients with cirrhosis and spontaneous bacterial peritonitis. N Engl J Med 1999;341(6):403–9.
18. Runyon BA, Greenblatt M, Ming RH. Hepatic hydrothorax is a relative contraindication to chest tube insertion. Am J Gastroenterol 1986;81(7):566–7.
19. Lieberman FL, Hidemura R, Peters RL, et al. Pathogenesis and treatment of hydrothorax complicating cirrhosis with ascites. Ann Intern Med 1966;64(2): 341–51.
20. Kiafar C, Gilani N. Hepatic hydrothorax: current concepts of pathophysiology and treatment options. Ann Hepatol 2008;7(4):313–20.
21. Fathy O, Zeid MA, Abdallah T, et al. Laparoscopic cholecystectomy: a report on 2000 cases. Hepatogastroenterology 2003;50(52):967–71.
22. Lazaridis KN, Frank JW, Krowka MJ, et al. Hepatic hydrothorax: pathogenesis, diagnosis, and management. Am J Med 1999;107(3):262–7.
23. Strauss RM, Boyer TD. Hepatic hydrothorax. Semin Liver Dis 1997;17(3): 227–32.
24. Tamano M, Hashimoto T, Kojima K, et al. Diagnosis of hepatic hydrothorax using contrast-enhanced ultrasonography with intraperitoneal injection of Sonazoid. J Gastroenterol Hepatol 2010;25(2):383–6.
25. Rubinstein D, McInnes IE, Dudley FJ. Hepatic hydrothorax in the absence of clinical ascites: diagnosis and management. Gastroenterology 1985;88(1 Pt 1): 188–91.
26. Truninger K, Frey LD. Hepatic hydrothorax without ascites. Schweiz Med Wochenschr 2000;130(44):1706.
27. Bhattacharya A, Mittal BR, Biswas T, et al. Radioisotope scintigraphy in the diagnosis of hepatic hydrothorax. J Gastroenterol Hepatol 2001;16(3): 317–21.
28. Ajmi S, Hassine H, Guezguez M, et al. Isotopic exploration of hepatic hydrothorax: ten cases. Gastroenterol Clin Biol 2004;28(5):462–6.
29. Runyon BA, Committee AP. Management of adult patients with ascites due to cirrhosis: an update. Hepatology 2009;49(6):2087–107.

30. Strauss RM, Martin LG, Kaufman SL, et al. Transjugular intrahepatic portal systemic shunt for the management of symptomatic cirrhotic hydrothorax. Am J Gastroenterol 1994;89(9):1520–2.
31. Jeffries MA, Kazanjian S, Wilson M, et al. Transjugular intrahepatic portosystemic shunts and liver transplantation in patients with refractory hepatic hydrothorax. Liver Transpl Surg 1998;4(5):416–23.
32. Chalasani N, Clark WS, Martin LG, et al. Determinants of mortality in patients with advanced cirrhosis after transjugular intrahepatic portosystemic shunting. Gastroenterology 2000;118(1):138–44.
33. Dhanasekaran R, West JK, Gonzales PC, et al. Transjugular intrahepatic portosystemic shunt for symptomatic refractory hepatic hydrothorax in patients with cirrhosis. Am J Gastroenterol 2010;105(3):635–41.
34. Gordon FD, Anastopoulos HT, Crenshaw W, et al. The successful treatment of symptomatic, refractory hepatic hydrothorax with transjugular intrahepatic portosystemic shunt. Hepatology 1997;25(6):1366–9.
35. Malinchoc M, Kamath PS, Gordon FD, et al. A model to predict poor survival in patients undergoing transjugular intrahepatic portosystemic shunts. Hepatology 2000;31(4):864–71.
36. Xiol X, Tremosa G, Castellote J, et al. Liver transplantation in patients with hepatic hydrothorax. Transpl Int 2005;18(6):672–5.
37. Lee WJ, Kim HJ, Park JH, et al. Chemical pleurodesis for the management of refractory hepatic hydrothorax in patients with decompensated liver cirrhosis. Korean J Hepatol 2011;17(4):292–8.
38. Kilburn JP, Hutchings J, Misselhorn D, et al. Use of indwelling tunneled pleural catheters for the management of hepatic hydrothorax. Chest J 2010; 138(4_MeetingAbstracts):418A.
39. Ferrante D, Arguedas MR, Cerfolio RJ, et al. Video-assisted thoracoscopic surgery with talc pleurodesis in the management of symptomatic hepatic hydrothorax. Am J Gastroenterol 2002;97(12):3172–5.
40. Milanez de Campos JR, Filho LO, de Campos Werebe E, et al. Thoracoscopy and talc poudrage in the management of hepatic hydrothorax. Chest 2000; 118(1):13–7.
41. Hadsaitong D, Suttithawil W. Pleurovenous shunt in treating refractory nonmalignant hepatic hydrothorax: a case report. Respir Med 2005;99(12):1603–5.
42. Park SZ, Shrager JB, Allen MS, et al. Treatment of refractory, nonmalignant hydrothorax with a pleurovenous shunt. Ann Thorac Surg 1997;63(6):1777–9.
43. Perera E, Bhatt S, Dogra VS. Complications of denver shunt. J Clin Imaging Sci 2011;1:6.
44. Saito R, Rai T, Saito H, et al. Two cases of intractable hepatic hydrothorax successfully treated with nasal CPAP. Nihon Shokakibyo Gakkai Zasshi 2006; 103(10):1146–51.
45. Borchardt J, Smirnov A, Metchnik L, et al. Treating hepatic hydrothorax. BMJ 2003;326(7392):751–2.
46. Takahashi K, Chin K, Sumi K, et al. Resistant hepatic hydrothorax: a successful case with treatment by nCPAP. Respir Med 2005;99(3):262–4.
47. Barreales M, Saenz-Lopez S, Igarzabal A, et al. Refractory hepatic hydrothorax: successful treatment with octreotide. Rev Esp Enferm Dig 2005;97(11):830–5.
48. Kalambokis G, Economou M, Fotopoulos A, et al. The effects of chronic treatment with octreotide versus octreotide plus midodrine on systemic hemodynamics and renal hemodynamics and function in nonazotemic cirrhotic patients with ascites. Am J Gastroenterol 2005;100(4):879–85.

49. Ibrisim D, Cakaloglu Y, Akyuz F, et al. Treatment of hepatic hydrothorax with terlipressin in a cirrhotic patient. Scand J Gastroenterol 2006;41(7):862–5.
50. Xiol X, Guardiola J. Hepatic hydrothorax. Curr Opin Pulm Med 1998;4(4): 239–42.

Non-cirrhotic Portal Hypertension

Shiv K. Sarin, MD, DM, FNA, DSc[a],*, Rajeev Khanna, MD, PDCC[b]

KEYWORDS

- Portal hypertension • Non-cirrhotic portal fibrosis
- Extrahepatic portal venous obstruction • Endotherapy • Shunt surgery
- Portal biliopathy

KEY POINTS

- NCPH includes a wide range of disorders presenting with PHT, preserved liver synthetic functions and normal or mildly elevated hepatic venous pressure gradient (HVPG).
- NCPF/IPH and EHPVO are two distinct diseases – former is a disorder of young adults, whereas later is a disease of childhood.
- Likely pathogenesis in both of them relates to recurrent infections in a prothrombotic individual.
- Diagnosis needs exclusion of cirrhosis in NCPF/IPH and presence of a cavernoma in EHPVO.
- Effective management focused on PHT results in good long term survival.

Non-cirrhotic portal hypertension (NCPH) encompasses a wide range of vascular conditions leading to portal hypertension (PHT) associated with normal or mildly elevated hepatic venous pressure gradient (HVPG), whereas the portal venous pressure gradient between the portal vein (PV) and inferior vena cava is comparable or higher than cirrhotic PHT. The diseases leading to NCPH are classified anatomically by the site of resistance to blood flow as prehepatic, hepatic, and posthepatic; hepatic causes are further subdivided into presinusoidal, sinusoidal, and postsinusoidal.[1–3] **Fig. 1** gives an approach and classifies various disorders listed under the category of NCPH. In most of the conditions leading to NCPH, PHT is a late manifestation of the primary disease, except for NCPF and extrahepatic PV obstruction (EHPVO) whereby PHT is the only or predominant manifestation.[1,3,4] The present review describes these 2 entities in detail with a brief discussion on some other causes. Some of the contrasting differences between NCPF and EHPVO have been highlighted in **Table 1**.

Financial Support: Nil.

The authors have nothing to disclose.

[a] Department of Hepatology, Institute of Liver and Biliary Sciences, D-1 Vasant Kunj, New Delhi 110070, India; [b] Department of Pediatric Hepatology, Institute of Liver and Biliary Sciences, D-1 Vasant Kunj, New Delhi 110070, India

* Corresponding author.

E-mail address: shivsarin@gmail.com

1089-3261/14/$ – see front matter © 2014 Elsevier Inc. All rights reserved.

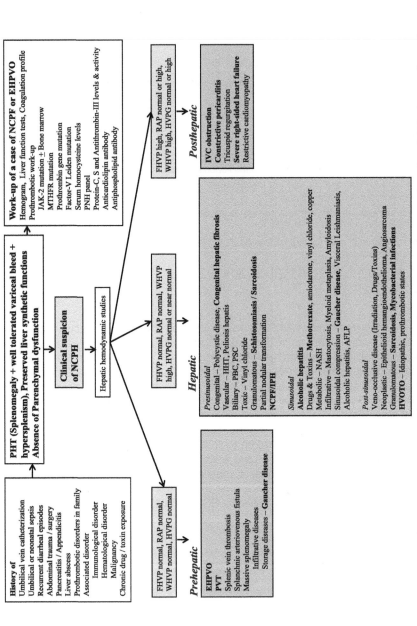

Fig. 1. Approach to a patient of NCPH. NCPH is suspected on clinical grounds and various causes are then classified by hepatic hemodynamic studies as shown. AFLP, acute fatty liver of pregnancy; EHPVO, extrahepatic portal venous obstruction; FHVP, free hepatic venous pressure; HHT, hereditary hemorrhagic telangiectasia; HVOTO, hepatic venous outflow tract obstruction; IPH, idiopathic portal hypertension; IVC, inferior vena cava; JAK-2, Janus kinase-2; MTHFR, methylene tetrahydrofolate reductase deficiency; PBC, primary biliary cirrhosis; PNH, paroxysmal nocturnal hemoglobinuria; PSC, primary sclerosing cholangitis; PVT, portal vein thrombosis; RAP, right atrial pressure; WHVP, wedge hepatic venous pressure. (*Data from* Refs.[1,3,26])

Table 1
Differences between NCPF/IPH and EHPVO

	NCPF/IPH	EHPVO
Epidemiology	Developing > developed[a]	Developing >> developed
Age of onset	Third–fourth decade (India)[b]	First–second decade
First variceal bleed (mean age)	30 y	5 y
Male/female	1.0–2.5:1.0 (1:3 in Japan)	Variable 1–2:1
Etiologic factors	Infections[c] Prothrombotic states Drugs & toxins Immunologic Genetic	Infections[c] Prothrombotic states Congenital
Pathogenetic theories	Unifying hypothesis Dual theory Endothelial-mesenchymal transition	Unifying hypothesis
Pathology		
Liver parenchymal architecture	Maintained Differential atrophy	Maintained
Characteristic hallmark	Obliterative portal venopathy Portal angiomatosis	Cavernomatous transformation of PV
Fibrosis	Periportal and perisinusoidal	None or portal
Presenting features		
Liver size – normal/shrunken	Normal in two-thirds, shrunken in one-third	Normal
Splenomegaly	28%–97%	90%–100%
Variceal bleeding	32%–84%	85%
Number of bleeds before presentation	Median 1 (range 1–20)	Mean 1.8–3.1
Jaundice	9%–31%[d]	Rare[e]
Ascites	10%–34%	10% (after variceal bleeding)
Laboratory parameters/alterations		
Elevation of AST/ALT	2%–73%	Absent
Elevation of SAP/GGT	Not seen	With portal biliopathy
Hypoalbuminemia	17%	During variceal bleeding episodes
Hypoprothrombinemia	4%–81%	83%
Reduced platelet aggregation	78%	89%
Hypofibrinogenemia	+	+ (89%)
Hypersplenism	27%–87%	22%–70%
Transient elastography	7.8–10.2 kPa	5.9 kPa
Prothrombotic states	30%–52%	0%–55%
Immune disorders	17%	Absent
Immunologic alterations	Reduced and altered CMI	Abnormal CMI
Hyperdynamic circulation	+	++

(continued on next page)

	NCPF/IPH	EHPVO
Table 1 *(continued)*		
Autonomic dysfunction	25%	67%
Radiological features		
Ultrasound Doppler	Prominent SPA, dilated PV with thick walls, cutoff of intrahepatic second- and third-degree PV branches (withered-tree appearance)	Cavernoma formation (PV replaced by a bunch of collaterals)
Endoscopic findings		
Esophageal varices	33%–97%	80%–100%
Gastric varices	22%–31%	10%–33%
GOV1	—	19%–64%
GOV2	—	9%–13%
IGV1	—	1%–6%
Gastropathy	2%	12%–40%
Colopathy	40%	54%
Anorectal varices	—	63%–95%
Hemodynamics		
Intravariceal pressure	High	High
WHVP	Normal or mildly elevated	Normal
FHVP	Normal	Normal
HVPG	Normal or up to 6–8 mm Hg	Normal (≤5 mm Hg)
Natural history		
Long-term prognosis	Good	Good
Parenchymal extinction	9%–19%	21%
Portal biliopathy	9%–40%	80%–100%
Minimal hepatic encephalopathy	Not known	32%–35%
Growth retardation	Not studied	31%–57%
Quality of life	Not studied	Impaired

Abbreviations: ALT, alanine transaminase; AST, aspartate transaminase; CMI, cell mediated immunity; FHVP, free hepatic venous pressure; GGT, gamma-glutamyl transpeptidase; GOV, gastroesophageal varices; HVPG, hepatic venous pressure gradient; IGV, isolated gastric varices; IPH, idiopathic PHT; SAP, serum alkaline phosphatase; TNF-R, tumor necrosis factor receptor; VCAM, vascular cell adhesion molecule; WHVP, wedge hepatic venous pressure.

[a] Prevalence in the developed world era is increasing in patients with HIV/AIDS.
[b] Fourth to fifth decade in Japan.
[c] Plausible hypothesis is that severe gastrointestinal infections in infancy or early childhood lead to EHPVO, whereas milder ones at a later age lead to NCPF.
[d] Seen with parenchymal extinction after fourth to fifth decades of life.
[e] Seen with development of portal biliopathy or parenchymal extinction.
Adapted from Refs.[1–3,5–12,14,15,20–22,24–28,32,35,37,40–42,51,53–62,66–70,72–75]; and DM Tripathi and SK Sarin, 2014, unpublished data.

NON-CIRRHOTIC PORTAL FIBROSIS

Non-cirrhotic portal fibrosis (NCPF), variously called *idiopathic PHT* (IPH) in Japan, *hepatoportal sclerosis*, *obliterative venopathy*, and *idiopathic non-cirrhotic PHT* in the West, is a disorder of unknown cause clinically characterized by features of PHT: moderate to massive splenomegaly with or without hypersplenism, preserved liver functions, and patent hepatic and PVs.[1,5–12] Epidemiologically, NCPF/IPH has been reported world-wide, more so from the developing countries, especially in young men in the third to fourth decade belonging to low socioeconomic status.[8–11] NCPF accounts for approximately 10% to 30% of all patients of variceal bleeding in several parts of the world, including India.[12] In Japan and in the Western world, there is a female preponderance of the disease, with presentation at around the fifth decade.[5–7] Such variations may be attributed to differences in living conditions, ethnicity, average life span, reporting bias, as well as the diagnostic criteria used. The declining trend in the East is probably related to improvement in perinatal care and hygiene leading to reduction in incidences of umbilical sepsis and diarrheal episodes, respectively, in early childhood.[13] In the West, on the other hand, there has been an upsurge in the patients of NCPF/IPH in individuals who are human immunodeficiency virus (HIV) positive.[12]

Etiopathogenesis

The precise etiopathogenesis of NCPF/IPH is still unclear, and various hypotheses have been suggested (DM Tripathi and SK Sarin, 2014, unpublished data) (**Fig. 2**).[1,3,14]

Etiologic factors

Infections and *prothrombotic states* are commonly incriminated in Eastern and Western patients, respectively.[1,2] The association with recurrent diarrheal illnesses, umbilical sepsis, and HIV points toward an infectious cause, whereas the presence of prothrombotic disorders and PV thrombosis (PVT) indicates the role of thrombotic predisposition in the disease pathogenesis. Although the former one has been widely supported by various animal models,[14,15] the latter one is negated by the facts that PVT is not universally present and blood flow in the splenic vein is increased rather than decreased.[16] Prolonged exposure to several *medications and toxins*, especially arsenic, has also been incriminated as a cause.[1,3,17,18] The *immunologic* basis is propagated because of the female preponderance, association with autoimmune disorders, and presence in serum of various autoantibodies.[1,16] Lastly, familial clustering and the association with human leukocyte antigen (HLA)-DR3 and with certain genetic syndromes suggest a *genetic* basis.[1,3]

Pathology

Liver pathology is characterized by phlebosclerosis, fibroelastosis, periportal and perisinusoidal fibrosis, aberrant vessels in portal tract (portal angiomatosis), preserved lobular architecture, nodular regenerative hyperplasia, and differential atrophy.[6,16,19,20] The main PV trunk is dilated with thickened sclerosed walls, along with thrombosis in medium and small PV branches, the histologic hallmark termed *obliterative portal venopathy*.[19] A staging system based on the presence of parenchymal atrophy and PVT has been proposed.[20]

Immunologic and cellular changes

Total peripheral T lymphocytes and suppressor/cytotoxic phenotype (T8) cells are reduced. There are increased levels of vascular cell adhesion molecule-1, connective tissue growth factor, and soluble tumor necrosis factor (TNF)-receptor I and II in blood and of endothelin-1 in PV and liver. Mixed autologous lymphocytic reaction is defective.[1,21,22]

Spleen The spleen is disproportionately enlarged in patients with NCPF/IPH (weighing up to 1500 g) in comparison with patients with cirrhosis (weighing ∼700 g).[23] Histopathology reveals hyperplasia of the lymphatic tissue within the white pulp of the spleen (splenadenoma) and sinusoidal ectasia. Increased availability of vasodilator nitric

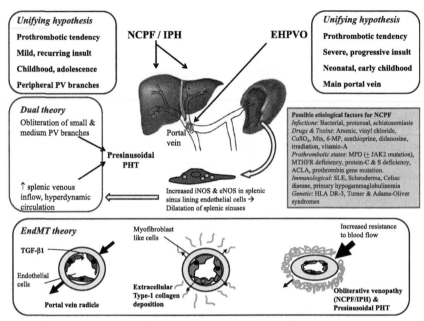

Fig. 2. Pathogenetic theories for NCPF/IPH and EHPVO. *Unifying hypothesis* proposed by Sarin and Kumar[2] explains the pathogenesis of both NCPF/IPH and EHPVO. According to this, a major thrombotic event occurring at a young age involves main PV and results in EHPVO, whereas repeated microthrombotic events later in life involve small or medium branches of PV leading to NCPF. *Dual theory* proposed by Schouten and colleagues[3] takes into account the role of increased splenic blood flow and intrahepatic obstruction. High levels of inducible nitric oxide synthase (iNOS) as well as endothelial NO synthase (eNOS) in splenic endothelial cells lead to dilatation of splenic sinuses and increased splenic venous inflow. *Endothelial-mesenchymal transition* (EndMT) *theory* by Sato and Nakanuma says that vascular endothelial cells of portal venules acquire myofibroblastic features leading to increased synthesis of type I collagen causing obliterative portal venopathy and presinusoidal PHT. This transformation is evidenced by the change from endothelial (vascular endothelial cell marker CD34) to mesenchymal markers (S100A4, alpha-smooth muscle actin, COL1A1 and pSmad2) and is induced by transforming growth factor-β1 (TGF-β1).[14] 6-MP, 6-mercaptopurine; ACLA, anticardiolipin antibody; $CuSO_4$, copper sulfate; HLA, human leukocyte antigen; JAK, Janus kinase; MPD, myeloproliferative disorders; MTHFR, methylene tetrahydrofolate reductase; Mtx, methotrexate; SLE, systemic lupus erythematosus.

oxide (NO) in the spleen and low levels of Endothelin-1 (ET-1) may lead to the dilatation of splenic sinuses, leading to splenomegaly and subsequent PHT.[23]

Diagnosis

The diagnosis of NCPF is largely on clinical ground i.e. presentation with PHT but without any evidence of liver dysfunction. Demonstration of patency of hepatic and PVs is necessary to establish the diagnosis.[1,13]

Clinical Presentation

A proportion of patients are asymptomatic. The duration of symptoms at presentation could vary from 15 days to 18 years; well-tolerated episodes of variceal bleeding, long-standing splenomegaly, and anemia are common. The frequency of variceal bleeding episodes increases with age, with a median of 1 bleeding episode (range 1–20) before presentation.[9,10] Bleeding from nongastrointestinal sites is reported in about 20%.[11] Ascites is seen in 10% to 34% of patients.[8–10,12] Other common presentations are repeated attacks of left upper quadrant pain caused by perisplenitis or splenic infarction.[8] Clinically, there is moderate to massive splenomegaly (average size 11 cm below costal margin).[9] Jaundice and hepatic encephalopathy are rare (~2%) and usually seen either after a major bleed or shunt surgery.[8,10] Associated immunologic and hematologic disorders are seen in 10% and 9% of patients, respectively.[12]

Laboratory Evaluation

Hypersplenism is seen in 27% to 87%, with anemia being the most common abnormality followed by thrombocytopenia and leucopenia. In most of the patients, liver function tests are normal; but a proportion may have derangements in liver enzymes, prothrombin time, and albumin.[6–11] Autonomic dysfunction and coagulation and platelet abnormalities are also seen.[24,25]

Hemodynamics

Intrasplenic (ISP) and intravariceal pressures (IVP) are significantly elevated in NCPF/IPH as compared with wedge hepatic venous pressures (WHVP) and intrahepatic pressures (IHP), suggesting a presinusoidal level of block. There are 2 independent pressure gradients, one between ISP and IHP and another between IHP and WHVP.[26] The median HVPG is 7 mm Hg, but values more than 10 mm Hg are present in 40%.[12] IVP is the investigative tool of choice for PHT. Hyperdynamic circulation, similar to cirrhosis, is seen.[26]

Endoscopic Findings

Esophageal varices are seen in 80% to 90% of patients.[9,10,27] In comparison with patients with cirrhosis, esophageal varices are more often large (90% vs 70%), gastroesophageal varices (GOV1 and GOV2) more common (31%–44% vs 22%), portal hypertensive gastropathy (PHG) less common (10.9% vs 5.4%), and anorectal varices larger and more common (89% vs 56%).[27–30]

Radiological Features

Doppler ultrasound (USG) is the first step in the radiology evaluation of NCPF/IPH patients. The liver is normal in size and echotexture. The spleen is enlarged; the splenoportal axis is dilated and patent. The PV is thickened (>3 mm) with echogenic walls, and its intrahepatic radicles are smooth and regular with a sudden cutoff of its second- and third-degree PV branches—a withered-tree appearance. The splenic index and PV inflow are high.[1,9] Spontaneous shunts (paraumbilical and gastroadrenorenal) are seen in 16%.[9] Intrahepatic PV abnormalities (nonvisualization, reduced caliber, occlusive thrombosis), focal nodular hyperplasialike nodules, and perfusion defects on contrast-enhanced computed tomography (CT) help in differentiating NCPF/IPH from cirrhosis.[31] Radionuclide scintigraphy using 99m-Technetium-Tin (Tc-Sn) colloid shows the absence of increased bone marrow uptake.[32]

Role of Liver Biopsy

Liver biopsy is indicated in all NCPF/IPH patients to exclude cirrhosis and other causes of PHT.[13]

HIV and NCPF/IPH

There has been an abrupt increase in patients of NCPF/IPH, and nearly one-fifth of NCPF/IPH patients in the West are related to HIV.[12,33] Patients with HIV-related

NCPF/IPH are predominantly men (50%–100%), homosexuals (50%–75%), and have prolonged infection (median 11.5 years) and immune reconstitution.[33–36] Recurrent opportunistic gut infections; prolonged usage of highly active antiretroviral therapy, especially didanosine; hypercoagulability; direct effect of HIV; and an underlying pro-thrombotic state may contribute to the development of NCPH.[18,33,34,36] The direct role of HIV is indicated by its ability to infect hepatic stellate cells and cause endothelial injury via cytokines like endothelin-1, inerleukins-1 and -6, and platelet-derived growth factor.[36] The presentation is with features of PHT. Liver decompensation requiring liver transplantation (LTx) has been reported.[12]

Natural History and Prognosis of NCPF

The natural course of NCPF/IPH is good except for the development of PVT and hep-atopulmonary syndrome (HPS) in a minority.[37] Patients with absent varices develop them at rates of 10%, 20%, and 65%; those patients with small ones show progression at rates of 13%, 35%, and 44%, respectively.[12] Liver functions usually remain well preserved; but with the course of time in 20% to 33% of patients, the liver slowly undergoes parenchymal atrophy with subsequent decompensation, development of HPS, and need for LTx.[38–40] Ascites, seen in 26%, is not always a terminal event and is mostly transient.[12]

PVT in NCPF/IPH

The overall incidence of PVT in NCPF/IPH ranges from 13% to 36% over a mean period of 7 years.[6,12,38] Actuarial probability of PVT is around 9%, 16%, 33%, and 42% at 1, 2, 5, and 10 years, respectively, and is associated with the presence of HIV infection, variceal bleeding at diagnosis, and elevated bilirubin levels. The usage of an anticoagulant has been shown to recanalize PV in half of these patients.[12] Over a period of time, preexisting PHT worsens in half and new PVT develops in almost one-third of patients, a proportion requiring LTx.[7] The development of PVT is, thus, a serious complication in the natural history of NCPF/IPH leading to further increased risk of variceal bleeding, progression of liver disease, and eventual decompensation and increased mortality. However, the same findings have not been reproduced in the transplant or autopsy series.[7,40]

The 10-year survival in patients with NCPF/IPH is around 86% to 95%.[12,13] However, in a recent contrary report, the 1-, 5-, and 10-year survival has been reported as 100%, 78%, and 56%, respectively.[38] The discrepancy is explainable by the retrospective nature of these studies; different patient populations; and contribution by associated disorders, especially HIV. There are limited data on the need and outcome of LTx in NCPF/IPH. Patients with PVT, decompensation, HPS, and refractory variceal bleeding may be considered for LTx; but their candidature is not guided by HVPG, the Model for End-stage Liver Disease (MELD), or MELD-Sodium (Na) scores.[1,12]

EHPVO

EHPVO is a childhood disorder characterized by a chronic blockage of PV blood supply leading to PHT and its sequelae in the setting of well-preserved liver function.[4] EHPVO is a major cause of PHT (54%) and upper gastrointestinal bleeding in children (68%–84%) from the developing world,[41,42] whereas in the West, it constitutes a small proportion (11%).[43]

Definition

EHPVO is a vascular disorder of liver characterized by obstruction of the extrahepatic PV with or without involvement of intrahepatic PV radicles or splenic or superior mesenteric veins.[44] This definition, in contrast to the Baveno V consensus, excludes all patients of acute PVT as well as chronic PVT, which develops in a cirrhotic liver or secondary to hepatocellular carcinoma.[45] EHPVO is, in fact, a distinct disease rather an event in the natural history or an extension or association of a primary liver disease. Also, isolated splenic vein or superior mesenteric vein thrombosis is not included in the present definition because of the differences in the etiologic spectrum.[1]

Etiopathogenesis

Etiologic factors

Like other venous thrombosis states, various etiologic factors leading to EHPVO can be divided into those within the vessel lumen (prothrombotic states), within the wall (injury, inflammation, infiltration), or outside the wall (external compression). A small proportion of patients are secondary to developmental *anomalies* like PV stenosis, atresia, or agenesis, which are mostly seen in association with other major malformations, particularly cardiac. Pediatric and adult patients differ in their etiologic spectrum, and approximately 70% of patients may remain idiopathic.[1,2,46–48] Methylene tetrahydrofolate reductase deficiency (C677T) and prothrombin gene mutations (G20201A) are commonly seen in children, whereas primary myeloproliferative disorders (MPD) (with or without Janus kinase 2 [JAK2] mutation V617F) are common in adults with EHPVO. Overall, a single or more prothrombotic state is seen in 28% to 62% of patients.[1] In a recent meta-analysis, the prevalence of MPD and JAK2 mutations in PVT was found to be 31.5% and 27.7%, respectively.[49] In patients with nonmalignant non-cirrhotic PVT, the odds ratios of the usage of oral contraceptives, or the presence of prothrombin gene mutation, factor-V Leiden, or deficiencies of protein-C, protein-S, and antithrombin-III are 50.0, 7.0, 1.5, 5.0, 3.0, and 1.0, respectively.[50] But extrapolation of these results to EHPVO is dubious.

Pathogenesis

A unifying hypothesis proposed by Sarin and Kumar[2] explains the pathogenesis of EHPVO (see **Fig. 2**). Umbilical vein catheterization (UVC) and sepsis are independently present in 9% of EHPVO patients. Prospective ultrasonographic evaluation of such patients shows resolution of PVT in most of them. Progression to EHPVO is related to traumatic UVC or severe or inadequately treated umbilical sepsis.[51] The initial acute PVT event in EHPVO often goes unrecognized, and thrombus gradually becomes organized. Multiple hepatopetal collaterals develop around the PV within a span of 6 to 20 days, replace it, and form a bunch of vessels called *cavernoma* within 3 weeks.[52] These collaterals terminate in middle-sized intrahepatic PV branches, thus overcoming prehepatic obstruction and compensating for a reduction of total hepatic blood flow. But, as a result of high pressure in the splanchnic bed, hepatofugal vessels develop at sites of portosystemic communications and transform into varices, hemorrhoids, and collaterals, some of which become spontaneous shunts.[1,4]

Pathology

PV is replaced by cavernoma, which may extend for a variable length inside and outside the liver. Liver architecture is well preserved. Mild periportal fibrosis may be seen.[1,4]

Diagnosis

EHPVO presents similarly as NCPF/IPH: predominant PHT without any liver dysfunction but from early childhood to adolescence. The presence of portal cavernoma on ultrasound (USG) Doppler clinches the diagnosis.[44]

Clinical Features

There is a bimodal age of presentation: 3 years for those secondary to UVC or umbilical sepsis and more than 8 years for the idiopathic ones or those following intraabdominal infections.[1,4] Growth retardation is frequent.[53] The mean ages of the first bleeding episode and the initial presentation are 5.3 years and 6.3 to 9.3 years, respectively. Children present with a mean of 1.8 to 3.1 bleeding episodes before presentation,[42,54–61] which are recurrent, mostly related to febrile illnesses, and become more frequent and severe with increasing age of onset. However, the recurrences tend to decrease after puberty. Splenic size and portal pressure do not correlate with the incidence or severity of the bleed. Asymptomatic hypersplenism is common, and the proportion increases with age. Ascites develops in 13% to 21% of EHPVO patients, usually after a bleeding episode, and is related to hypoalbuminemia or, in late stages, to parenchymal extinction.[4,62] Perisplenitis and splenic infarction are common. Mesenteric vein thrombosis, bowel ischemia, hemoperitoneum, hemobilia, and pulmonary emboli are rarely seen.[1,4] Clinical examination reveals moderate to massive splenomegaly with normal or shrunken liver and absence of stigmata of chronic liver disease. Jaundice is seen secondary to the development of portal biliopathy or late in the course of the disease because of parenchymal extinction.[1,62]

Laboratory Findings

Hypersplenism is common. Liver function tests are essentially normal, but elevations of alkaline phosphatase and gamma-glutamyl transpeptidase are seen with the development of portal biliopathy. Hypoalbuminemia is frequently seen during bleeding episodes.[1,4] Splenic stiffness is high, and a value more than 42.8 kPa predicts variceal bleeding with fairly good accuracy.[63] Coagulation and platelet abnormalities along with a state of low-grade disseminated intravascular coagulation secondary to portosystemic shunting have been demonstrated.[25] Autonomic dysfunction secondary to a hyperdynamic circulatory state is seen in two-thirds of patients.[24] Cell-mediated immunity is reduced secondary to splenic sequestration of lymphocytes.[4]

Hemodynamics

Like NCPF, EHPVO patients also have significantly elevated ISP and IVP, whereas WHVP and IHP are normal. HVPG is normal. IVP reliably predicts the severity of PHT.[1] Hepatic blood flow is normal or decreased, depending on collateral flow and hepatic arterial buffer response. Hyperdynamic circulatory state is seen, possibly related to elevated NO levels.[64,65]

Endoscopic Findings

Similar to NCPF in comparison with patients with cirrhosis, esophageal and gastric varices are more common, whereas PHG is less common. Esophageal varices are more often large. Isolated gastric varices (IGV1) are present in up to 6% of patients with EHPVO and IGV2, which indicates ectopic or duodenal varices, are also common.[27,28,57–59] Anorectal varices and colopathy are also frequent and rarely may bleed profusely.[29,30]

Radiological Features

Doppler USG of the splenoportal axis (SPA) reveals cavernoma and is the diagnostic investigation of choice, with a sensitivity and specificity more than 95%.[4] Splenoportography or arterial portography have been replaced by noninvasive methods, CT and magnetic resonance (MR) angiography and portography, the later ones also provide an anatomic road map before shunt surgery.[66]

Role of Liver Biopsy

Liver biopsy is not essential for the diagnosis of EHPVO unless underlying chronic liver disease is suspected.[44]

Natural History and Prognosis of EHPVO

Unlike NCPF/IPH, the natural history of EHPVO is rather more complex. This complexity is because of the early insult and the presence of growth failure, parenchymal extinction, impaired quality of life (QoL), minimal hepatic encephalopathy (MHE) and portal biliopathy. Overall prognosis of EHPVO after control of variceal bleed is good with long-term (>10-year) survival nearly 100%.[4]

Growth retardation

Stunting and wasting is present in 37% to 54% and 31% to 57% of children with EHPVO, respectively. Impairment depends on the duration of PHT and is unrelated to caloric intake.[1,53,67] Reduced portal blood supply with concomitant deprivation of hepatotropic factors, poor substrate utilization, and/or malabsorption caused by portal hypertensive enteropathy, growth hormone (GH) resistance evidenced by high levels of GH and low levels of insulinlike growth factor-1 (IGF-1) and IGF binding protein-3, along with the presence of anemia and hypersplenism are certain factors contributing to growth failure.[1]

Impaired QoL

Children with EHPVO have poor health-related QoL with regard to physical, social, emotional, and school functioning; this is unaffected by esophageal eradication but shows an improving trend after shunt surgery.[68]

Portal biliopathy

Portal biliopathy, variously named as portal hypertensive biliopathy, pseudosclerosing cholangitis, or more recently portal cavernoma associated cholangiopathy, refers to biliary ductal (extrahepatic and intrahepatic) and gall-bladder wall abnormalities in patients with PHT developing secondary to cavernomatous transformation of PV.[69,70] Portal biliopathy takes the form of intrahepatic biliary radicles dilatation, indentations, caliber irregularities, displacements, angulations, ectasias, strictures, stones, filling defects, compressions, gall-bladder and pericholedochal varices, or mass. The frequency of these changes in patients with EHPVO, cirrhosis, and NCPF is 80% to 100%, 0% to 33% and 9% to 40%, respectively.[69–72] The changes are produced by compressive and ischemic effects of portal cavernoma in the biliary and peribiliary region, some of which are irreversible even after shunt surgery.[69,70] The left hepatic duct is involved more commonly (38%–100%) and severely. Most of the patients are asymptomatic (62%–95%). Common symptoms are jaundice, biliary colic, abdominal pain, and recurrent cholangitis and are seen with old age, long-standing disease, presence of stones, and abnormal liver function tests.[69–72] Endoscopic retrograde cholangiopancreatography (ERCP) is the diagnostic gold standard; but, being invasive, it has been replaced by the equally efficacious modality MR cholangiopancreatography (MRCP). MRCP with portography also helps in differentiating choledochal varices from stones. Overall, approximately 4% to 10% of these patients succumb to these sequelae despite endoscopic treatments.[69–71]

MHE

MHE has been described in the setting of EHPVO with or without shunt surgery.[74–78] After shunt surgery, toxic substances directly enter into systemic circulation bypassing the liver; prevalence is more with nonselective as compared with selective shunts. MHE is also seen in 32% to 35% of EHPVO patients without a surgical shunt from abnormalities in critical flicker frequency, psychometric tests, and P300 auditory event-related potential.[74–76] This finding is related to the presence of spontaneous shunts, elevated brain glutamine, and the glutamine/creatine ratio on ^{1}H-MR spectroscopy, high blood ammonia, and proinflammatory cytokines (TNF-alpha and interleukin [IL]-6); changes tend to worsen after shunt surgery.[75–77] MHE persists in 75% and new-onset MHE develops in 5% over 1 year.[78]

Liver dysfunction

Parenchymal extinction caused by long-standing deprivation of PV blood supply occurs with increasing age leading to progressive deterioration of liver functions and ascites.[62] Untreated portal biliopathy also leads to progression to secondary biliary cirrhosis.[1]

HEPATIC SCHISTOSOMIASIS

Liver involvement in schistosomiasis is seen in 4% to 8% of patients. Two trematode flukes, namely, Schistosoma mansoni and japonicum, are implicated in disease pathogenesis. Although the former is seen predominantly in Africa and South America, the latter is common in Eastern Asia, especially Mainland China. Liver disease develops as a result of entrapment of eggs in portal venules (<50 mm in diameter), with granulomatous inflammation leading to fibrosis (termed Symmers pipestem fibrosis) and concomitant presinusoidal followed by perisinusoidal PHT.[79] The intense granulomatous inflammatory response elicited by live eggs is T-helper 1 (Th1)-type, which is subsequently replaced by the Th2 response with the development of fibrosis.[79] The deposition of procollagens I, III, and IV, as well as its markers (fibronectin and glycosaminoglycans) is increased; this is positively regulated by IL-13 and negatively by gamma-interferon.[80,81] The Foxp3 gene, necessary for the generation of CD4+CD25+ T-regulatory cells, is overexpressed and ameliorates granuloma formation in such livers.[82] HLA-A5 and a gene closely linked to the interferon-gamma receptor are related to disease severity.[79]

The clinical presentation is similar to NCPF and EHPVO. The diagnosis is based on the demonstration of eggs in stools or rectal biopsy by the Kato-Katz method. Serologic tests, particularly immunoassays with soluble antigen of the Schistosoma mansoni egg, are helpful in the diagnosis.[79,83] The natural history of schistosomal PHT is closely related to the number of eggs deposited in the liver, which roughly parallels the number of eggs excreted in stool.[79]

CONGENITAL HEPATIC FIBROSIS

Congenital hepatic fibrosis (CHF) is a rare autosomal recessive developmental disorder primarily affecting the renal and hepatobiliary systems. The underlying abnormality is ductal plate malformation (DPM), leading to PHT. The majority (64%) is associated with autosomal recessive polycystic kidney disease (ARPKD), secondary to mutations in the PKHD1 gene encoding for fibrocystin/polycystin protein essential for maintenance of 3-dimensional tubular architecture of renal and biliary epithelia, thus, leading to fusiform dilatations of the renal collecting duct and DPM.[84] Another 26% of CHF is associated with Caroli disease or syndrome and less than 1% with type V choledochal cyst; the remaining 10% is isolated CHF.[84] Several other mutations and genetic syndromes have been described.[85] The median age at diagnosis is 0 to 20; ARPKD and Caroli phenotypes present early with renal insufficiency (74%).[84,86] Presentation with PHT and cholangitis, although not mutually exclusive, is seen in 52% to 86% and 34% of patients, respectively. Esophageal varices and hypersplenism are present in 40% to 78% and 44% to 75%, respectively.[84–87] Rarely, patients present with ascites, hepatic encephalopathy, and HPS. There is increased predisposition to cholangiocarcinoma.[84] Liver involvement is unrelated to the degree of renal impairment.[86,87] Liver functions are essentially preserved except in the setting of cholangitis and variceal bleeding.[87] Imaging (USG and MRCP) reveals dilatation of the biliary system (70%), enlargement of the left lobe, and splenomegaly with or without hepatic and renal cysts.[84,85] Mortality is primarily related to sepsis, cholangiocarcinoma, variceal bleeding, and very rarely liver failure.[84] Neonatal presentation is associated with poor prognosis and an early need for combined liver/kidney transplantation (CLKT).[86]

NODULAR REGENERATIVE HYPERPLASIA

Nodular regenerative hyperplasia (NRH) constitutes around 27% and 14% of patients of NCPH in Europe and Japan, respectively.[88] The overall incidence in the general population as per autopsy studies is 2.6% to 7.0 times more in people older than 80 years.[89] Various etiological factors of NRH comprise chemotherapeutic and immunosuppressant drugs, hematologic, autoimmune, inflammatory and neoplastic disorders. Pathogenesis seems to be related to adaptive hyperplastic reaction of hepatocytes in response to mechanical or functional abnormalities of portal hepatic blood flow.[88–91] Pathologically, there are regenerative nodules but with absence of fibrous septa between them. Hypertrophied hepatocytes are located at the center, whereas atrophic ones are at the periphery.[88] HVPG is less than 12 mm Hg in 75%, whereas PV pressure is high.[91] Clinically, the majority is asymptomatic; symptoms are related to PHT.[88] Imaging features are nonspecific; on USG, nodules appear hypoechoic or isoechoic with a sonolucent rim. On contrast-enhanced CT, they are isodense or hypodense in both arterial and portal venous phases, whereas on contrast-enhanced MR, they are hyperintense on T1-weighted and isointense to hypointense on T2-weighted images.[88] Survival primarily depends on the underlying disease and is not related to PHT or varices.[90]

MANAGEMENT

Key management issues in almost all the patients of NCPH are primarily related to control and prophylaxis of acute variceal bleeding, massive splenomegaly, and hypersplenism; 3 additional areas of concern in EHPVO are portal biliopathy, growth failure, and MHE. Management differs from PHT in a cirrhotic patient because of well-preserved liver functions, tolerated bleeding episodes, absence of decompensation, and overall a fairly good prognosis. Three pillars of management include medical, endoscopic, and surgical (**Fig. 3**).[1]

Medical and Endoscopic Management: Control and Prophylaxis of Variceal Bleeding

As per the Baveno V consensus, in view of a paucity of controlled trials, the principles related to vasoconstrictor drugs, endotherapy, and propanolol applicable to cirrhotic PHT should be applied in patients with NCPH with variceal bleeding.[45,55–59,92,93] After esophageal variceal eradication, GOV1 decreases, whereas IGV1, PHG, and ectopic varices increase (**Table 2, Fig. 3**).[57–59,61,92] The usage of beta-blockers for secondary prophylaxis in a single randomized controlled trial (RCT) in NCPF and EHPVO showed comparable efficacy with endoscopic variceal ligation (EVL); 18% had minor adverse

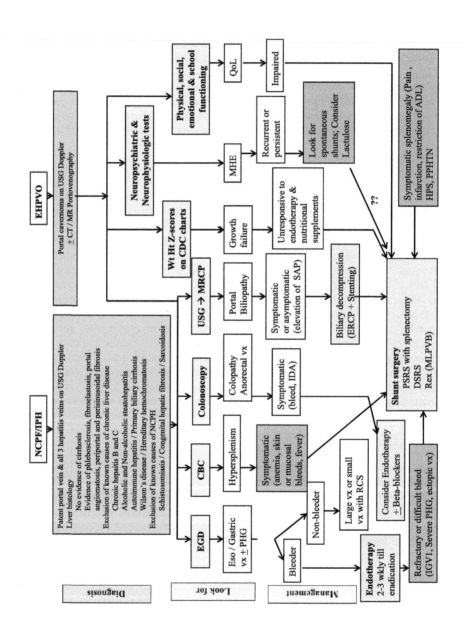

events.[93] A small proportion (8%–12%) of patients whereby medical and endoscopic measures fail to control variceal bleeding, surgical ablative procedures, transjugular intrahepatic portosystemic shunt, or balloon-occluded retrograde transvenous obliteration may be needed.[44,45] There is no consensus on the usage of anticoagulants in NCPH, except in those with a known prothrombotic state when they may be used judicially considering bleeding risk from varices.[1]

Role of Surgery

Surgery is indicated in those NCPH patients that fail to respond to endoscopic management; other indications are highlighted in **Fig. 3**.[44,94–101] Nonphysiologic portosystemic shunts are the most common surgeries done, which are either total (or nonselective) or partial (or selective); the prototype shunts in these categories are the proximal splenorenal shunt (PSRS) or central splenorenal shunt with splenectomy and the distal splenorenal shunt (DSRS), respectively. Ablative procedures like esophagogastric devascularization and splenectomy, previously done in patients with failed shunts, or absent shuntable veins, or with refractory variceal bleed, have become obsolete nowadays.[1,4,94,95] In NCPF, after shunt surgery, PHT improves but with an associated risk of rebleeding, MHE, glomerulonephritis, pulmonary arteriovenous fistula, and ascites.[37,96] In EHPVO, long-term surgical results are excellent but with issues of technical difficulty and shunt thrombosis in small children, most of which have been overcome with improvement in surgical techniques (**Table 3**).[1,4,97] The physiologic or Rex shunt, or mesenterico-left PV bypass (MLPVB), bypasses the level of obstruction in EHPVO by decompressing the superior mesenteric vein to the left branch of the PV via an autologous graft, thus, maintaining the hepatic portal blood flow.[97–99] In view of the long-term advantages, this shunt has become the initial procedure of choice in EHVPO patients (**Table 4**).[1,66,98,99] A single RCT has compared shunt surgery (PSRS) with endotherapy and found comparable mortality and treatment failure but with a high rebleeding rate and transfusion requirement in the EST group.[60] However, most experts think that in the presence of shuntable veins and adequate surgical expertise, it is better to perform shunt surgery in EHPVO, thus, dealing with all the issues in a holistic manner while simultaneously preventing the future development of gastric varices and portal biliopathy.[4,44,98]

Management of Portal Biliopathy

It is one of the consequences of long-standing EHPVO. Although asymptomatic patients do not require any treatment, symptomatic ones or those with persistently raised alkaline phosphatase need to be intervened by ERCP with biliary decompression. Those with severe abnormalities, persistent symptoms, or young age require a

◄────────────────

Fig. 3. Algorithmic approach for diagnosis and management of NCPF and EHPVO. For the diagnosis of NCPF, patency of PV and hepatic veins is essential along with suggestive biopsy and exclusion of other known causes of chronic liver disease or NCPH.[1,3,12] Presence of cavernoma clinches the diagnosis in EHPVO in appropriate setting.[42] All the patients need to be looked up for varices, hypersplenism, and portal biliopathy; EHPVO patients, in addition, need careful attention toward growth, minimal hepatic encephalopathy, and QoL. Indications of shunt surgery have been shown.[98] ADL, activities of daily living; CBC, complete blood counts; CDC, Centers for Disease Control and Prevention; DSRS, distal splenorenal shunt; EGD, esophagogastroduodenoscopy; HPS, hepatopulmonary syndrome; Ht, height; IDA, iron deficiency anemia; MLPVB, mesenterico-left portal vein bypass; PPHTN, portopulmonary hypertension; PSRS, proximal splenorenal shunt with splenectomy; RCS, red color signs; SAP, serum alkaline phosphatase; vx, varix; Wt, weight.

Table 2
Long-term results of endotherapy (EST and EVL) in EHPVO

Study,[Ref.] Year	No. of Subjects	EST/EVL	Eso Vx Eradication (%)	Vx Recurrence (%)	Rebleed (%)	Mortality (%)	Complications (%)	Others
Ittha,[58] 2006	183	EST	89	40	7	0	NA	GOV1 decreased (50%–34%) GOV2 increased (9%–14%) IGV increased (1%–9%) PHG increased (12%–41%)
Poddar,[42] 2008	278	EST	95	14	3	1.7	Eso ulcer 16 Stricture 17 Perforation 2	—
Thomas,[59] 2009	198	EST	NA	20	17	1.5	Stricture 14.6	GOV1 decreased (19.0%–2.5%) GOV2 decreased (13%–11%) IGV same
Sarin,[92] 1997 (RCT)	48 47	EST EVL	NA NA	8 29	21 6	6 6	Stricture 10 vs 0	Obliteration of GOV1 in 52% vs 59%
Zargar,[55] 2002 (RCT)	24 25	EST EVL	92 96	10 17	25 4	0 0	25 4	—
Poddar,[57] 2004	274	EST	95	4.3	3	2	NA	GOV decreased (64%–45%) IGV increased (1%–14%) PHG increased (25%–52%)
Poddar,[61] 2011	101 60	EVL → EST EST	100 95	26 39	4 10	NA NA	7 28	GOV1 decreased (52%–30%) GOV2 increased (9%–22%) IGV increased (3%–11%)

Abbreviations: Eso vx, esophageal varix; NA, not available; Vx, varix.

Table 3
Long-term results of shunt surgeries in patients with EHPVO

Study,Ref. Year	No. of Subjects	Type of Shunt	Follow-up Interval	Patency of Shunt (%)	Rebleed (%)	Mortality (%)	HE (Overt or Minimal) (%)	Others
Alvarez,[102] 1983	76	PSRS MCS	Mean 43 mo	92	8	0	0	Resolution of variceal bleeding and growth recovery in 100%
Warren,[103] 1988	70	DSRS Other shunts Splenectomy Devascularization	NA	96 17 — —	4 67 4 50	0 0 20 30	0 17 NA NA	Following DSRS, improvement in liver blood flow, reduction in spleen size, and increase in platelets
Mitra,[104] 1993	81	LRS without splenectomy	Mean 54 mo	84	10	NA	0	Growth recovery, disappearance of vx, reduction in spleen size & pulp pressure, improvement in hypersplenism
Prasad,[94] 1994	160	PSRS	12–156 mo	NA	11	4	0	15-y Survival 95% Pneumococcal meningitis 1 (0.6%) Recurrent malaria 24%
Orloff,[95] 1994	162	PSRS, MCS	5–35 y	98	2	1.9	NA	Survival at 5 y 99% & 10 y 96% Improvement in QoL & social functioning
Wani,[60] 2011 (RCT)	31 30	PSRS EST	NA NA	97 —	3 23	3 3	NA	—
Lautz,[105] 2009	45	Rex shunt	5–24 mo	100	0	0	NA	Improvement in weight, height, and BMI Z-scores
Superina,[97] 2006	34	Rex shunt	1–7 y	91	0	0	0	Improvement in hypersplenism, coagulopathy, liver volume and flow in SPA Reduction in spleen size
Chaves,[66] 2012	92	Rex shunt	NA	75	NA	0	NA	—

(continued on next page)

Table 3
(continued)

Study,[Ref.] Year	No. of Subjects	Type of Shunt	Follow-up Interval	Patency of Shunt (%)	Rebleed (%)	Mortality (%)	HE (Overt or Minimal) (%)	Others
Lautz,[99] 2013	65 16	Rex shunt DSRS + MCS	Median 4.5 y Median 1.8 y	NA	4 0	NA	NA	Improvement in growth indices in both groups; Rex group has significantly more increase in platelets; INR and ammonia improved after Rex but worsened after other shunts
Agarwal,[100] 2011	37	PSRS	Mean 32 mo	97	0	0	NA	Reversal of portal biliopathy by PSRS alone in 65%; second stage biliary decompression required in 35%
Chattopadhyay,[101] 2012	56	PSRS Splenectomy + devascularization	NA	88	NA	NA	NA	Reversal of portal biliopathy in 88% Biliary decompression procedures following PSRS in 15%

Abbreviations: BMI, body mass index; INR, international normalized ratio; LRS, lienorenal shunt; MCS, mesocaval shunt; NA, not available.

Table 4
Comparison between standard shunt (PSRS and DSRS) and Rex shunt

	Splenorenal Shunt	Rex (MLPVB) Shunt
Type	Nonphysiologic	Physiologic
Cures	PHT only	PHT as well as basis defect
Shunt anatomy	SV to LRV	SMV to left branch of PV
Indication	Any cause of PHT (Child A cirrhotic + NCPH)	Chronic PVT (EHPVO)
Hepatic blood flow	Compromised	Maintained
Requirement	Patent SV and LRV Adequate length of SV Adequate diameter ≥6.5 mm Minimum age 8 y	Patency of SMV & left branch of PV Contiguity of right and left branches of PV Diameter ≥2 mm No minimum age limit (reported at 1 mo of age)
Preoperative assessment	Doppler & CT/MR portovenography	Doppler & CT/MR portovenography ± CTAP, ± wedge hepatic venous portography
Patency	80%–100%	70%–80%
Improvement in growth indices	+++	+++
Improvement in liver volume	Not known	+
Reduction of spleen size	+++	++
Correction of hypersplenism	+++	++
Improvement of hepatic encephalopathy	May worsen	++
Improvement of neurocognitive ability	Not known	++
Reduction of esophageal varices	++	++
Resolution of portal biliopathy	++	+ (Theoretically prevents)
Special expertise	Not required	Required

Abbreviations: CTAP, computerized tomographic arterial portography; LRV, left renal vein; SMV, superior mesenteric vein; SV, splenic vein.
   Adapted from Refs.[1,42,92–101,103,104]

shunt surgery. If symptoms of biliary obstruction persist after surgery, patients are considered for a second surgical procedure (ie, biliary diversion).[1,69,100,101]

Surveillance

It is advisable to follow all NCPF/IPH and EHPVO patients at 6 and 3 monthly intervals, respectively, for clinical and laboratory evaluation, close surveillance for growth, QoL, school performance, learning abilities, spleen size, evidence of decompensation, development of PVT, hepatopulmonary syndrome, and biliopathy.[1]

Management of Schistosomiasis, CHF, and NRH

For the management of these disorders, the basic principles are common as mentioned earlier. In addition, the usage of praziquantel in hepatic schistosomiasis helps in reversion of PHT.[83] In CHF, the option of CLKT should be considered in an appropriate setting.[84,86] On the other hand, in NRH, treatment is primarily directed toward the underlying disease state rather than the management of PHT.[90]

SUMMARY

The term *NCPH* comprises a heterogeneous group of liver disorders, vascular in origin, leading to PHT with near normal HVPG. NCPF/IPH is a disorder of young adults or middle-aged women, whereas EHPVO is a disorder of childhood. The likely pathogenesis in both the conditions is explainable by recurrent infections at a young age in individuals with a thrombotic predisposition. Clinically, both the disorders present with features of PHT in the absence of parenchymal dysfunction. The diagnosis is mostly clinical, supported by imaging modalities. Management centers on control and prophylaxis of variceal bleeding. Both of the disorders otherwise have a fairly good prognosis but need regular and careful surveillance. Hepatic schistosomiasis, CHF, and NRH present similarly and have a comparable prognosis; but the treatment strategies are marginally different.

REFERENCES

1. Khanna R, Sarin SK. Non-cirrhotic portal hypertension- diagnosis and management. J Hepatol 2013. http://dx.doi.org/10.1016/j.jhep.2013.08.013. pii: S0168–8278(13) 00607-7.
2. Sarin SK, Kumar A. Noncirrhotic portal hypertension. Clin Liver Dis 2006;10: 627–51.
3. Schouten JN, Garcia-Pagan JC, Valla DC, et al. Idiopathic noncirrhotic portal hypertension. Hepatology 2011;54:1071–81.
4. Sarin SK, Agarwal SR. Extrahepatic portal vein obstruction. Semin Liver Dis 2002;22(1):43–58.
5. Aoki H, Hasumi A, Yoshida K. A questionnaire study on treatment of idiopathic portal hypertension and extrahepatic portal obstruction. In: Kameda H, editor. Annual report on portal portal hemodynamics abnormalities. Tokyo: Japan Ministry of Health and Welfare; 1988. p. 179–89 [in Japanese].
6. Hillaire S, Bonte E, Denninger MH, et al. Idiopathic non-cirrhotic intrahepatic portal hypertension in the West: a re-evaluation in 28 patients. Gut 2002; 51(2):275–80.
7. Cazals-Hatem D, Hillaire S, Rudler M, et al. Obliterative portal venopathy: portal hypertension is not always present at diagnosis. J Hepatol 2011;54(3): 455–61.
8. Sarin SK, Agarwal SR. Idiopathic portal hypertension. Digestion 1998;59:420–3.
9. Dhiman RK, Chawla Y, Vasishta RK, et al. Non-cirrhotic portal fibrosis (idiopathic portal hypertension): experience with 151 patients and a review of the literature. J Gastroenterol Hepatol 2002;17:6–16.
10. Pande C, Kumar A, Sarin SK. Non-cirrhotic portal fibrosis: a clinical profile of 366 patients. Am J Gastroenterol 2006;101:S2, 191 (abstract No. 439).
11. Madhu K, Avinash B, Ramakrishna B, et al. Idiopathic non-cirrhotic intrahepatic portal hypertension: common cause of cryptogenic intrahepatic portal hypertension in a Southern Indian tertiary hospital. Indian J Gastroenterol 2009;28(3): 83–7.
12. Siramolpiwat S, Seijo S, Miquel R, et al. Idiopathic portal hypertension: natural history and long-term outcome. Hepatology 2013. http://dx.doi.org/10.1002/hep.26904.

13. Sarin SK, Kumar A, Chawla YK, et al. Noncirrhotic portal fibrosis/idiopathic portal hypertension: APASL recommendations for diagnosis and treatment. Hepatol Int 2007;1:398–413.
14. Sato Y, Nakanuma Y. Role of endothelial-mesenchymal transition in idiopathic portal hypertension. Histol Histopathol 2013;28(2):145–54.
15. Omanwar S, Rizvi MR, Kathayat R, et al. A rabbit model of non-cirrhotic portal hypertension by repeated injections of E. coli through indwelling cannulation of the gastrosplenic vein. Hepatobiliary Pancreat Dis Int 2004;3:417–22.
16. Okudaria M, Ohbu M, Okuda K. Idiopathic portal hypertension and its pathology. Semin Liver Dis 2002;22:59–71.
17. Sarin SK, Sharma G, Banerjee S, et al. Hepatic fibrogenesis using chronic arsenic ingestion: studies in a murine model. Indian J Exp Biol 1999;37:147–51.
18. Maida I, Garcia-Gasco P, Sotgiu G, et al. Antiretroviral-associated portal hypertension: a new clinical condition? Prevalence, predictors, and outcome. Antivir Ther 2008;13:103–7.
19. Nayak NC, Ramalingaswami B. Obliterative portal venopathy of the liver. Arch Pathol 1969;87:359–69.
20. Nakanuma Y, Tsuneyama K, Ohbu M, et al. Pathology and pathogenesis of idiopathic portal hypertension with an emphasis on the liver. Pathol Res Pract 2001; 197:65–76.
21. Nayyar AK, Sharma BK, Sarin SK, et al. Characterization of peripheral blood lymphocytes in patients with non-cirrhotic portal fibrosis: a comparison with cirrhotic and healthy controls. J Gastroenterol Hepatol 1990;5:554–9.
22. Yamaguchi N, Tokushige K, Haruta I, et al. Analysis of adhesion molecules in patients with idiopathic portal hypertension. J Gastroenterol Hepatol 1999;14: 364–9.
23. Däbritz J, Worch J, Materna U, et al. Life-threatening hypersplenism due to idiopathic portal hypertension in early childhood: case report and review of the literature. BMC Gastroenterol 2010;10:122.
24. Rangari M, Sinha S, Kapoor D, et al. Prevalence of autonomic dysfunction in cirrhotic and non-cirrhotic portal hypertension. Am J Gastroenterol 2002;97(3): 707–13.
25. Bajaj JS, Bhattacharjee J, Sarin SK. Coagulation profile and platelet function in patients with extrahepatic portal vein obstruction and non-cirrhotic portal fibrosis. J Gastroenterol Hepatol 2001;16:641–6.
26. Sarin SK, Sethi KK, Nanda R. Measurement and correlation of wedged hepatic, intrahepatic, intrasplenic and intravariceal pressure in patients with cirrhosis of liver and non-cirrhotic portal fibrosis. Gut 1987;28:260–6.
27. Sarin SK, Lahoti D, Saxena SP, et al. Prevalence, classification and natural history of gastric varices: a long-term follow up study in 568 portal hypertension patients. Hepatology 1992;16:1343–9.
28. Sarin SK, Shahi HM, Jain M, et al. The natural history of portal hypertensive gastropathy: influence of variceal eradication. Am J Gastroenterol 2000;95: 2888–93.
29. Chawla Y, Dilawari JB. Anorectal varices—their frequency in cirrhotic and non-cirrhotic portal hypertension. Gut 1991;32:309–11.
30. Ganguly S, Sarin SK, Bhatia V, et al. The prevalence and spectrum of colonic lesions in patients with cirrhosis and noncirrhotic portal hypertension. Hepatology 1995;21:1226–31.
31. Glatard AS, Hillaire S, d'Assignies G, et al. Obliterative portal venopathy: findings at CT imaging. Radiology 2012;263(3):741–50.

32. Qureshi H, Kamal S, Khan RA, et al. Differentiation of cirrhotic vs idiopathic portal hypertension using 99mTc-Sn colloid dynamic and static scintigraphy. J Pak Med Assoc 1991;41:126–9.
33. Vispo E, Moreno A, Maida I, et al. Noncirrhotic portal hypertension in HIV-infected patients: unique clinical and pathological findings. AIDS 2010;24:1171–6.
34. Chang PE, Miquel R, Blanco JL, et al. Idiopathic portal hypertension in patients with HIV infection treated with highly active antiretroviral therapy. Am J Gastroenterol 2009;104:1707–14.
35. Schouten JN, Van der Ende ME, Koëter T, et al. Risk factors and outcome of HIV-associated idiopathic noncirrhotic portal hypertension. Aliment Pharmacol Ther 2012;36(9):875–85.
36. Tuyama A, Hong F, Saiman Y, et al. Human immunodeficiency virus (HIV)-1 infects human hepatic stellate cells and promotes collagen I and monocyte chemoattractant protein-1 expression: implications for the pathogenesis of HIV/hepatitis C virus-induced liver fibrosis. Hepatology 2010;52:612–22.
37. Pal S, Desai PR, Rao G, et al. Non-cirrhotic portal fibrosis: results of surgery in 317 consecutive cases over a 25-year period from an Indian center [abstract]. Gastroenterology 2002;123(Suppl 1). T1454:88.
38. Schouten JN, Nevens F, Hansen B, et al. Idiopathic noncirrhotic portal hypertension is associated with poor survival: results of a long-term cohort study. Aliment Pharmacol Ther 2012;35(12):1424–33.
39. Krasinskas AM, Eghtesad B, Kamath PS, et al. Liver transplantation for severe intrahepatic noncirrhotic portal hypertension. Liver Transpl 2005;11(6):627–34.
40. Sawada S, Sato Y, Aoyama H, et al. Pathological study of idiopathic portal hypertension with an emphasis on cause of death based on records of Annuals of Pathological Autopsy Cases in Japan. J Gastroenterol Hepatol 2007;22(2):204–9.
41. Yachha SK. Portal hypertension in children: an Indian perspective. J Gastroenterol Hepatol 2002;17:S228–31.
42. Poddar U, Thapa BR, Rao KL, et al. Etiological spectrum of esophageal varices due to portal hypertension in Indian children: is it different from the West? J Gastroenterol Hepatol 2008;23:1354–7.
43. Fagundes ED, Ferreira AR, Roquete ML, et al. Clinical and laboratory predictors of esophageal varices in children and adolescents with portal hypertension syndrome. J Pediatr Gastroenterol Nutr 2008;46(2):178–83.
44. Sarin SK, Sollano JD, Chawla YK, et al, Members of the APASL Working Party on Portal Hypertension. Consensus on extra-hepatic portal vein obstruction. Liver Int 2006;26(5):512–9.
45. de Franchis R, On behalf of the Baveno V Faculty. Revising consensus in portal hypertension: report of the Baveno V consensus workshop on methodology of diagnosis and therapy in portal hypertension. J Hepatol 2010;53:762–8.
46. Abd El-Hamid N, Taylor RM, Marinello D, et al. Aetiology and management of extrahepatic portal vein obstruction in children: King's College Hospital experience. J Pediatr Gastroenterol Nutr 2008;47:630–4.
47. Weiss B, Shteyer E, Vivante A, et al. Etiology and long-term outcome of extrahepatic portal vein obstruction in children. World J Gastroenterol 2010;16:4968–72.
48. Ferri PM, Rodrigues Ferreira A, Fagundes ED, et al. Evaluation of the presence of hereditary and acquired thrombophilias in Brazilian children and adolescents

with diagnoses of portal vein thrombosis. J Pediatr Gastroenterol Nutr 2012; 55(5):599–604.

49. Smalberg JH, Arends LR, Valla DC, et al. Myeloproliferative neoplasms in Budd-Chiari syndrome and portal vein thrombosis: a meta-analysis. Blood 2012;120(25):4921–8.

50. Valla DC. Thrombosis and anticoagulation in liver disease. Hepatology 2008; 47(4):1384–93.

51. Yadav S, Dutta AK, Sarin SK. Do umbilical vein catheterization and sepsis lead to portal vein thrombosis? A prospective, clinical and sonographic evaluation. J Pediatr Gastroenterol Nutr 1993;17:392–6.

52. De Gaetano AM, Lafortune M, Patriquin H, et al. Cavernous transformation of the portal vein: patterns of intrahepatic and splanchnic collateral circulation detected with Doppler sonography. AJR Am J Roentgenol 1995;165:1151–5.

53. Sarin SK, Bansal A, Sasan S, et al. Portal-vein obstruction in children leads to growth retardation. Hepatology 1992;15:229–33.

54. Webb LJ, Sherlock S. The aetiology, presentation and natural history of extrahepatic portal venous obstruction. Q J Med 1979;192:627–39.

55. Zargar SA, Javid G, Khan BA, et al. Endoscopic ligation compared with sclerotherapy for bleeding esophageal varices in children with extrahepatic portal venous obstruction. Hepatology 2002;36:666–72.

56. Zargar SA, Yattoo GN, Javid G, et al. Fifteen-year follow up of endoscopic injection sclerotherapy in children with extrahepatic portal venous obstruction. J Gastroenterol Hepatol 2004;19:139–45.

57. Poddar U, Thapa BR, Singh K. Frequency of gastropathy and gastric varices in children with extrahepatic portal venous obstruction treated with sclerotherapy. J Gastroenterol Hepatol 2004;19:1253–6.

58. Itha S, Yachha SK. Endoscopic outcome beyond esophageal variceal eradication in children with extrahepatic portal venous obstruction. J Pediatr Gastroenterol Nutr 2006;42(2):196–200.

59. Thomas V, Jose T, Kumar S. Natural history of bleeding after esophageal variceal eradication in patients with extrahepatic portal venous obstruction: a 20-year follow-up. Indian J Gastroenterol 2009;28:206–11.

60. Wani AH, Shah OJ, Zargar SA. Management of variceal hemorrhage in children with extrahepatic portal venous obstruction – shunt surgery versus endoscopic sclerotherapy. Indian J Surg 2011;73(6):409–13.

61. Poddar U, Bhatnagar S, Yachha SK. Endoscopic band ligation followed by sclerotherapy: is it superior to sclerotherapy in children with extrahepatic portal venous obstruction? J Gastroenterol Hepatol 2011;26:255–9.

62. Rangari M, Gupta R, Jain M, et al. Hepatic dysfunction in patients with extrahepatic portal venous obstruction. Liver Int 2003;23(6):434–9.

63. Sharma P, Mishra SR, Kumar M, et al. Liver and spleen stiffness in patients with extrahepatic portal vein obstruction. Radiology 2012;263(3):893–9.

64. Jha SK, Kumar A, Sharma BC, et al. Systemic and pulmonary hemodynamics in patients with extrahepatic portal vein obstruction is similar to compensated cirrhotic patients. Hepatol Int 2009;3:384–91.

65. Goel P, Srivastava K, Das N, et al. The role of nitric oxide in portal hypertension caused by extrahepatic portal vein obstruction. J Indian Assoc Pediatr Surg 2010;15(4):117–21.

66. Chaves IJ, Rigsby CK, Schoeneman SE, et al. Pre- and postoperative imaging and interventions for the meso-Rex bypass in children and young adults. Pediatr Radiol 2012;42:220–32.

67. Nihal N, Bapat MR, Rathi P, et al. Relation of insulin-like growth factor-1 and insulin-like growth factor binding protein-3 levels to growth retardation in extrahepatic portal vein obstruction. Hepatol Int 2009;3:305–9.

68. Krishna YR, Yachha SK, Srivastava A, et al. Quality of life in children managed for extrahepatic portal venous obstruction. J Pediatr Gastroenterol Nutr 2010; 50(5):531–6.

69. Chandra R, Kapoor D, Tharakan A, et al. Portal biliopathy. J Gastroenterol Hepatol 2001;16:1086–92.

70. Condat B, Vilgrain V, Asselah T, et al. Portal cavernoma associated cholangiopathy: a clinical and MR cholangiography coupled with MR portography imaging study. Hepatology 2003;37:1302–8.

71. Dhiman RK, Behera A, Chawla YK, et al. Portal hypertensive biliopathy. Gut 2007;56:1001–8.

72. Khuroo MS, Yattoo GN, Zargar SA, et al. Biliary abnormalities associated with extrahepatic portal venous obstruction. Hepatology 1993;17:807–13.

73. Walser EM, Runyan BR, Heckman MG, et al. Extrahepatic portal biliopathy: proposed etiology on the basis of anatomic and clinical features. Radiology 2011; 258(1):146–53.

74. Sharma P, Sharma BC, Puri V, et al. Minimal hepatic encephalopathy in patients with extrahepatic portal vein obstruction. Am J Gastroenterol 2008;103(6): 1406–12.

75. Yadav SK, Srivastava A, Srivastava A, et al. Encephalopathy assessment in children with extra-hepatic portal vein obstruction with MR, psychometry and critical flicker frequency. J Hepatol 2010;52:348–54.

76. Srivastava A, Yadav SK, Yachha SK, et al. Pro-inflammatory cytokines are raised in extrahepatic portal venous obstruction with minimal hepatic encephalopathy. J Gastroenterol Hepatol 2011;26(6):979–86.

77. Srivastava A, Yadav SK, Lal R, et al. Effect of surgical portosystemic shunt on prevalence of minimal hepatic encephalopathy in children with extrahepatic portal venous obstruction: assessment by magnetic resonance imaging and psychometry. J Pediatr Gastroenterol Nutr 2010;51(6):766–72.

78. Sharma P, Sharma BC, Puri V, et al. Natural history of minimal hepatic encephalopathy in patients with extrahepatic portal vein obstruction. Am J Gastroenterol 2009;104(4):885–90.

79. Ross AG, Bartley PB, Sleigh AC, et al. Schistosomiasis. N Engl J Med 2002; 346(16):1212–20 [review].

80. Harvie M, Jordan WT, Flamme AC. Differential liver protein expression during schistosomiasis. Infect Immun 2007;75(2):736.

81. Czaja MJ, Weiner FR, Takahashi S, et al. Gamma-interferon treatment inhibits collagen deposition in murine schistosomiasis. Hepatology 1989;10(5): 795–800.

82. Singh KP, Gerard HC, Hudson AP, et al. Retroviral Foxp3 gene transfer ameliorates liver granuloma pathology in Schistosoma mansoni infected mice. Immunology 2005;114:410–7.

83. Ruiz-Guevara R, de Noya BA, Valero SK, et al. Clinical and ultrasound findings before and after praziquantel treatment among Venezuelan schistosomiasis patients. Rev Soc Bras Med Trop 2007;40:505–11.

84. Srinath A, Shneider BL. Congenital hepatic fibrosis and autosomal recessive polycystic kidney disease. J Pediatr Gastroenterol Nutr 2012;54(5):580–7.

85. Shorbagi A, Bayraktar Y. Experience of a single center with congenital hepatic fibrosis: a review of literature. World J Gastroenterol 2010;16(6):683–90.

86. Rawat D, Kelly DA, Milford DV, et al. Phenotypic variation and long term outcome of children with congenital hepatic fibrosis. J Pediatr Gastroenterol Nutr 2013; 57(2):161–6.
87. Gunay-Aygun M, Font-Montgomery E, Lukose L, et al. Characteristics of congenital hepatic fibrosis in a large cohort of patients with autosomal recessive polycystic kidney disease. Gastroenterology 2013;144:112–21.
88. Hartleb M, Gutkowski K, Milkiewicz P. Nodular regenerative hyperplasia: evolving concepts on underdiagnosed cause of portal hypertension. World J Gastroenterol 2011;17(11):1400–9.
89. Wanless IR. Micronodular transformation (nodular regenerative hyperplasia) of the liver: a report of 64 cases among 2,500 autopsies and a new classification of benign hepatocellular nodules. Hepatology 1990;11(5):787–97.
90. Morris JM, Oien KA, McMahon M, et al. Nodular regenerative hyperplasia of the liver: survival and associated features in a UK case series. Eur J Gastroenterol Hepatol 2010;22(8):1001–5.
91. Bissonnette J, Généreux A, Côté J, et al. Hepatic hemodynamics in 24 patients with nodular regenerative hyperplasia and symptomatic portal hypertension. J Gastroenterol Hepatol 2012;27(8):1336–40.
92. Sarin SK, Govil A, Jain AK, et al. Prospective randomized trial of endoscopic sclerotherapy versus variceal band ligation for esophageal varices: influence on gastropathy, gastric varices and variceal recurrence. J Hepatol 1997;26(4): 826–32.
93. Sarin SK, Gupta N, Jha SK, et al. Equal efficacy of endoscopic variceal ligation and propranolol in preventing variceal bleeding in patients with noncirrhotic portal hypertension. Gastroenterology 2010;139(4):1238–45.
94. Prasad AS, Gupta S, Kohli V, et al. Proximal splenorenal shunts for extrahepatic portal venous obstruction in children. Ann Surg 1994;219:193–6.
95. Orloff MJ, Orloff MS, Rambotti M. Treatment of bleeding esophagogastric varices due to extrahepatic portal hypertension: results of portal-systemic shunts during 35 years. J Pediatr Surg 1994;29:142–51 [discussion: 151–4].
96. Sharma BC, Singh RP, Chawla YK, et al. Effect of shunt surgery on spleen size, portal pressure and oesophageal varices in patients with non-cirrhotic portal hypertension. J Gastroenterol Hepatol 1997;12(8):582–4.
97. Superina R, Bambini DA, Lokar J, et al. Correction of extrahepatic portal vein thrombosis by the mesenteric to left portal vein bypass. Ann Surg 2006;243: 515–21.
98. Superina R, Shneider B, Emre S, et al. Surgical guidelines for the management of extra-hepatic portal vein obstruction. Pediatr Transplant 2006;10:908–13.
99. Lautz TB, Keys LA, Melvin JC, et al. Advantages of the meso-Rex bypass compared with portosystemic shunts in the management of extrahepatic portal vein obstruction in children. J Am Coll Surg 2013;216(1):83–9.
100. Agarwal AK, Sharma S, Singh S, et al. Portal biliopathy: a study of 39 surgically treated patients. HPB (Oxford) 2011;13:33–9.
101. Chattopadhyay S, Govindasamy M, Singla P, et al. Portal biliopathy in patients with non-cirrhotic portal hypertension: does the type of surgery affect outcome? HPB (Oxford) 2012;14(7):441–7.
102. Alvarez F, Bernard O, Brunell F, et al. Portal obstruction in children. II. Results of surgical portosystemic shunts. J Pediatr 1983;103:703–7.
103. Warren WD, Henderson JM, Millikan WJ, et al. Management of variceal bleeding in patients with noncirrhotic portal vein thrombosis. Ann Surg 1988 May;207(5): 623–34.

104. Mitra SK, Rao KLN, Narasimhan KL, et al. Side-to-side lienorenal shunt without splenectomy in noncirrhotic portal hypertension in children. J Pediatr Surg 1993; 28:398–401; discussion 401–2.

105. Lautz TB, Sundaram SS, Whitington PF, et al. Growth impairment in children with extrahepatic portal vein obstruction is improved by mesenterico-left portal vein bypass. J Pediatr Surg 2009;44:2067–70.

Surgery in Patients with Portal Hypertension

A Preoperative Checklist and Strategies for Attenuating Risk

Gene Y. Im, MD, Nir Lubezky, MD, Marcelo E. Facciuto, MD,
Thomas D. Schiano, MD*

KEYWORDS

- Surgery • MELD • Child-Turcotte-Pugh • Ascites • Cirrhosis • Portal hypertension
- Variceal bleeding • TIPS • Checklist

KEY POINTS

- Patients with liver disease and portal hypertension, usually as a result of advanced fibrosis or cirrhosis, are at increased risk of complications when undergoing surgery.
- Acute or fulminant liver failure and acute viral and alcoholic hepatitis are contraindications to elective surgery.
- The model for end-stage liver disease score is likely more accurate than the Child-Turcotte-Pugh score in predicting perioperative morbidity and mortality.
- Improved assessment of surgical risk can improve informed consent as well as surgical decision making and thus lead to the implementation of medical and surgical strategies, including preoperative transjugular intrahepatic portosystemic shunt, to mitigate risks.
- Use of a preoperative liver assessment checklist (POLA) may be useful as a guideline for assessing surgical risk.

INTRODUCTION

Patients with liver disease and portal hypertension, usually as a result of advanced fibrosis or cirrhosis, are at increased risk of complications when undergoing surgery. Recent advances in hepatology, intensive care medicine, radiology, surgery, and liver transplantation have allowed better optimization of cirrhotic patients before surgery and the reduction of postoperative complications. Despite this progress, the estimation of surgical risk in a patient with cirrhosis is challenging, often involving more art

Disclosures: The authors have no disclosures to report.
Icahn School of Medicine at Mount Sinai, The Mount Sinai Medical Center, Recanati/Miller Transplantation Institute, One Gustave Levy Place, Box 1104, New York, NY 10029-6574, USA
* Corresponding author.
E-mail address: thomas.schiano@mountsinai.org

than science. This article addresses current concepts in the perioperative evaluation of patients with liver disease and portal hypertension with a focus on medical and surgical strategies to mitigate perioperative complications, including a preoperative liver assessment (POLA) checklist.

PATHOPHYSIOLOGY

Understanding about the effects of anesthesia and surgery on the liver has not changed significantly in the past decade.[1] The liver is responsible for the synthesis of most serum proteins, metabolism of nutrients and drugs, detoxification of toxins, and filtering of portal venous blood.[1] Hepatic dysfunction can significantly impair any or all of these functions.[2,3] In particular, the duration of action of many drugs can be increased as a result of altered metabolism by cytochrome P450 enzymes, decreased plasma-binding proteins, and decreased biliary excretion.[4] As a result, opioids like morphine and oxycodone and benzodiazepines like midazolam and diazepam should be avoided to reduce the risk of central nervous system depression and hepatic encephalopathy (HE).[5,6] The metabolism of fentanyl, oxazepam, and temazepam do not seem to be affected by hepatic dysfunction.[7,8]

In healthy patients, the induction of anesthesia with neuromuscular blocking agents and volatile anesthetics reduced hepatic blood flow by up to 36% during the first 30 minutes, but it improves thereafter.[9] Halothane can cause a severe hepatitis and, like enflurane, can also reduce hepatic arterial blood flow. Isoflurane, desflurane, and sevoflurane undergo minimal hepatic metabolism and are preferred.[1] Although propofol is metabolized extensively by the liver, it does not alter hepatic blood flow significant or require dose adjustment in cirrhosis.[10–12] In contrast, spinal or epidural anesthetics may reduce mean arterial pressure and impose significant bleeding risks in patients with cirrhosis and portal hypertension.[13]

Cirrhosis and portal hypertension lead to a hyperdynamic circulation and splanchnic vasodilation, with subsequent activation of the sympathetic nervous system and neurohormonal axis to maintain arterial perfusion pressure.[14] This carefully compensated milieu becomes easily disrupted by the hemodynamic shifts that occur during surgery such as induction of anesthesia, hemorrhage, hypotension, and vasoactive medications.[5] Hypoxemia can occur from ascites, hepatic hydrothorax, hepatopulmonary syndrome, and portopulmonary hypertension.[15] Intermittent positive-pressure ventilation, pneumoperitoneum from laparoscopy, and even traction on abdominal viscera may reduce hepatic blood flow.[15,16] These insults lead to hepatic ischemia and increase the risk of hepatic decompensation.[17]

These various effects on the liver can explain why most surgical procedures are followed by minor increases in liver enzymes, regardless of anesthesia type.[18] However, these disturbances are usually transient and subclinical without consequence in patients without liver disease.[1]

PREOPERATIVE SCREENING FOR LIVER DISEASE

Routine assessment of liver function is not recommended unless suggested by a patient's history and physical examination.[5,19] In an older study of 7620 patients undergoing elective surgery over a period of 1 year, preoperative screening revealed abnormal liver enzymes in only 11 patients (0.14%).[20] If a patient's transaminase or alkaline phosphatase levels are increased to more than 3 times the upper limit of normal or with any increase of the total bilirubin, surgery should be delayed until a thorough work-up is performed.[5,21,22] Asymptomatic patients with this biochemical profile have an incidence of undiagnosed cirrhosis of 6% to 34% and are likely to have an increased risk of surgical complications.[21,22] In contrast, patients with milder forms of liver disease without cirrhosis or portal hypertension are probably at low risk for surgical complications.[23,24]

The impact of specific liver disease causes on surgical risk is largely unknown, but a few recommendations can be given.[15] Adequate preoperative sobriety in patients with excessive alcohol use or mild alcoholic hepatitis should be recommended to avoid perioperative withdrawal symptoms.[25] In patients with autoimmune hepatitis on prednisone, perioperative use of stress-dose hydrocortisone is recommended.[1] Patients with hemochromatosis should be evaluated for complications like diabetes and cardiomyopathy. Patients with Wilson disease may have neuropsychiatric involvement that may interfere with informed consent, with surgery being a precipitant of neurologic symptoms.[26] D-Penicillamine interferes with cross-linking of collagen and may impair wound healing, so the dose should be decreased in the first 1 to 2 postoperative weeks.[26] We recommend paying particular attention to a patient's platelet count as a surrogate marker of portal hypertension by splenic sequestration together with an isolated aspartate aminotransferase (AST) increase as subtle and early biochemical markers of cirrhosis.[27] Patients can have liver disease and even cirrhosis with normal liver enzymes, especially in patients with nonalcoholic steatohepatitis (NASH).[28–30]

ESTIMATING SURGICAL RISK

There is no such thing as a good cirrhotic patient (surgery proverb)[31]

The initial assessment of a patient with liver disease is similar in any setting. It starts with determining the cause of the liver disease and the severity of liver dysfunction manifested in a patient's symptoms and correlated with laboratory, endoscopic, and radiologic findings. Identifying the impact of comorbid conditions is also essential. The indication, urgency, and alternatives to surgery are additional elements to be considered in the surgical risk assessment. The more urgent the need for surgery, the less relevant a risk assessment is, especially in life-threatening situations. Thus, the estimation of risk plays a larger role in less urgent or elective surgeries, in which there is time to assess the patient and initiate strategies to mitigate risks or consider alternative treatments.[15] Accurate assessment of surgical risk can also enhance informed consent from the patient and may influence surgical decision making, especially when quantitative predictions of postoperative mortality are given.

Timing of Surgery

There is a general consensus in the literature that emergent surgeries performed in patients with cirrhosis have poorer outcomes than those with normal liver function and compared with elective surgery (**Table 1**).[32–40] This consensus is likely related to the

Table 1							
Mortality after elective and emergent surgery in patients with cirrhosis							
	Doberneck et al,[32] **1983**	**Garrison et al,**[33] **1984**	**Aranha et al,**[34] **1986**	**Mansour et al,**[35] **1997**	**Farnsworth et al,**[36] **2004**	**Telem et al,**[38] **2010**	**Neeff et al,**[37] **2011**
Elective (%)	11	10	10	18	17	6	9
Emergent (%)	45	57	86	50	19	25	47

effect of life-threatening presentations in sicker cirrhotic patients and the paucity of time to optimize patients before surgery.

Contraindications to Elective Surgery

There are several clinical situations in which elective or semielective surgeries should be strongly avoided in patients with liver disease (**Box 1**). Patients with acute or fulminant liver failure should not undergo any surgery unless involving liver transplantation. Other surgeries, like sleeve gastrectomy, umbilical herniorrhaphy and even coronary artery bypass graft (CABG), can sometimes be performed safely during liver transplantation, although experience is limited.[41–43] Studies predating modern serologic testing of patients with acute viral hepatitis undergoing diagnostic laparotomy report mortalities between 10% and 100%.[44,45] This observation extends to acute alcoholic hepatitis, in which patients undergoing various surgeries (open liver biopsy, portosystemic shunt surgery, exploratory laparotomy) have experienced mortalities of 55% to 100%.[45–49] Because most cases of acute hepatitis are self-limited, elective surgery should be delayed (usually >3 months) and reevaluated when the patient's clinical profile returns to its baseline.

A special consideration is the safety of surgery in patients with acute hepatic porphyrias, a group of rare inherited metabolic disorders of the heme biosynthetic pathway occurring in the liver.[50] General anesthesia has the porphyrinogenic qualities of cytochrome-mediated metabolism and high lipid solubility and, together with surgery, has been linked to precipitation of life-threatening porphyric crises.[51,52] Various surgeries have been shown to be safe in patients with acute hepatic porphyria, when liver enzymes are usually normal.[51,52] There is a consensus that, although propofol is safe, lidocaine and etomidate are not in patients with porphyria.[51,53,54] Before surgery, anesthesiologists should refer to websites containing updated databases to assess the safety of proposed anesthetic medications.[55]

Prediction Models of Surgical Risk

The preoperative evaluation of a patient with liver disease has long been considered more art than science.[56] Prospective studies are lacking and relevant studies are case series with inherent selection bias and reflecting different eras of medical, anesthetic, and surgical advances. It is difficult to accurately assess surgical risk for a patient who may have a unique clinical profile undergoing a specific surgery at a certain time that has not been characterized by prior studies. Reflecting the general trend in hepatology is the recent emergence of the Model for End-Stage Liver Disease (MELD) in favor of the Child-Turcotte-Pugh (CTP) score for assessing perioperative morbidity

---

Box 1
Contraindications to elective surgery in patients with liver disease

Acute liver failure

Fulminant liver failure

Acute viral hepatitis

Acute alcoholic hepatitis

ASA class V

Abbreviation: ASA, American Society of Anesthesiologists.

and mortality in patients with cirrhosis, eclipsing its standard-bearer status for more than 3 decades.[5,56]

Prediction Models: CTP

Since the 1970s, the standard for assessing perioperative morbidity and mortality in patients with cirrhosis has been the CTP scoring system, which is based on 3 laboratory values and 2 clinical variables (**Table 2**).[5,15] The CTP score was originally designed to predict outcome after portocaval shunt surgery, and was then modified for prediction in patients undergoing esophageal transection of bleeding varices.[5,57,58] There are numerous retrospective studies that have shown the good correlation of surgical outcomes with the CTP score (**Table 3**).[33,36–38,59–62] Although limited by their small numbers of highly selected, mostly Child class A patients, data from the 2 most often cited studies, by Garrison and colleagues[33] and Mansour and colleagues,[35] are highly concordant. Patients who were Child class A had a 10% risk of inpatient mortality after surgery, 30% to 31% for Child class B, and 76% to 82% for Child class C. **Table 2** also includes more recent studies for comparison that affirm the predictive value of the CTP score but with improved outcomes in Child class B and C patients. This finding likely reflects differences in the surgeries performed, institutional expertise, improvements in patient selection, and advances in hepatology and surgery.

The older study cohorts of Garrison and colleagues[33] and Mansour and colleagues[35] included surgery for complications of peptic ulcer disease and gastrointestinal (GI) bleeding, comprising 12% and 23% of the cohort, respectively. Such surgeries were often emergent, with ensuing high mortality, but are less relevant now because these types of surgeries are rarely performed today. We recently described a modern cohort of 100 patients with cirrhosis who underwent abdominal surgery at our institution, the Mount Sinai Medical Center. Although the CTP score correlated linearly with operative morbidity, both Child B and C classes had 12% 30-day postoperative mortality.[38]

The CTP scoring system has several limitations. The variables were selected empirically, 2 are subjective, all are weighted equally, they are categorized in a trichotomous fashion using arbitrary cutoff values, and they are not validated at defined time points.[56,63,64] Also, within each class there can be considerable heterogeneity. For example, there is a ceiling effect by which a serum bilirubin of 4 mg/dL garners the

Table 2
CTP classification for severity of cirrhosis

Parameter	Points		
	1	**2**	**3**
Ascites	None	Mild to moderate	Severe
Hepatic Encephalopathy	None	Mild to moderate (grade 1–2)	Severe (grade 3–4)
Total bilirubin (mg/dL)	<2	2–3	>3
Serum albumin (g/dL)	>3.5	2.8–3.5	<2.8
International Normalized Ratio	<1.7	1.7–2.3	>2.3

CTP score is obtained by adding the score for each parameter. CTP class A, 5–6 points; class B, 7–9 points; class C, 10–15 points.

Data from Child CG, Turcotte JG. Surgery and portal hypertension. Major Probl Clin Surg 1964;1:1–85; and Pugh RN, Murray-Lyon IM, Dawson JL, et al. Transection of the esophagus for bleeding esophageal varices. Br J Surg 1973;60(8):646–9.

Table 3
Performance of CTP in the prediction of mortality after surgery in patients with cirrhosis

	Garrison et al,[33] 1984	Mansour et al,[35] 1997	Costa et al,[62] 2009	Neeff et al,[37] 2011	Telem et al,[38] 2010
Number of patients	100	33	190	138	100
Liver disease	Mostly ALD	Unknown	87% ALD	60% ALD	50% HCV
Institution	Louisville	Texas A&M	Portugal	Germany	Mount Sinai
Surgery (%)	29 CC 23 PUD 9 Colon	100 CC	26 Hernia 17 Liver 17 CC	28 Hernia 22 PUD 17 Colon 11 CC	47 Hernia 17 Colon
Elective (%)	58	Unknown	59	51	68
CTP mortality (%)	A: 10 B: 31 C: 76	A: 10 B: 30 C: 82	A: 5 B: 14 C: 31	A: 10 B: 17 C: 63	A: 2 B: 12 C: 12

Abbreviations: ALD, alcoholic liver disease; Colon, colectomy; CC, cholecystectomy; HCV, hepatitis C virus infection; Hernia, herniorrhaphy; Liver, liver resection; PUD, peptic ulcer disease.

same 3 points as 40 mg/dL, although there is likely an outcome difference between these two values. Another example is a patient with Child class B cirrhosis (CTP score 7) with 3 points from massive ascites who is more likely to incur wound complications after abdominal surgery compared with another Child B cirrhotic with the same score and no ascites.

Prediction Models: MELD

The MELD score was originally designed to predict outcome in patients with cirrhosis after placement of a transjugular intrahepatic portosystemic shunt (TIPS).[65] The MELD score has been prospectively validated as a prediction model in patients with cirrhosis awaiting liver transplantation, and for patients with acute variceal bleeding and acute alcoholic hepatitis (**Table 4**).[63,66,67] There are several advantages of MELD compared with CTP. It is a continuous scoring system with weighted objective variables and has been validated to predict mortality at short-term and intermediate-term time points.[56,64] MELD also includes serum creatinine, which has been shown to be correlated with postoperative mortality.[68] Several recent retrospective studies have examined the MELD score as a prediction model for surgical risk in patients with cirrhosis (**Table 5**). Each has shown good correlation between MELD and surgical outcomes

Table 4
Modified MELD score

MELD Score	3-mo Mortality (%)
>40	71.3
30–39	52.6
20–29	19.6
10–19	6.0
<9	1.9

MELD = 3.78[Ln serum bilirubin (mg/dL)] + 11.2[Ln INR] + 9.57[Ln serum creatinine (mg/dL)] + 6.43.
Data from Wiesner R, Edwards E, Freeman R, et al. Model for end-stage liver disease (MELD) and allocation of donor livers. Gastroenterology 2003;124(1):91–6.

Table 5
Performance of CTP and MELD in the prediction of mortality after surgery in patients with cirrhosis

	Farnsworth, et al,[36] 2004	Perkins et al,[60] 2004	Befeler et al,[61] 2005	Northup et al,[59] 2005	Costa et al,[62] 2009	Telem et al,[38] 2010	Neeff et al,[37] 2011
Number of patients	40	33	53	140	190	100	138
Liver disease (%)	58 Viral	Unknown	47 Viral	28 ALD 14 HCV	87 ALD	50 HCV	60 ALD
Institution	Baylor	Texas A&M	Saint Louis	Virginia	Portugal	Mount Sinai	Germany
Surgery (%)	25 I&D 15 Liver 13 CC	100 CC	55 CC 45 Ex-lap	21 CC 10 Hip 9 Hernia 4 CABG	26 Hernia 17 Liver 17 CC	47 Hernia 17 Colon	28 Hernia 22 PUD 17 Colon 11 CC
Elective (%)	24	Unknown	Unknown	42	59	68	51
CTP mortality (%)	A: 15 B: 9 C: 60		A: 0 B: 22 C: 23	N/A	A: 5 B: 14 C: 31	A: 2 B: 12 C: 12	A: 10 B: 17 C: 63
MELD mortality	≤8: 8% 9–16: 10% ≥17: 57%	<8: 0 ≥8: 6%	<14: 9% ≥14: 77%	5–10: 5–8% 10–15: 8–14% 15–20: 14–25%	<14: 9% ≥14: 77%	<15: 5.5% ≥15: 36%	<10: 9% 10–15: 19% >15: 54%
Conclusions	MELD = CTP	MELD≥CTP	MELD>CTP	MELD AUC = 0.72	MELD = CTP = iMELD	MELD>CTP, especially with albumin <2.5 and ASA class	CTP + ASA class + sodium <130 > MELD

Abbreviations: ASA, American Society of Anesthesiologists; AUC, area under curve; CC, cholecystectomy; Ex-lap, exploratory laparotomy; Hip, orthopedic hip repair; I&D, incision and drainage; iMELD, integrative MELD.

with the equal or superior predictive performance of MELD compared with CTP.[36–38,59–62] The previously described limitations of retrospective case series again make it difficult to draw definite conclusions. For example, Perkins and colleagues[60] described a unique cohort of 33 cirrhotic patients who all underwent a single type of surgery, (cholecystectomy). There was likely significant selection bias given the low median CTP and MELD scores in the study. Without sufficient numbers of Child B and C and higher MELD patients, the outcomes of these sicker patients cannot be deduced from this study.

Although one of the putative strengths of the MELD score is that it is a continuous scoring system, there is a natural desire to ascertain the cutoff MELD score that marks a threshold beyond which the predicted surgical risk is unreasonable. Several of the studies in **Table 5** showed that a MELD score of $\sim$15 marks a divergence in outcomes after surgery. A MELD score of 15 is conveniently familiar to many practitioners and not likely by accident. Patients with MELD 15 to 34 have a higher mortality compared with MELD less than 15 (17.4% vs 8.8%) while awaiting liver transplantation.[69–71] At lower MELD scores, the morbidity from transplant surgery and immunosuppression is untenable, but when patients reach a MELD greater than or equal to 15 they are considered candidates for liver transplantation at most institutions.[38,69] This score is generally considered the upper limit at which a TIPS could be safely placed at our institution and is the basis for the so-called Share 15 National rule, whereby deceased adult donor livers are offered to all candidates in status 1A and 1B and those with MELD/Pediatric End-stage Liver Disease (PELD) greater than or equal to 15 locally, regionally, and nationally before being offered to candidates with lower MELD/PELD scores.[71]

Although not a prospective study, the case-control study by Teh and colleagues[64] is the largest and most useful study of the MELD score for surgical risk assessment in patients with cirrhosis to date. These investigators from the Mayo Clinic in Rochester, Minnesota, identified 772 patients with cirrhosis with a median MELD of 8 who underwent major digestive, orthopedic, or cardiac surgical procedures and were grouped into 2 cohorts based on surgical decade (1980–1990 and 1994–2004). The cirrhosis was caused by alcohol (24%), viral hepatitis (18%), cholestatic liver disease (18%), and others (40%). Laparoscopic cholecystectomy patients were excluded. The two control groups comprised 562 outpatients having cirrhosis without surgery and a group of 303 patients undergoing so-called minor surgeries like appendectomy and herniorrhaphy. Whether these surgeries are minor in the setting of advanced liver disease is patient dependent and debatable.

Multivariable analysis showed that a patient's age, American Society of Anesthesiologists (ASA) physical status class, and MELD score were statistically significant predictors of mortality at 30 and 90 days and long term after surgery (**Table 6**).[64] All patients with cirrhosis were at least ASA class III. Age greater than 70 years was associated with higher mortality, and ASA class alone was the strongest predictor of the 7-day mortality. The 10 ASA class V patients had 100% mortality, which suggests that ASA class V should be a contraindication to surgery other than liver transplantation in patients with cirrhosis.[56,64] In contrast with prior studies, emergent surgery was not an independent predictor of mortality because these patients had higher median MELD scores compared with elective surgery patients (and thus confounded by MELD score on multivariable analysis). Patients who underwent major surgery had higher 7-day, 30-day, and 90-day mortality compared with the controls but, as expected, there was no difference in mortality at 1 year between the 3 groups, because the impact of surgery likely dissipates after 90 days.[64]

The relationship between MELD score and relative risk of mortality after surgery was almost perfectly linear for MELD greater than 8, with a 14% increase in

Table 6
ASA physical status classification

ASA Class	Preoperative Health Status
I	Normal healthy patient
II	Patients with mild systemic disease
III	Patients with severe systemic disease
IV	Patients with severe systemic disease that is a constant threat to life
V	Moribund patients who are not expected to survive without the operation
VI	A declared brain-dead patient whose organs are being removed for donor purposes

30-day and 90-day mortality for every 1 point increase in MELD (**Fig. 1**).[64] This finding was higher than was previously estimated by Northup and colleagues.[59] With MELD scores less than or equal to 7, this point change effect was blunted by 75%. The addition of age and ASA class to the MELD score further enhanced the predictive accuracy of determining surgical risk in patients with cirrhosis and at specific time points, which can be easily calculated at http://www.mayoclinic.org/meld/mayomodel9.html. This modified MELD score for surgery is particularly useful in its ease of use and ability to provide quantitative probabilities of 7-day, 30-day, and 90-day mortality (**Table 7**), and this avoids the vagueness of low-risk, intermediate-risk, or high-risk predictions and avoids the pitfalls of poorly informed consent with patients thinking, "I was told it was no big deal."[31] In the acute setting, admission CTP and MELD scores can be inflated by transient delirium, hypotension, acute kidney injury, cholestasis of sepsis, hemolysis, and so forth, which may be misleading and not fully reflective of a patient's liver dysfunction. Thus, there is value in trending laboratory tests and predictive scores over time, with only MELD being validated for use at various time points.

As with prior studies, the cutoff MELD score was about 15 and likely should be as low as 12. This gray area of risk (MELD 12–15) conferring a predicted mortality of 25.4%, may give pause to patient and surgeon decision making and prompt stronger consideration of more conservative treatments (or palliative care) or transfer to a liver transplant center. We have described that the addition of serum albumin into the risk

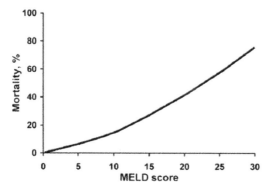

Fig. 1. Relationship between MELD score and relative risk of mortality at 30 days after surgery. (*From* Teh S, Nagorney DM, Stevens SR, et al. Risk factors for mortality after surgery in patients with cirrhosis. Gastroenterology 2007;132(4):1267; with permission.)

Table 7
Modified MELD for surgery (postoperative mortality risk in patients with cirrhosis)

MELD Score	Mortality (%)		
	7 d	30 d	90 d
0–7	1.9	5.7	9.7
8–11	3.3	10.3	17.7
12–15	7.7	25.4	32.3
16–20	14.6	44.0	55.8
21–25	23.0	53.8	66.7
≥26	30.0	90.0	90.0

assessment in these borderline patients (MELD≥15) can also be useful, because a level of less than 2.5 mg/dL was associated with a mortality or liver transplantation rate of 60% compared with 14% with albumin greater than 2.5 mg/dL.[38]

A disadvantage of using a MELD-based scoring system for surgical risk assessment is the well-recognized inability of MELD to reflect the severity of illness in some patients who are said to be sicker than their MELD. The MELD score has been shown not to correlate well with the severity of HE or ascites.[72] In patients with diuretic-resistant ascites but low MELD scores, use of the modified MELD for surgery predicting low mortality may not be as applicable to umbilical hernia surgery, in which wound healing and fluid management would be problematic compared with an orthopedic surgery not involving the abdomen. Clinical scenarios such as these suggest that the subjective variables in the CTP scoring system can be advantageous at times and is why determination of the CTP score in the preoperative evaluation of a patient with cirrhosis is still recommended.

TYPE OF SURGERY

There are many published case series about a single type of surgery in patients with cirrhosis. Several reviews have covered this area in detail so this article focuses on pertinent and more commonly encountered clinical scenarios pertaining to patients with cirrhosis and portal hypertension.[1,5,13,15,19,73–77] There are no data available on surgery in patients with noncirrhotic portal hypertension. In the interpretation of data presented in all of these case series, an emphasis needs to be placed on the presence or absence of the collective experience and expertise of the nurses, hepatologists, and surgeons in managing complicated patients with cirrhosis and portal hypertension. In addition, the impact of anesthesiologists during surgery and intensivists after surgery who are specialized in liver disease, such as those found at a liver transplant center, cannot be underestimated and is increasingly being recognized.[78,79]

Laparoscopic Versus Open Cholecystectomy

The prevalence of gallstones in patients with cirrhosis is 29.4%, more than twice that of the general population.[74] Most of these patients are asymptomatic, and should not be operated on. The advantages of laparoscopy compared with open cholecystectomy in healthy patients have been well described, with laparoscopy leading to shorter hospital stays and operative time, faster operative rehabilitation, and reduced wound complications.[74,80–83] Several studies have shown that cholecystectomy is safe in patients with Child A and B cirrhosis and MELD scores of up to 11 to 13, with mortalities of 0% to 6% and laparoscopy the preferred method.[84–92] The conversion rate of laparoscopy to open cholecystectomy is 5% to 12%. The advantages of laparoscopy are shorter operative time and length of hospitalization, and reduced morbidity and mortality.[84–92] Both CTP and MELD scores predict postoperative outcomes, with thrombocytopenia and intraoperative platelet transfusions also having statistical significance.[84–92] When the risks of surgery are prohibitive, alternative treatments should be considered, such as prolonged antibiotic treatment, percutaneous cholecystostomy (not preferred if ascites is present), and transpapillary cystic duct stenting.[93–95] The feasibility and efficacy of this type of stenting is generally low, as is for oral dissolution therapy for stones associated with cirrhosis with ursodiol. The benefits of laparoscopy in patients with cirrhosis have been shown to extend to other surgeries like splenectomy, colectomy, and appendectomy as well.[96–98]

Herniorrhaphy

Patients with both cirrhosis and ascites have a 20% risk of developing an umbilical hernia (UH).[99] Even though rupture and evisceration are rare occurrences, their association with 30% to 60% mortality is ominous while caring for a patient with a liver disorder with an UH.[100–104] Incarcerated UH is more common than rupture or evisceration.[105] Early surgical experience with UH repair in patients with cirrhosis was dismal and led to surgical dogma stipulating repair in only those who develop complications.[106] We stress the importance of good hernia care from the beginning with conservative measures like abdominal binders augmented by the well-placed tennis ball adjacent to UHs and the careful titration of diuretics and salt intake. The observation that incarceration can occur soon after large-volume paracentesis as a floating bowel loop is caught in the hernia during decompression must be noted.

Although the natural course of UH in the presence of concurrent ascites is largely unknown, in a study of 34 patients with cirrhosis, ascites, and UH, 17 had elective UH repair, 13 were managed conservatively, and 4 underwent hernia repair during liver transplantation. In the conservative treatment group, 69% became incarcerated and 1 ruptured.[107] Thus, elective surgery should be considered.

Several recent studies have shown excellent outcomes of patients, even with Child C cirrhosis, undergoing elective UH repair.[99,107–111] Elective surgery not only avoids incarceration or rupture, but is also associated with fewer complications and, in some studies, reduced mortality, likely in large part caused by the nonemergent timing of surgery.[99,107–111] In a study of almost 23,000 patients with cirrhosis undergoing UH repair identified by the American College of Surgeons National Surgical Quality Improvement Program, logistic regression analysis showed that age greater than 65 years, MELD greater than 15, serum albumin les than 3.0 mg/dL, and sepsis at presentation were associated with postoperative mortality.[110]

Although Teh and colleagues[64] considered herniorrhaphy and cholecystectomy as minor surgical procedures and included them in a control cohort compared with major abdominal surgery, in our experience they are not minor, especially in patients awaiting liver transplantation. Although repair of UH can be performed at the time of liver transplantation, concerns about potential incarceration and rupture must be balanced with the risk of surgery and decompensation in already tenuous patients with ascites and high CTP and MELD scores. Because of poor wound healing, dehiscence, infection, and hernia recurrence associated with postrepair ascites, there has been considerable interest in decreasing portal pressures over the year by several perioperative methods, including peritoneovenous shunting, temporary peritoneal dialysis catheters, closed-system peritoneal drainage without suction, and TIPS.[112–116]

Several multicenter, randomized controlled trials have shown TIPS to be superior to large-volume paracentesis in select patient populations by controlling ascites in

80% to 90%.[111,117–120] Several small case series have described the effect of preoperative TIPS in patients with portal hypertension.[111,117,121–123] In the largest series from the University of Michigan, Kim and colleagues[123] described 25 patients with a median MELD score of 15 (28% Child C) who underwent TIPS before abdominal or cardiothoracic surgery. The perioperative mortality risk was only 12%. This lower-than-expected mortality suggested that the portal pressure reduction of preoperative TIPS was protective beyond attenuating wound complications or ascites. The rapid control of ascites after TIPS without diuretics is unreasonable because it might take more than 4 to 6 weeks before the beneficial effects of TIPS are seen.

We described our experience with 21 patients with Child B and C cirrhosis mostly from hepatitis C and refractory ascites complicated by UH incarceration or rupture.[111] The overall mortality was 20% at a mean follow-up of 3 years, with UH rupture conferring a decreased transplant-free survival compared with incarceration despite a lack of perioperative mortality. A trend toward a decrease in wound complications (27% vs 17%) was noted in the 6 patients who underwent TIPS 1 day before surgery, but not with closed-suction drain placement alone. Although the sample size is small, we recommend semielective surgery with preoperative TIPS in patients with UH rupture when feasible.

Compared with UHs, inguinal herniorrhaphy in patients with cirrhosis seems to be safe. Perioperative complications were not higher in patients with cirrhosis and not associated with severity of liver disease by Child class in one case series.[124]

Colorectal Surgery

Two large series of colorectal surgery for mostly diverticular disease and colorectal cancer in patients with cirrhosis showed mortalities of 13% to 23% and morbidity sustained in about one-half.[74,125] Emergent surgery has been correlated with worse outcomes.[111,126] A population-based study in the United States of colorectal surgery performed from 1998 to 2005 showed greater than an 11-fold increase in adjusted mortality of cirrhotic patients with portal hypertension undergoing elective colorectal surgeries compared with patients with no cirrhosis.[126] Because of these risks, less-invasive alternatives such as decompression of large bowel obstruction by colonoscopy and stenting should be considered.

The need for colorectal surgery is often broached in patients with inflammatory bowel disease and primary sclerosing cholangitis. In a study of 23 patients with mostly Child A and B cirrhosis with mean MELD score of 9 undergoing restorative proctocolectomy, there was almost universal postoperative morbidity (83%), comprising mostly bleeding and worsening liver function.[127] However, perioperative mortality was low (9%), and was attributed to pelvic abscesses with shock. There were no outcomes differences between an ileoanal pouch procedure or colectomy with ileostomy.

Thoracic Procedures

There is a considerable literature on thoracoscopic procedures for the treatment of refractory hepatic hydrothorax, a complication with a prevalence of 5% in patients with cirrhosis.[128,129] Chest tubes are occasionally placed as treatment of symptomatic hepatic hydrothorax. We have described our experience with 59 patients with mostly Child B and C cirrhosis who had chest tubes placed for various reasons, but predominantly for hepatic hydrothorax.[130] Chest tubes were only able to be removed two-thirds of the time because of high-volume output with nearly all (80%) having one or more of these complications: renal dysfunction, electrolyte imbalances, and infection. Serum total bilirubin levels, presence of HE, and Child class C were predictors of mortality, with an overall mortality of 25%. As a result, we think that placement of chest tubes is contraindicated in hepatic hydrothorax, except in special situations like parapneumonic effusions (true empyema) or aiding in extubation from ventilator support by reducing lung compression or atelectasis. Chest tubes can be avoided in most patients with hepatic hydrothorax if meticulous attention to sodium intake, titration of diuretics, and possibly TIPS are performed. More recently, video-assisted thoracoscopic surgery with closure of diaphragmatic defects and/or mechanical or chemical pleurodesis have been described in selected patients to successfully allow prolonged symptomatic relief in 48% to 75% with no mortality in many case series.[131–133]

Bariatric Surgery

Patients with cirrhosis are not immune from the epidemic of obesity in the United States. NASH is now the third or fourth leading indication for liver transplantation in the United States and is likely to overtake hepatitis C in the next several decades.[134,135] The consideration of bariatric surgery will become increasingly commonplace in patients with NASH because it has been shown to decrease steatosis, inflammation, and fibrosis and improve hyperlipidemia and diabetes.[136,137] NASH without advanced fibrosis does not increase the risk of bariatric surgery.[15,138] The incidence of unexpected cirrhosis at the time of bariatric surgery is estimated in the range of 2% to 6%.[15,23] In a questionnaire to 126 bariatric surgeons, biopsy-proven cirrhosis was noted in 125 patients during surgery, with the surgeons proceeding with surgery in 73% and a perioperative mortality of 3.2%.[23] This is about 5 times higher than in patients without cirrhosis. However, the incidence of cirrhosis was only 0.14%.

Although controversial, several studies have shown that morbid obesity is associated with an increase in mortality and primary graft nonfunction after liver transplantation.[139] As a result, some transplant centers have adopted body mass index limits that require weight loss that is difficult for candidates and may jeopardize candidacy. There is little literature evaluating the safety of bariatric surgery in cirrhosis. Wu and colleagues[136] gathered data from 3 studies of a total of 44 patients with Child A and B cirrhosis undergoing bariatric surgery (one-third unexpectedly) of mostly laparoscopic Roux-en-Y gastric bypass (RYGB) with a complication rate of 32% and 1 perioperative death.

The 3 most widely used laparoscopic modalities are RYGB, gastric banding, and sleeve gastrectomy (SG), each of which has advantages and disadvantages.[136] RYGB renders the stomach remnant accessible only by deep enteroscopy and is complicated by malabsorption and vitamin deficiencies. Gastric banding is the least invasive and effective, but carries an infection risk with ascites and is contraindicated by the US Food and Drug Administration in patients with cirrhosis.[140] Sleeve gastrectomy may have the best profile for patients with cirrhosis and portal hypertension, but carries a risk of gastric variceal hemorrhage because a portion of the stomach is removed.[136] As a result, there has been interest in SG in the pretransplant, intratransplant, and posttransplant settings. Lin and colleagues[141] from the University of California, San Francisco, reviewed records of 26 pretransplant patients who underwent laparoscopic SG with 23% complications but no perioperative mortalities, with excellent weight loss response and eventual transplantation in 31%. Heimbach and colleagues[42] performed 7 SGs at the time of liver transplantation with 2 complications, no mortality or graft loss, and all with substantial weight loss. Further study is needed before SG can be recommended routinely in morbidly obese pretransplant patients with cirrhosis from NASH.

Cardiac Surgery

The hemodynamic shifts in cardiac surgery cause it to be particularly perilous for patients with cirrhosis and portal hypertension. Published studies are small, but they all report increased postoperative morbidity and mortality compared with other surgeries (**Table 8**).[142–144] Klemperer and colleagues[142] showed good safety of cardiac surgery in patients with Child A cirrhosis, but poor outcomes in Child B. More recent studies show an improvement in survival of patients with Child B cirrhosis, with Filsoufi and colleagues[144] identifying that the time of cardiopulmonary bypass (CPB), the type of CPB (pulsatile vs nonpulsatile), and perioperative pressor support were associated with hepatic decompensation.[143] Macaron and colleagues[145] confirmed the findings of Suman and colleagues[143] that CTP score greater than or equal to 8 was highly predictive of 90-day mortality after CABG with or without valve surgery with CPB. Cirrhosis conferred a 5 times increased risk of mortality compared with matched controls.

Liver Resection

Both primary and metastatic cancers can occur in patients with cirrhosis. Patients with cirrhosis are at increased risk to develop hepatocellular cancer (HCC), with an overall prevalence of approximately 1% to 4% per year.[146–148] Screening of patients with cirrhosis has resulted in a growing number of patients diagnosed with HCCs that are amenable to resection. Patients with cirrhosis who undergo liver resection are at significant risk for morbidity and mortality related mainly to decompensation of their liver disease, caused by loss of liver parenchyma, and the limited ability of the cirrhotic liver to undergo regeneration. The main factors that determine risk for postoperative morbidity and mortality are the extent of the required liver resection, and severity of hepatic dysfunction. Patients with decompensated liver disease or evidence of portal hypertension (thrombocytopenia, splenomegaly, presence of varices on imaging, or increased pressures on transhepatic measurements) are typically excluded from consideration of liver resection, and are referred for evaluation for liver transplantation. Patients with Child A cirrhosis or MELD score less than 9 to 10, normal bilirubin and albumin, and no portal hypertension can be considered for liver resection.[149] Other markers of limited liver functional reserve that have been used to assess surgical risk include high retention of indocyanine green, and uptake of radioactive technetium-marked albumin.[150,151]

Several perioperative techniques have been developed to improve outcome in cirrhotic patients undergoing liver resection. Before surgery, nutritional status should be optimized. Patients considered for hemiliver resection should undergo percutaneous portal vein embolization (PVE) of the lobe planned for resection. PVE results in atrophy of the embolized lobe, and compensatory hypertrophy of the contralateral lobe. Failure of the contralateral lobe to undergo hypertrophy is a sign that the liver has poor capacity to regenerate, and surgery should be carefully reconsidered. PVE has been shown to significantly reduce postoperative morbidity secondary to liver decompensation in cirrhotic patients undergoing major liver resections.[152]

During surgery, care should be taken by the anesthesia team to minimize alteration in hepatic blood flow by avoiding hypotension. Patients should have a central line placed to actively monitor central venous pressure, which should be kept low

Table 8 Mortality after cardiac surgery in patients with cirrhosis			
Child Class	Klemperer et al,[142] 1998	Suman et al,[143] 2004	Filsoufi et al,[144] 2007
A (%)	0/8 (0)	1/31 (3)	1/10 (10)
B (%)	4/5 (80)	5/12 (42)	2/11 (18)
C (%)	—	1/1 (100)	4/6 (67)

($\sim$5 cm H_2O) in order to minimize bleeding from hepatic veins during parenchymal dissection. Pressors can be used to maintain blood pressure (to avoid hepatic ischemia) and hypovolemia corrected following the completion of the resection. There is some debate as to the safety of using the Pringle maneuver during parenchymal dissection in patients with cirrhosis. Our experience has been that it is probably safe to clamp the liver hilum for intermittent short intervals (10–15 minutes), separated by 5-minute intervals of unclamping. Drains should be placed at the end of the case for possible bile leaks and to aid in draining ascites that may develop after surgery and can result in wound dehiscence. Drains should be removed when the drained volume is low, and in all cases up to 5 to 7 days after surgery, to prevent intra-abdominal infections.

STRATEGIES FOR ATTENUATING PERIOPERATIVE RISK

Our institution has a long tradition of caring for patients with liver disease. More than 3800 liver transplants have been performed at our institution. As an institution specializing in liver medicine and transplantation, we have implemented specific pathways and protocols pertaining to the perioperative care of patients with cirrhosis.[111] We have previously described our experience and management approach in the care of hospitalized patients with cirrhosis.[153] Several preoperative, intraoperative, and postoperative strategies have been developed to minimize the perioperative risk in cirrhotic patients undergoing abdominal surgery. Many of our recommendations are not governed by results of randomized clinical trials, but are based on collective and institutional experience.

Preoperative Strategies

Preoperative checklist in patients with cirrhosis or portal hypertension
In an attempt to simplify the process of assessing surgical risk in patients with liver disease, we propose the use of a preoperative liver assessment (POLA) checklist that could not only be privy to consultants but could be embedded into increasingly prevalent electronic medical records in appropriate patient situations, allowing access by other providers as well. Similar preoperative checklists have been shown to be valuable and can reduce morbidity and mortality.[154–156] The POLA checklist is meant to be filled out in chronologic order, and is shown in **Fig. 2**. Further investigation is required to determine whether implementation of the POLA checklist has any effects on patient and provider decision making, patient care, and outcomes. The discussion presented later informs the salient points included on the POLA checklist.

Optimizing medical therapy: compensate the decompensated Consultants must tailor their approach to the particular patient whom they are assessing for surgical risk. When time is available and surgery is semielective or elective, the potential of the consultant to effect mitigating strategies is greatest. First, the type, chronicity, and severity of liver disease must be evaluated, with mild liver disease proceeding to surgery and near-absolute contraindications like fulminant hepatic failure and acute alcohol or viral hepatitis ruled out or delayed. Significant comorbid conditions must also be considered, especially conditions conferring added cardiovascular risks, like diabetes mellitus.

Obtaining a thorough history of prior hepatic decompensation is important because it may portend the future decompensation symptoms after anesthesia and surgery with the opportunity for troubleshooting. If there is a history of ascites, the threshold to use postoperative diuretics may be lower. If HE has been a problem, reduced sedation and analgesia, strict monitoring of bowel movements, and aspiration precautions

☐ **Emergent or elective**

- If surgery is potentially life-saving, proceed with surgery with adequate informed consent, but also consider nonsurgical alternatives like such as ongoing medical therapy or interventional radiologic procedures or palliative care as appropriate.

☐ **Characterize liver disease**

- Determine cause and chronicity of liver disease.
  - If acute viral or alcoholic hepatitis or severe drug-induced injury, postpone surgery for at least 3 months
  - If chronic but mild liver disease, proceed with surgery
  - If there is evidence of cirrhosis or noncirrhotic portal hypertension, continue with liver assessment

☐ **Identify significant comorbid conditions**

- Focus on presence of diabetes, chronic kidney disease, and cardiovascular disease
- If moderate or severe nutrition is present, optimize nutrition by oral, enteral, or even parenteral means before surgery

☐ **Perform liver imaging**

- MRI or CT are preferred to evaluate for liver appearance, vessel patency, hepatocellular carcinoma, and evidence of portal hypertension (eg, intra-abdominal varices, spleen size)
- Ultrasound with Doppler is sufficient if there is contraindication to CT or MRI such as acute kidney injury

☐ **Obtain history of prior hepatic decompensation**

- Ascites: if yes, consider future impact on wound healing with postoperative recurrence
- Encephalopathy: if yes, adjust planned sedation and analgesia, and monitor for regular bowel movements.
  - Do not restrict dietary protein (give 1.2–1.5 g/kg protein daily)
- Variceal bleeding: if yes, perform upper endoscopy and initiate variceal hemorrhage prophylaxis

☐ **Evaluate for current hepatic decompensation**

- Ascites: if yes, perform diagnostic paracentesis to evaluate for SBP
  - If moderate or severe, perform LVP before surgery
  - Consider preoperative TIPS if diuretic resistant and MELD <15, but not typically for emergent cases
  - Give 2 g sodium diet, 35–45 kcal/g daily
- Encephalopathy: if yes, optimize lactulose to achieve 2–4 bowel movements/day (even by NGT) and give rifaximin
  - Do not restrict dietary protein (give 1.2–1.5 g/kg protein daily)
  - Order aspiration precautions
- Variceal bleeding: if yes, perform upper endoscopy and initiate variceal hemorrhage prophylaxis
- Hypoxemia or CHF: if yes, consider hepatopulmonary syndrome or portopulmonary hypertension
  - Perform ABG, contrast-enhanced echocardiography

Fig. 2. Preoperative Liver Assessment (POLA) checklist. ABG, arterial blood gas; CHF, congestive heart failure; CT, computed tomography; ddAVP, desamino-D-arginine vasopressin; INR, International Normalized Ratio; LVP, large volume paracentesis; MRI, magnetic resonance imaging; NGT, nasogastric tube; NSAIDs, nonsteroidal antiinflammatory drugs; SBP, spontaneous bacterial peritonitis; TMP/SMX, trimethoprim/sulfamethoxazole.

☐ **Estimate liver function and likelihood of portal hypertension**

- Check serum total bilirubin, albumin, INR, creatinine, platelets, hepatic venous pressure gradient, if available

☐ **Calculate CTP, MELD, and modified MELD for surgery at several time points**

(postoperative mortality risk in patients with:

(cirrhosis calculator found at http://www.mayoclinic.org/meld/mayomodel9.html); note: all

cirrhotics are ≥ASA class III)

- If Child C or MELD >12 or high risk, consider alternatives to surgery or transfer to liver transplant center
- If Child C or MELD >12 or high risk, consider completing liver transplant evaluation before surgery

☐ **Evaluate coagulopathy and anemia**

- Give subcutaneous vitamin K supplementation leading up to surgery
- Give DDAVP/desmopressin if renal insufficiency present
- Consider use of recombinant factor VIIa for refractory hemorrhage
- In the absence of hemorrhage, do not transfuse platelets if count >50 × 10^3/µL or cryoprecipitate if fibrinogen >50 mg/dL
- Avoid overtransfusion to correct anemia (use hemoglobin goal of 7 g/dL) to avoid increasing portal pressures

☐ **Review medications**

- Avoid hepatotoxic medications like herbal supplements and acetaminophen >2 g per day.
- Avoid nephrotoxic medications like NSAIDs (ie, ketorolac, ibuprofen) or aminoglycosides (ie, gentamicin)
- Avoid all benzodiazepines for anxiety/insomnia and narcotics or administer those with short half-lives
- Monitor and correct for electrolyte and acid-base disturbances that may precipitate encephalopathy
- Avoid prophylactic antibiotics with greater risks of drug-induced liver injury like amoxicillin-clavulanate (Augmentin), nitrofurantoin, TMP/SMX (Bactrim), ciprofloxacin, and levofloxacin

Fig. 2. (continued)

could be planned. An upper endoscopy should be performed before surgery if not done recently (>1 year) or if a patient has a history of varices or variceal bleeding.

In patients with cirrhosis who are moderately or severely malnourished, optimizing nutritional status before elective surgery can reduce negative postoperative outcomes.[33] If oral or enteral nutrition is inadequate or fasting lasts longer than 72 hours, the use of parenteral nutrition is recommended, even in cirrhosis.[157]

The evaluation for early active signs and symptoms of hepatic decompensation is paramount. If ascites is present, a diagnostic paracentesis must be performed to evaluate for spontaneous bacterial peritonitis (SBP). In the case of moderate or severe ascites, performance of a large-volume paracentesis with intravenous albumin replacement may reduce lung restriction from intra-abdominal pressure that may affect the induction of anesthesia. We use a liberal replacement strategy of 12.5 g of 25% albumin for every 1 to 2 L of ascites removed depending the presence of renal insufficiency.[153] A preoperative TIPS should be considered if a patient has diuretic-resistant ascites and MELD less than 15. Before surgery, a 2 g sodium diet is preferred. If HE is present, optimization of lactulose dosing to 2 to 4 bowel movements per day and administration of rifaximin are recommended. If HE is severe, we place a soft, small-caliber nasogastric tube regardless of the presence of esophageal varices for the administration of oral lactulose.[153] We find that lactulose enemas are less effective, but can also be used. Consistent with recently published guidelines, we do not restrict dietary protein and give 1.2 to 1.5 g/kg of protein daily.[158] If there is evidence of active or recent variceal bleeding, an urgent upper endoscopy must be done with a low threshold to perform esophageal variceal band ligation in an attempt to reduce the risk of perioperative variceal bleeding. If hypoxemia or congestive heart failure symptoms are present, a consideration of hepatopulmonary syndrome or portopulmonary hypertension should lead to the minimum performance of an arterial blood gas and contrast-enhanced echocardiography. The presence of these special conditions, depending on severity, may be contraindications to surgery or even liver transplantation.

As a general rule, we recommend an abdominal CT or MRI with IV contrast to evaluate for the liver appearance (whether there is a nodular appearance), vessel patency (whether there is portal vein or mesenteric thrombosis), hepatic masses (undiagnosed HCC or nodular regenerative hyperplasia), and spleen size (indirect evidence of portal hypertension). If a patient's renal function precludes a contrast-enhanced study, we routinely obtain an abdominal ultrasound with Doppler evaluation.

Next, liver function and the likelihood of portal hypertension are estimated by gathering the aforementioned data and reviewing blood work, paying particular attention to serum total bilirubin, albumin, International Normalized Ratio (INR), creatinine, and platelets. The patient's CTP, MELD, and modified MELD for surgery should be calculated and clearly documented in the medical record. The quantitative operative risk prediction should be discussed in detail with the patient and the surgical providers for shared informed consent. If a patient has Child C cirrhosis or MELD greater than 12, or has high surgical risk for other reasons, alternative treatments, completion of liver transplant evaluation before surgery, or transfer to a liver transplant center should be considered (**Fig. 3**).

An evaluation of hematologic disturbances should be performed. We usually give routine subcutaneous vitamin K, 10 mg daily, for 3 days to correct any underlying deficiency and effects on INR that may alter CTP or MELD scores. We avoid rote administration of fresh frozen plasma (FFP) to correct coagulopathic numbers if there is no evidence of bleeding, but give FFP if INR is greater than 1.5 just before a nontransplant surgery. In patients with renal dysfunction, administration of desamino-D-arginine vasopressin/desmopressin is advocated to help correct quantitative platelet dysfunction (at a dose of 0.3 μg/kg). As supported by a recent study, we avoid overtransfusion and have used a restrictive resuscitation strategy of red cells to a goal of hemoglobin 7 g/dL (including all blood products and crystalloid) to avoid increasing portal pressures.[159] Platelets are often administered by our surgeons just before surgery if the platelet count is less than $50 \times 10^3/\mu L$.

A review of the patient's medications should be done to avoid hepatotoxic medications like unnecessary over-the-counter or herbal supplements and acetaminophen greater than 2 g/d. Nephrotoxic medications like nonsteroidal antiinflammatory drugs (NSAIDs), especially intravenous ketorolac, should be avoided. The "as needed" orders for NSAIDs are often embedded within electronic order sets and should be reviewed and adjusted carefully before implementation. All benzodiazepines and narcotics should be avoided or administered carefully. Avoidance of electrolyte (especially hypokalemia) and acid-base disturbances to avoid precipitating HE and

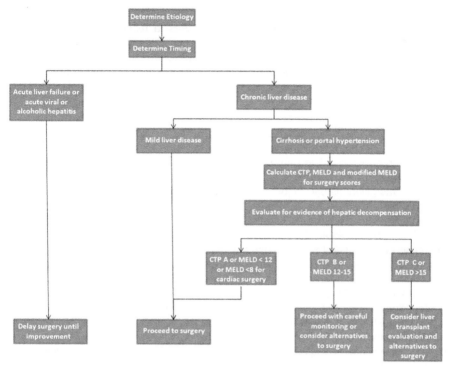

Fig. 3. Preoperative risk assessment and decision algorithm.

cardiac arrhythmias is stressed. The QT interval is prolonged in many patients with cirrhosis, so medications that potentially lengthen it further should be avoided.

Successful completion of the POLA checklist and preoperative evaluation should not prompt the consultant to "sign off" because the immediate postoperative period often is the most critical time in which reevaluation is required and mitigating strategies effected.

Intraoperative strategies

During surgery, the anesthesia team has an important role in determining outcome in cirrhotic patients. Having a dedicated liver disease–oriented team of anesthesiologists is important. Administration of anesthesia invariably reduces blood flow to the liver, which is well tolerated by patients with normal liver function, but can precipitate liver decompensation in cirrhotic patients. Alterations in liver perfusion during surgery should therefore be minimized, and avoidance of hypotension is crucial. Normovolemia should be maintained, especially in circumstances of potential large-volume losses, such as bleeding, clamping of large vessels, or aspiration of large volume of ascites when opening the abdomen. Ascites should be replaced by albumin, usually at a ratio of 12.5 g of 25% albumin for every 1 L of ascites removed during surgery.

The surgeon should attempt to avoid significant blood loss during surgery. Extreme care should be taken when handling varices, because these vessels have a thin wall and high pressure, which can result in massive bleeding if injured. Meticulous hemostasis is important, because postoperative coagulopathy and thrombocytopenia can precipitate significant bleeding from even minor potential sources. When performing emergent UH repairs, we always prefer to perform primary repair of the fascial defect, to avoid possible mesh infection.[160] In most cases, a tension-free repair can be completed, because the fascia is lax from the chronic distention caused by the ascites. At the end of the case, placing a drain to avoid wound complications caused by tense ascites should be considered. Controversy exists as to whether the drain reduces risk of wound dehiscence, and whether it may increase risk for intra-abdominal infection.

Postoperative Strategies

If oral or enteral nutrition is inadequate after surgery, patients with cirrhosis should receive early postoperative parenteral nutrition. After abdominal surgery in patients with cirrhosis, a lower complication rate was observed when postoperative parenteral nutrition was given instead of just intravenous fluid and electrolytes.[161] Maintenance fluids should be based on 5% albumin to increase oncotic pressure. If drains were placed, they should not remain longer than 5 to 7 days after surgery in order to reduce the risk of infection. As an alternative to drains, interval, preemptive, large-volume paracentesis can be used to avoid tense ascites and minimize wound complications.

In the event of ascites leaking from a wound or wound dehiscence, we recommend early large-volume paracentesis and the subsequent use of short-term 25% intravenous albumin infusions and diuresis with furosemide and spironolactone. However, acute kidney injury often accompanies this clinical scenario, which limits diuresis. In this case, we try to reverse the kidney injury and sometimes request our interventional radiology colleagues to place an intra-abdominal drain to divert ascites away from the wound. Careful monitoring of ascites output to achieve equal fluid balance using 25% albumin and crystalloid is also important. Meticulous wound care is then initiated, without vacuum-assisted wound closure, which may cause fistula formation, to allow for the formation of granulation tissue in a drier environment and removal of the drain as soon as possible.

Measures to avoid postoperative complications are similar to preoperative measures: avoidance of narcotics, benzodiazepines, and electrolyte or acid-base disturbances for reducing HE and lactulose to avoid opioid-related constipation. We have observed that lactulose can cause gas with abdominal distension that can mimic ileus or obstruction before and after surgery. Substitution with MiraLax (polyethylene glycol 3350) to achieve the same bowel movement goal is usually effective. In addition, overuse of lactulose causing excessive diarrhea can lead to dehydration and electrolyte disturbances, and may precipitate HE. Prophylactic measures against venous thromboembolism should be taken, including early mobilization, compression stockings, and/or subcutaneous heparin injections if the INR is less than 2 and the platelet count is greater than $50 \times 10^3/\mu L$. In addition, antiviral medications for patients with human immunodeficiency virus or chronic hepatitis B should be restarted immediately after surgery with attention to dosing for any renal impairment that may occur. Patients on hepatitis C virus treatment going into surgery usually stop treatment after surgery to allow for recovery.

SUMMARY

Patients with liver disease and portal hypertension, usually as a result of advanced fibrosis or cirrhosis, are at increased risk of complications when undergoing surgery. MELD is likely more accurate than the CTP score in predicting perioperative morbidity and mortality, although there is still value in calculation of CTP. Improved assessment of surgical risk can improve informed consent as well as surgical decision making and implementation of medical and surgical strategies to mitigate risks. A POLA checklist may be useful as a guideline for assessing surgical risk. Further studies are needed to enhance the preoperative risk assessment of patients with cirrhosis and portal hypertension and evaluate the usefulness of strategies like preoperative TIPS.

REFERENCES

1. Friedman LS. The risk of surgery in patients with liver disease. Hepatology 1999; 29(6):1617–23.
2. Friedman LS, Maddrey WC. Surgery in the patient with liver disease. Med Clin North Am 1987;71(3):453–76.
3. Gholson CF, Provenza JM, Bacon BR. Hepatologic considerations in patients with parenchymal liver disease undergoing surgery. Am J Gastroenterol 1990; 85(5):487–96.
4. Delcò F, Tchambaz L, Schlienger R, et al. Dose adjustment in patients with liver disease. Drug Saf 2005;28(6):529–45.
5. Hanje AJ, Patel T. Preoperative evaluation of patients with liver disease [review]. Nat Clin Pract Gastroenterol Hepatol 2007;4(5):266–76 Erratum in: Nat Clin Pract Gastroenterol Hepatol. 2007 Jul;4(7):409.
6. Ochs HR, Greenblatt DJ, Verburg-Ochs B, et al. Temazepam clearance unaltered in cirrhosis. Am J Gastroenterol 1986;81(1):80–4.
7. Pentikäinen PJ, Välisalmi L, Himberg JJ, et al. Pharmacokinetics of midazolam following intravenous and oral administration in patients with chronic liver disease and in healthy subjects. J Clin Pharmacol 1989;29(3):272–7.
8. Ghabrial H, Desmond PV, Watson KJ, et al. The effects of age and chronic liver disease on the elimination of temazepam. Eur J Clin Pharmacol 1986;30(1):93–7.
9. Cowan RE, Jackson BT, Grainger SL, et al. Effects of anesthetic agents and abdominal surgery on liver blood flow. Hepatology 1991;14(6):1161–6.
10. Servin F, Desmonts JM, Haberer JP, et al. Pharmacokinetics and protein binding of propofol in patients with cirrhosis. Anesthesiology 1988;69(6):887–91.
11. Costela JL, Jiménez R, Calvo R, et al. Serum protein binding of propofol in patients with renal failure or hepatic cirrhosis. Acta Anaesthesiol Scand 1996; 40(6):741–5.
12. Mandell MS, Durham J, Kumpe D, et al. The effects of desflurane and propofol on portosystemic pressure in patients with portal hypertension. Anesth Analg 2003;97(6):1573–7.
13. Martin P. Perioperative considerations for patients with liver disease. Cleve Clin J Med 2009;76(Suppl 4):S93–7.
14. Groszmann RJ, Atterbury CE. The pathophysiology of portal hypertension: a basis for classification. Semin Liver Dis 1982;2(3):177–86.
15. Friedman LS. Surgery in the patient with liver disease. Trans Am Clin Climatol Assoc 2010;121:192–204 [discussion: 205].
16. Sato K, Kawamura T, Wakusawa R. Hepatic blood flow and function in elderly patients undergoing laparoscopic cholecystectomy. Anesth Analg 2000;90(5): 1198–202.
17. Gelman SI. Disturbances in hepatic blood flow during anesthesia and surgery. Arch Surg 1976;111(8):881–3.
18. Clarke RS, Doggart JR, Lavery T. Changes in liver function after different types of surgery. Br J Anaesth 1976;48(2):119–28.
19. Millwala F, Nguyen GC, Thuluvath PJ. Outcomes of patients with cirrhosis undergoing non-hepatic surgery: risk assessment and management. World J Gastroenterol 2007;13(30):4056–63.

20. Schemel WH. Unexpected hepatic dysfunction found by multiple laboratory screening. Anesth Analg 1976;55(6):810–2.

21. Hay JE, Czaja AJ, Rakela J, et al. The nature of unexplained chronic aminotransferase elevations of a mild to moderate degree in asymptomatic patients. Hepatology 1989;9(2):193–7.

22. Hultcrantz R, Glaumann H, Lindberg G, et al. Liver investigation in 149 asymptomatic patients with moderately elevated activities of serum aminotransferases. Scand J Gastroenterol 1986;21(1):109–13.

23. Brolin RE, Bradley LJ, Taliwal RV. Unsuspected cirrhosis discovered during elective obesity operations. Arch Surg 1998;133(1):84–8.

24. Runyon BA. Surgical procedures are well tolerated by patients with asymptomatic chronic hepatitis. J Clin Gastroenterol 1986;8(5):542–4.

25. Oppedal K, Møller AM, Pedersen B, et al. Preoperative alcohol cessation prior to elective surgery. Cochrane Database Syst Rev 2012;(7):CD008343.

26. Yarze JC, Martin P, Muñoz SJ, et al. Wilson's disease: current status. Am J Med 1992;92(6):643–54.

27. Lok AS, Ghany MG, Goodman ZD, et al. Predicting cirrhosis in patients with hepatitis C based on standard laboratory tests: results of the HALT-C cohort. Hepatology 2005;42(2):282–92.

28. Wai CT, Greenson JK, Fontana RJ, et al. A simple noninvasive index can predict both significant fibrosis and cirrhosis in patients with chronic hepatitis C. Hepatology 2003;38:518–26.

29. Shah AG, Lydecker A, Murray K, et al. Comparison of noninvasive markers of fibrosis in patients with nonalcoholic fatty liver disease. Clin Gastroenterol Hepatol 2009;7:1104–12.

30. Harrison SA, Oliver D, Arnold HL, et al. Development and validation of a simple NAFLD clinical scoring system for identifying patients without advanced disease. Gut 2008;57:1441–7.

31. Henderson JM. What are the risks of general surgical abdominal operations in patients with cirrhosis? Clin Gastroenterol Hepatol 2010;8(5):399–400.

32. Doberneck RC, Sterling WA Jr, Allison DC. Morbidity and mortality after operation in nonbleeding cirrhotic patients. Am J Surg 1983;146(3):306–9.

33. Garrison RN, Cryer HM, Howard DA, et al. Clarification of risk factors for abdominal operations in patients with hepatic cirrhosis. Ann Surg 1984;199(6):648–55.

34. Aranha GV, Greenlee HB. Intra-abdominal surgery in patients with advanced cirrhosis. Arch Surg 1986;121(3):275–7.

35. Mansour A, Watson W, Shayani V, et al. Abdominal operations in patients with cirrhosis: still a major surgical challenge. Surgery 1997;122(4):730–5 [discussion: 735–6].

36. Farnsworth N, Fagan SP, Berger DH, et al. Child-Turcotte-Pugh versus MELD score as a predictor of outcome after elective and emergent surgery in cirrhotic patients. Am J Surg 2004;188(5):580–3.

37. Neeff H, Mariaskin D, Spangenberg HC, et al. Perioperative mortality after non-hepatic general surgery in patients with liver cirrhosis: an analysis of 138 operations in the 2000s using Child and MELD scores. J Gastrointest Surg 2011;15(1):1–11.

38. Telem DA, Schiano T, Goldstone R, et al. Factors that predict outcome of abdominal operations in patients with advanced cirrhosis. Clin Gastroenterol Hepatol 2010;8(5):451–7 [quiz: e58].

39. Wahlstrom K, Ney AL, Jacobson S, et al. Trauma in cirrhotics: survival and hospital sequelae in patients requiring abdominal exploration. Am Surg 2000;66(11):1071–6.

40. Christmas AB, Wilson AK, Franklin GA, et al. Cirrhosis and trauma: a deadly duo. Am Surg 2005;71(12):996–1000.
41. Axelrod D, Koffron A, Dewolf A, et al. Safety and efficacy of combined orthotopic liver transplantation and coronary artery bypass grafting. Liver Transpl 2004; 10(11):1386–90.
42. Heimbach JK, Watt KD, Poterucha JJ, et al. Combined liver transplantation and gastric sleeve resection for patients with medically complicated obesity and end-stage liver disease. Am J Transplant 2013;13(2):363–8.
43. de Goede B, van Kempen BJ, Polak WG, et al. Umbilical hernia management during liver transplantation. Hernia 2013;17(4):515–9.
44. Harville DD, Summerskill WH. Surgery in acute hepatitis. Causes and effects. JAMA 1963;184:257–61.
45. Powell-Jackson P, Greenway B, Williams R. Adverse effects of exploratory laparotomy in patients with unsuspected liver disease. Br J Surg 1982;69(8):449–51.
46. Greenwood SM, Leffler CT, Minkowitz S. The increased mortality rate of open liver biopsy in alcoholic hepatitis. Surg Gynecol Obstet 1972;134(4):600–4.
47. Mikkelsen WP. Therapeutic portacaval shunt. Preliminary data on controlled trial and morbid effects of acute hyaline necrosis. Arch Surg 1974;108(3):302–5 No abstract available.
48. Mikkelsen WP, Turrill FL, Kern WH. Acute hyaline necrosis of the liver. A surgical trap. Am J Surg 1968;116(2):266–72.
49. Mikkelsen WP, Kern WH. The influence of acute hyaline necrosis on survival after emergency and elective portacaval shunt. Major Probl Clin Surg 1974;14: 233–42.
50. Goldberg A, Moore MR, McColl KE, et al. Porphyrin metabolism and the porphyrias. In: Wetherall DJ, Ledingham JG, Warrell DA, editors. Oxford textbook of medicine. 2nd edition. Oxford (United Kingdom): Oxford University Press; 1987.
51. James MF, Hift RJ. Porphyrias. Br J Anaesth 2000;85(1):143–53.
52. Dover SB, Plenderleith L, Moore MR, et al. Safety of general anaesthesia and surgery in acute hepatic porphyria. Gut 1994;35(8):1112–5.
53. Meissner PN, Harrison GG, Hift RJ. Propofol as an IV anaesthetic induction agent in variegate porphyria. Br J Anaesth 1991;66:60–5.
54. Weir PM, Hodkinson BP. Is propofol a safe agent in porphyria? Anaesthesia 1988;43:1022–3.
55. American Porphyria Foundation. Available at: http://www.porphyriafoundation.com/drug-database. Accessed September 22, 2013.
56. O'Leary JG, Friedman LS. Predicting surgical risk in patients with cirrhosis: from art to science. Gastroenterology 2007;132(4):1609–11.
57. Child CG, Turcotte JG. Surgery and portal hypertension. Major Probl Clin Surg 1964;1:1–85.
58. Pugh RN, Murray-Lyon IM, Dawson JL, et al. Transection of the oesophagus for bleeding oesophageal varices. Br J Surg 1973;60(8):646–9.
59. Northup PG, Wanamaker RC, Lee VD, et al. Model for End-Stage Liver Disease (MELD) predicts nontransplant surgical mortality in patients with cirrhosis. Ann Surg 2005;242:244–51.
60. Perkins L, Jeffries M, Patel T. Utility of preoperative scores for predicting morbidity after cholecystectomy in patients with cirrhosis. Clin Gastroenterol Hepatol 2004;2(12):1123–8.
61. Befeler AS, Palmer DE, Hoffman M, et al. The safety of intra-abdominal surgery in patients with cirrhosis: model for end-stage liver disease score is superior to

Child-Turcotte-Pugh classification in predicting outcome. Arch Surg 2005; 140(7):650–4 [discussion: 655].

62. Costa BP, Sousa FC, Serôdio M, et al. Value of MELD and MELD-based indices in surgical risk evaluation of cirrhotic patients: retrospective analysis of 190 cases. World J Surg 2009;33(8):1711–9.

63. Kamath PS, Wiesner RH, Malinchoc M, et al. A model to predict survival in patients with end-stage liver disease. Hepatology 2001;33(2):464–70.

64. Teh SH, Nagorney DM, Stevens SR, et al. Risk factors for mortality after surgery in patients with cirrhosis. Gastroenterology 2007;132(4):1261–9.

65. Malinchoc M, Kamath PS, Gordon FD, et al. A model to predict poor survival in patients undergoing transjugular intrahepatic portosystemic shunts. Hepatology 2000;31(4):864–71.

66. Wiesner R, Edwards E, Freeman R, et al. Model for end-stage liver disease (MELD) and allocation of donor livers. Gastroenterology 2003;124(1):91–6.

67. Chalasani N, Kahi C, Francois F, et al. Model for end-stage liver disease (MELD) for predicting mortality in patients with acute variceal bleeding. Hepatology 2002;35(5):1282–4.

68. Wait RB, Kahng KU. Renal failure complicating obstructive jaundice [review]. Am J Surg 1989;157(2):256–63.

69. Merion RM, Schaubel DE, Dykstra DM, et al. The survival benefit of liver transplantation. Am J Transplant 2005;5:307–13.

70. Available at: http://optn.transplant.hrsa.gov/PublicComment/pubcommentProp Sub_287.pdf. Accessed September 22, 2013.

71. Washburn K, Pomfret E, Roberts J. Liver allocation and distribution: possible next steps. Liver Transpl 2011;17(9):1005–12.

72. Yoo HY, Edwin D, Thuluvath PJ. Relationship of the model for end-stage liver disease (MELD) scale to hepatic encephalopathy, as defined by electroencephalography and neuropsychometric testing, and ascites. Am J Gastroenterol 2003;98(6):1395–9.

73. de Goede B, Klitsie PJ, Lange JF, et al. Morbidity and mortality related to nonhepatic surgery in patients with liver cirrhosis: a systematic review. Best Pract Res Clin Gastroenterol 2012;26(1):47–59.

74. Bhangui P, Laurent A, Amathieu R, et al. Assessment of risk for non-hepatic surgery in cirrhotic patients. J Hepatol 2012;57(4):874–84.

75. Nicoll A. Surgical risk in patients with cirrhosis. J Gastroenterol Hepatol 2012; 27(10):1569–75.

76. Rai R, Nagral S, Nagral A. Surgery in a patient with liver disease. J Clin Exp Hepatol 2012;2(3):238–46.

77. Muir AJ. Surgical clearance for the patient with chronic liver disease. Clin Liver Dis 2012;16(2):421–33.

78. Hevesi ZG, Lopukhin SY, Mezrich JD, et al. Designated liver transplant anesthesia team reduces blood transfusion, need for mechanical ventilation, and duration of intensive care. Liver Transpl 2009;15(5):460–5.

79. Mandell MS, Pomfret EA, Steadman R, et al. Director of anesthesiology for liver transplantation: existing practices and recommendations by the United Network for Organ Sharing. Liver Transpl 2013;19(4):425–30.

80. Neri V, Ambrosi A, Di Lauro G, et al. Difficult cholecystectomies: validity of the laparoscopic approach. JSLS 2003;7:329–33.

81. Curet MJ, Contreras M, Weber DM, et al. Laparoscopic cholecystectomy. Surg Endosc 2002;16:453–7.

82. Fernando R. Laparoscopic cholecystectomy. World J Surg 2002;26:1401.

83. Johnston SM, Kidney S, Sweeney KJ, et al. Changing trends in the management of gallstone disease. Surg Endosc 2003;17:781–6.
84. Schiff J, Misra M, Rendon G. Laparoscopic cholecystectomy in cirrhotic patients. Surg Endosc 2005;19(9):1278–81.
85. Quillin RC 3rd, Burns JM, Pineda JA. Laparoscopic cholecystectomy in the cirrhotic patient: predictors of outcome. Surgery 2013;153(5):634–40.
86. Delis S, Bakoyiannis A, Madariaga J, et al. Laparoscopic cholecystectomy in cirrhotic patients: the value of MELD score and Child-Pugh classification in predicting outcome. Surg Endosc 2010;24(2):407–12.
87. Puggioni A, Wong LL. A metaanalysis of laparoscopic cholecystectomy in patients with cirrhosis. J Am Coll Surg 2003;197(6):921–6.
88. Chmielecki DK, Hagopian EJ, Kuo YH, et al. Laparoscopic cholecystectomy is the preferred approach in cirrhosis: a nationwide, population-based study. HPB (Oxford) 2012;14(12):848–53.
89. Laurence JM, Tran PD, Richardson AJ, et al. Laparoscopic or open cholecystectomy in cirrhosis: a systematic review of outcomes and meta-analysis of randomized trials. HPB (Oxford) 2012;14(3):153–61.
90. de Goede B, Klitsie PJ, Hagen SM, et al. Meta-analysis of laparoscopic versus open cholecystectomy for patients with liver cirrhosis and symptomatic cholecystolithiasis. Br J Surg 2013;100(2):209–16.
91. Fernandes NF, Schwesinger WH, Hilsenbeck SG, et al. Laparoscopic cholecystectomy and cirrhosis: a case-control study of outcomes. Liver Transpl 2000;6(3):340–4.
92. Ji W, Li LT, Wang ZM, et al. A randomized controlled trial of laparoscopic versus open cholecystectomy in patients with cirrhotic portal hypertension. World J Gastroenterol 2005;11(16):2513–7.
93. Aranha GV, Sontag SJ, Greenlee HB. Cholecystectomy in cirrhotic patients: a formidable operation. Am J Surg 1982;143:55–60.
94. Aranha GV, Kruss D, Greenlee HB. Therapeutic options for biliary tract disease in advanced cirrhosis. Am J Surg 1988;155:374–7.
95. Schlenker C, Trotter JF, Shah RJ, et al. Endoscopic gallbladder stent placement for treatment of symptomatic cholelithiasis in patients with end-stage liver disease. Am J Gastroenterol 2006;101:278–83.
96. Zhou J, Wu Z, Pankaj P, et al. Long-term postoperative outcomes of hypersplenism: laparoscopic versus open splenectomy secondary to liver cirrhosis. Surg Endosc 2012;26(12):3391–400.
97. Cobb WS, Heniford BT, Burns JM, et al. Cirrhosis is not a contraindication to laparoscopic surgery. Surg Endosc 2005;19(3):418–23.
98. Tsugawa K, Koyanagi N, Hashizume M, et al. A comparison of an open and laparoscopic appendectomy for patients with liver cirrhosis. Surg Laparosc Endosc Percutan Tech 2001;11(3):189–94.
99. Eker HH, van Ramshorst GH, de Goede B, et al. A prospective study on elective umbilical hernia repair in patients with liver cirrhosis and ascites. Surgery 2011; 150(3):542–6.
100. Tracy GD, Reeve TS, Thomas ID, et al. Spontaneous umbilical rupture in portal hypertension with massive ascites. Ann Surg 1965;161:623–6.
101. MacLellan DG, Watson KJ, Farrow HC, et al. Spontaneous paracentesis following rupture of an umbilical hernia. Aust N Z J Surg 1990;60:555–6.
102. Granese J, Valaulikar G, Khan M, et al. Ruptured umbilical hernia in a case of alcoholic cirrhosis with massive ascites. Am Surg 2002;68:733–4.
103. Ginsburg BY, Sharma AN. Spontaneous rupture of an umbilical hernia with evisceration. J Emerg Med 2006;30:155–7.

104. Lemmer JH, Strodel WE, Knol JA, et al. Management of spontaneous umbilical hernia disruption in the cirrhotic patient. Ann Surg 1983;198:30–4.
105. Trotter JF, Suhocki PV. Incarceration of umbilical hernia following transjugular intrahepatic portosystemic shunt for the treatment of ascites. Liver Transpl Surg 1999;5:209–10.
106. Perkins JD. Another patient with an umbilical hernia and massive ascites: what to do? Liver Transpl 2008;14(1):110–1.
107. Marsman HA, Heisterkamp J, Halm JA, et al. Management in patients with liver cirrhosis and an umbilical hernia. Surgery 2007;142(3):372–5.
108. McKay A, Dixon E, Bathe O, et al. Umbilical hernia repair in the presence of cirrhosis and ascites: results of a survey and review of the literature. Hernia 2009;13(5):461–8.
109. Choi SB, Hong KD, Lee JS, et al. Management of umbilical hernia complicated with liver cirrhosis: an advocate of early and elective herniorrhaphy. Dig Liver Dis 2011;43(12):991–5.
110. Cho SW, Bhayani N, Newell P, et al. Umbilical hernia repair in patients with signs of portal hypertension: surgical outcome and predictors of mortality. Arch Surg 2012;147(9):864–9.
111. Telem DA, Schiano T, Divino CM. Complicated hernia presentation in patients with advanced cirrhosis and refractory ascites: management and outcome. Surgery 2010;148(3):538–43.
112. Leonetti JP, Aranha GV, Wilkinson WA, et al. Umbilical herniorrhaphy in cirrhotic patients. Arch Surg 1984;119:442–5.
113. Belghiti J, Desgrandchamps F, Farges O, et al. Herniorrhaphy and concomitant peritoneovenous shunting in cirrhotic patients with umbilical hernia. World J Surg 1990;14:242–6.
114. Slakey DP, Benz CC, Joshi S, et al. Umbilical hernia repair in cirrhotic patients: utility of temporary peritoneal dialysis catheter. Am Surg 2005;71:58–61.
115. Fagan SP, Awad SS, Berger DH. Management of complicated umbilical hernias in patients with end-stage liver disease and refractory ascites. Surgery 2004; 135:679–82.
116. Elsebae MM, Nafeh AI, Abbas M, et al. New approach in surgical management of complicated umbilical hernia in the cirrhotic patient with ascites. J Egypt Soc Parasitol 2006;36(Suppl):11–20.
117. Azoulay D, Buabse F, Damiano I, et al. Neoadjuvant transjugular intrahepatic portosystemic shunt: a solution for extrahepatic abdominal operation in cirrhotic patients with severe portal hypertension. J Am Coll Surg 2001;193: 46–51.
118. Rossle M, Ochs A, Gulberg V, et al. A comparison of paracentesis and transjugular intrahepatic portosystemic shunting in patients with ascites. N Engl J Med 2000;342:1701–7.
119. Gines P, Tito L, Arroyo V, et al. Randomized study of therapeutic paracentesis with and without intravenous albumin in cirrhosis. Gastroenterology 1988;94: 1493–502.
120. Sanyal AJ, Genning C, Reddy RK, et al, North American Study for the Treatment of Refractory Ascites Group. The North American Study for the Treatment of Refractory Ascites. Gastroenterology 2003;124:634–41.
121. Vinet E, Perreault P, Bouchard L, et al. Transjugular intrahepatic portosystemic shunt before abdominal surgery in cirrhotic patients: a retrospective, comparative study. Can J Gastroenterol 2006;20(6):401–4.

122. Schlenker C, Johnson S, Trotter JF. Preoperative transjugular intrahepatic porto-systemic shunt (TIPS) for cirrhotic patients undergoing abdominal and pelvic surgeries. Surg Endosc 2009;23(7):1594–8.
123. Kim JJ, Dasika NL, Yu E, et al. Cirrhotic patients with a transjugular intrahepatic portosystemic shunt undergoing major extrahepatic surgery. J Clin Gastroenterol 2009;43(6):574–9.
124. Oh HK, Kim H, Ryoo S, et al. Inguinal hernia repair in patients with cirrhosis is not associated with increased risk of complications and recurrence. World J Surg 2011;35(6):1229–33 [discussion: 1234].
125. Gervaz P, Pak-art R, Nivatvongs S, et al. Colorectal adenocarcinoma in cirrhotic patients. J Am Coll Surg 2003;196(6):874–9.
126. Nguyen GC, Correia AJ, Thuluvath PJ. The impact of cirrhosis and portal hypertension on mortality following colorectal surgery: a nationwide, population-based study. Dis Colon Rectum 2009;52(8):1367–74.
127. Lian L, Menon KV, Shen B, et al. Inflammatory bowel disease complicated by primary sclerosing cholangitis and cirrhosis: is restorative proctocolectomy safe? Dis Colon Rectum 2012;55(1):79–84.
128. Hessheimer AJ, Earl TM, Chapman WC. Nonhepatic surgery in the cirrhotic patient. In: Jarnagin WR, Blumgart LH, editors. Blumgart's surgery of the liver, pancreas and biliary tract. London: Saunders; 2012. p. 1092–8.
129. Alberts WM, Salem AJ, Solomon DA, et al. Hepatic hydrothorax. Cause and management. Arch Intern Med 1991;151(12):2383–8.
130. Liu LU, Haddadin HA, Bodian CA, et al. Outcome analysis of cirrhotic patients undergoing chest tube placement. Chest 2004;126(1):142–8.
131. Assouad J, Barthes Fle P, Shaker W, et al. Recurrent pleural effusion complicating liver cirrhosis. Ann Thorac Surg 2003;75(3):986–9.
132. Mouroux J, Perrin C, Venissac N, et al. Management of pleural effusion of cirrhotic origin. Chest 1996;109(4):1093–6.
133. Cerfolio RJ, Bryant AS. Efficacy of video-assisted thoracoscopic surgery with talc pleurodesis for porous diaphragm syndrome in patients with refractory hepatic hydrothorax. Ann Thorac Surg 2006;82(2):457–9.
134. Afzali A, Berry K, Ioannou GN. Excellent posttransplant survival for patients with nonalcoholic steatohepatitis in the United States. Liver Transpl 2012;18(1):29–37.
135. Charlton MR, Burns JM, Pedersen RA, et al. Frequency and outcomes of liver transplantation for nonalcoholic steatohepatitis in the United States. Gastroenterology 2011;141(4):1249–53.
136. Wu R, Ortiz J, Dallal R. Is bariatric surgery safe in cirrhotics? Hepat Mon 2013; 13(2):e8536.
137. Hafeez S, Ahmed MH. Bariatric surgery as potential treatment for nonalcoholic fatty liver disease: a future treatment by choice or by chance? J Obes 2013; 2013:839275.
138. Weingarten TN, Swain JM, Kendrick ML, et al. Nonalcoholic steatohepatitis (NASH) does not increase complications after laparoscopic bariatric surgery. Obes Surg 2011;21(11):1714–20.
139. Nair S, Verma S, Thuluvath PJ. Obesity and its effect on survival in patients undergoing orthotopic liver transplantation in the United States. Hepatology 2002; 35(1):105–9.
140. Food and Drug Administration. 2012. Available at: http://www.accessdata.fda.gov/cdrh_docs/pdf7/P070009b.pdf. Accessed September 22, 2013.

141. Lin MY, Mehdi Tavakol M, Sarin A, et al. Laparoscopic sleeve gastrectomy is safe and efficacious for pretransplant candidates. Surg Obes Relat Dis 2013; 9(5):653–8.

142. Klemperer JD, Ko W, Krieger KH, et al. Cardiac operations in patients with cirrhosis. Ann Thorac Surg 1998;65(1):85–7.

143. Suman A, Barnes DS, Zein NN, et al. Predicting outcome after cardiac surgery in patients with cirrhosis: a comparison of Child-Pugh and MELD scores. Clin Gastroenterol Hepatol 2004;2(8):719–23.

144. Filsoufi F, Salzberg SP, Rahmanian PB, et al. Early and late outcome of cardiac surgery in patients with liver cirrhosis. Liver Transpl 2007;13(7):990–5.

145. Macaron C, Hanouneh IA, Suman A, et al. Safety of cardiac surgery for patients with cirrhosis and Child-Pugh scores less than 8. Clin Gastroenterol Hepatol 2012;10(5):535–9.

146. Serfaty L, Aumaitre H, Chazouilleres O, et al. Determinants of outcome of compensated hepatitis C virus related cirrhosis. Hepatology 1998;27:1435–40.

147. Fattovich G, Giustina G, Degos F, et al. Morbidity and mortality in compensated cirrhosis type C: a retrospective follow-up study of 384 patients. Gastroenterology 1997;112:463–72.

148. El-Serag HB. Hepatocellular carcinoma: recent trends in the United States. Gastroenterology 1994;127(5 Suppl 1):S27–34.

149. Cucchetti A, Ercolani G, Vivarelli M, et al. Impact of Model for End-stage Liver Disease (MELD) score on prognosis after hepatectomy for hepatocellular carcinoma on cirrhosis. Liver Transpl 2006;12:966–71.

150. Yasui M, Harada A, Torii A, et al. Impaired liver function and long-term prognosis after hepatectomy for hepatocellular carcinoma. World J Surg 1995;19: 439–43.

151. Kim YK, Nakano H, Yamagochi M, et al. Prediction of postoperative decompensated liver function by technetium-99m galactosyl-human serum albumin liver scintigraphy in patients with hepatocellular carcinoma complicating chronic liver disease. Br J Surg 1997;84:793–6.

152. Truty MJ, Vauthey JN. Uses and limitations of portal vein embolization for improving perioperative outcomes in hepatocellular carcinoma. Semin Oncol 2010;37:102–9.

153. Perumalswami PV, Schiano TD. The management of hospitalized patients with cirrhosis: the Mount Sinai experience and a guide for hospitalists. Dig Dis Sci 2011;56(5):1266–81.

154. Haynes AB, Weiser TG, Berry WR, et al. A surgical safety checklist to reduce morbidity and mortality in a global population. N Engl J Med 2009;360(5):491–9.

155. Morrow R. Perioperative quality and improvement. Anesthesiol Clin 2012;30(3): 555–63.

156. Böhmer AB, Wappler F, Tinschmann T, et al. The implementation of a perioperative checklist increases patients' perioperative safety and staff satisfaction. Acta Anaesthesiol Scand 2012;56(3):332–8.

157. Plauth M, Cabré E, Campillo B, et al. ESPEN guidelines on parenteral nutrition: hepatology. Clin Nutr 2009;28(4):436–44.

158. Amodio P, Bemeur C, Butterworth R, et al. The nutritional management of hepatic encephalopathy in patients with cirrhosis: International Society for Hepatic Encephalopathy and Nitrogen Metabolism consensus. Hepatology 2013;58(1):325–36.

159. Villanueva C, Colomo A, Bosch A, et al. Transfusion strategies for acute upper gastrointestinal bleeding. N Engl J Med 2013;368(1):11–21.

160. Ammar SA. Management of complicated umbilical hernias in cirrhotic patients using permanent mesh: randomized clinical trial. Hernia 2010;14(1):35–8.
161. Fan ST, Lo CM, Lai EC, et al. Perioperative nutritional support in patients undergoing hepatectomy for hepatocellular carcinoma. N Engl J Med 1994;331: 1547–52.

Index

Note: Page numbers of article titles are in **boldface** type.

Clin Liver Dis 18 (2014) 507–517
http://dx.doi.org/10.1016/S1089-3261(14)00019-1
1089-3261/14/$ – see front matter © 2014 Elsevier Inc. All rights reserved.

liver.theclinics.com

Moving?

Make sure your subscription moves with you!

To notify us of your new address, find your **Clinics Account Number** (located on your mailing label above your name), and contact customer service at:

Email: **journalscustomerservice-usa@elsevier.com**

800-654-2452 (subscribers in the U.S. & Canada)
314-447-8871 (subscribers outside of the U.S. & Canada)

Fax number: **314-447-8029**

Elsevier Health Sciences Division
Subscription Customer Service
3251 Riverport Lane
Maryland Heights, MO 63043

*To ensure uninterrupted delivery of your subscription, please notify us at least 4 weeks in advance of move.

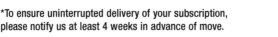

Moving?

Make sure your subscription moves with you!

Printed and bound by CPI Group (UK) Ltd, Croydon, CR0 4YY

03/10/2024

01040487-0009